Neurological Disorders and Pregnancy

Neurological Disorders and Pregnancy

Edited by

Alireza Minagar

ELSEVIER

AMSTERDAM • BOSTON • HEIDELBERG • LONDON • NEW YORK • OXFORD
PARIS • SAN DIEGO • SAN FRANCISCO • SINGAPORE • SYDNEY • TOKYO

Elsevier
32 Jamestown Road London NW1 7BY
30 Corporate Drive, Suite 400, Burlington, MA 01803, USA

First edition 2011

British Library Cataloguing-in-Publication Data
A catalogue record for this book is available from the British Library

Library of Congress Cataloging-in-Publication Data
A catalog record for this book is available from the Library of Congress

ISBN: 978-0-12-384911-3

This book has been manufactured using Print On Demand technology. Each copy is produced to order and is limited to black ink. The online version of this book will show color figures where appropriate.

Transferred to Digital Printing in 2010

Contents

Preface

The diagnosis and treatment of neurologic and psychiatric diseases during pregnancy and the postpartum period pose significant challenges to neurologists, psychiatrists, and other health care professionals. Pregnancy is associated with significant physiologic and particularly hormonal changes that can set the stage for manifestation of new neurologic or psychiatric diseases, may cause temporary remissions, or may cause their relapse. Differential diagnosis of these conditions must include certain diseases that present almost exclusively during pregnancy and the puerperium such as Sydenham's chorea and pituitary apoplexy. In addition, every diagnostic test must be arranged with the fetus' and mother's safety as the main concern. Any therapeutic decisions must be made with careful consideration of the risks and benefits of therapy versus withholding therapy for the developing fetus and pregnant mother, and these facts must be explained to the pregnant woman. Under ideal conditions, any pregnancy in the context of neurologic or psychiatric diseases must be planned in advance. A multidisciplinary team should be involved in management of these patients to best secure the safety of mother and fetus. Treatments with the highest safety index for mother and fetus should be selected and carefully administered.

However, in many cases pregnancies are unplanned, and in some of these cases the fetus already has been exposed to neurologic or psychiatric medications. Indeed, management of these patients poses a formidable challenge to the treating physician. Factors that assist in better treatment of these patients are familiarity with the nature of pregnancy, learning about physiologic changes associated with pregnancy, as well as being aware of the available literature about the impact of medications on pregnancy and their teratogenic properties. In addition, gaining knowledge about the safety of breast-feeding while patients are taking these medications is necessary. In general, it is better to use monotherapy and avoid using multiple medications. Pregnant patients with neurologic or psychiatric disorders who are under treatment should be started on folic acid and other pregnancy vitamin supplements to reduce the risk of certain congenital malformations.

This book covers major neurologic and psychiatric diseases in relation to pregnancy and the contributors present the most recent information on each subject. I very much appreciate the dedication of these authors from various countries of the world who provided their significant contributions. Without them, this book would have never been published and I am greatly indebted to their kindness. I also would like to express my appreciation to Mr. Paul Prasad Chandramohan and the other wonderful employees of the Elsevier publishing production team who provided their support and expertise. I hope that this book will raise awareness for this significant issue and will assist health care professionals in better management of their pregnant patients.

Alireza Minagar, MD, FAAN
Department of Neurology
Louisiana State University Health Sciences Center
Shreveport, LA, USA
E-mail: aminag@isuhsc.edu

Contributors

Laura Airas Department of Neurology, University of Turku, Turku, Finland

Nadejda Alekseeva Department of Neurology, Louisiana State University Health Sciences Center, Shreveport, LA, USA; Overton Brooks VA Medical Center, Shreveport, LA, USA

Renato Augusto Moreira de Sá PhD. Universidade Federal Fluminense, Niterói, Brazil; Grupo Perinatal, Rio de Janeiro, Brazil

Maike Tiede Blaya Department of Neurology, Tulane University School of Medicine, New Orleans, LA, USA

Aimee Borazanci Department of Neurology, Louisiana State University Health Sciences Center, Shreveport, LA, USA

Fernanda Campos da Silva MD. Universidade Federal Fluminense, Niterói, Brazil; Hospital Geral de Bonsucesso, Rio de Janeiro, Brazil; Grupo Perinatal, Rio de Janeiro, Brazil

Luciana Carneiro do Cima MD. Grupo Perinatal, Rio de Janeiro, Brazil; Instituto Fernandes Figueira, Rio de Janeiro, Brazil

Patricia Colon Department of Neurology, Tulane University School of Medicine, New Orleans, LA, USA

Debra Elliott Louisiana State University Health Sciences Center, Shreveport, LA, USA

Masoud Etemadifar Isfahan Research Committee of Multiple Sclerosis (IRCOMS), Isfahan, Iran; Department of Neurology, Isfahan University of Medical Sciences, Isfahan, Iran

Jennifer E. Fugate Department of Neurology, Mayo Clinic, Rochester, MN, USA

Emil Gaitour Department of Neurology, Louisiana State University Health Sciences Center, Shreveport, LA, USA

Felix Geller Department of Psychiatry, Louisiana State University Health Sciences Center, Shreveport, LA, USA

Eduardo Gonzalez-Toledo Department of Neurology, Louisiana State University Health Sciences Center, Shreveport, LA, USA; Department of Radiology, Louisiana State University Health Sciences Center, Shreveport, LA, USA

Rita Horton Department of Psychiatry, Louisiana State University Health Sciences Center, Shreveport, LA, USA

Stephen L. Jaffe Department of Neurology, Louisiana State University Health Sciences Center, Shreveport, LA, USA

Roger E. Kelley Department of Neurology, Tulane University School of Medicine, New Orleans, LA, USA

John W. Kevill Department of Neurology, Louisiana State University Health Sciences Center, Shreveport, LA, USA

Xiangping Li Louisiana State University Health Sciences Center, Shreveport, LA, USA

Amir-Hadi Maghzi Isfahan Research Committee of Multiple Sclerosis (IRCOMS), Isfahan, Iran; Isfahan Neurosciences Research Center, Isfahan University of Medical Sciences, Isfahan, Iran; Neuroimmunology Unit, Centre for Neuroscience and Trauma, Blizard Institute of Cell and Molecular Science, Barts and the London School of Medicine and Dentistry, London, UK

Jeanie McGee Department of Neurology, Louisiana State University Health Sciences Center, Shreveport, LA, USA

Alireza Minagar Department of Neurology, Louisiana State University Health Sciences Center, Shreveport, LA, USA

Alejandro A. Rabinstein Department of Neurology, Mayo Clinic, Rochester, MN, USA

Aronkumar Reddy Department of Neurology, Louisiana State University Health Sciences Center, Shreveport, LA, USA

Kourosh Rezania Department of Neurology, The University of Chicago Medical Center, Chicago, IL, USA

Natalya Shneyder Department of Neurology, Louisiana State University Health Sciences Center, Shreveport, LA, USA

Ahmet Ursavas Uludag University Medical Faculty, Respiratory Medicine Department, Bursa, Turkey

Peimin Zhu Louisiana State University Health Sciences Center, Shreveport, LA, USA

1 Pregnancy and Multiple Sclerosis

Laura Airas[1], *Masoud Etemadifar*[2,3], *Amir-Hadi Maghzi*[2,4,5]

[1]Department of Neurology, University of Turku, Turku, Finland
[2]Isfahan Research Committee of Multiple Sclerosis (IRCOMS), Isfahan, Iran
[3]Department of Neurology, Isfahan University of Medical Sciences, Isfahan, Iran
[4]Isfahan Neurosciences Research Center, Isfahan University of Medical Sciences, Isfahan, Iran
[5]Neuroimmunology Unit, Centre for Neuroscience and Trauma, Blizard Institute of Cell and Molecular Science, Barts and the London School of Medicine and Dentistry, London, UK

Introduction

Multiple sclerosis (MS) is the most common debilitating disease of the central nervous system (CNS) of young adults, with a prevalence of approximately 1 per 1000 in the Western world. About 80% of people with MS are diagnosed between the ages of 20 and 45 and, in adults, the female-to-male ratio is about 2.5 to 1. Hence, the majority of individuals obtaining the diagnosis of MS are women of childbearing age [1]. These women are naturally concerned as to how a pregnancy will affect their disease, how the disease might modify the outcome of the pregnancy and influence the developing child, and how the medication they are using might affect the child. Several studies have been performed to answer these questions and a consensus has been reached about how pregnancy affects MS activity; the relapse rate is typically reduced during late pregnancy but increases in the postpartum period [2–6]. The reasons for the increased postpartum activity are not entirely clear, but factors such as the abrupt decrease in estrogen levels immediately following delivery and the loss of immunosuppressive state of pregnancy are likely of importance [7–9]. There is a general view that MS does not affect the course or outcome of pregnancy, but all original studies addressing these questions are either retrospective and register-based [10–12], or conclusions have been drawn from very small cohorts [13]. In this chapter, we will review the following: (1) how pregnancy affects the disease activity; (2) pregnancy outcome among MS mothers; (3) treatment of MS mothers during pregnancy and lactation; and (4) immunologic basis of pregnancy-induced disease remission.

Neurological Disorders and Pregnancy. DOI: 10.1016/B978-0-12-384911-3.00001-4

How Pregnancy Affects the Disease Activity

Relapses

Pregnancy typically is a stabilizing period in the clinical course of MS. During the third trimester, relapse rate can be 70% lower than the time before pregnancy, but aggravation of the disease commonly is observed after delivery.

Several early retrospective studies suggested that pregnancy has a beneficial effect on the clinical course of MS [2,14], but this view was not shared by all investigators [15,16]. Uncertainty about how to advise young women with MS on family planning was resolved after the publication of the PRISMS study [5]. In the largest prospective study so far to evaluate the effect of pregnancy on the clinical activity of MS, Confavreux et al. [5] followed 254 women with MS through 269 pregnancies. The study was conducted as a multicenter study in 12 European countries. The enrollment was performed between 4 and 36 gestational weeks, and follow-up was continued for 1 year after delivery. Data were collected on relapse frequency and disability. During the year before pregnancy, 164 relapses occurred among the 227 women who were followed for the entire observation period, resulting in an annual relapse rate of 0.7. During pregnancy the relapse frequency steadily declined and reached the minimum annual relapse rate of 0.2 during the third trimester of pregnancy (meaning that during the third trimester only 12 of 225 women [=5%] experienced a relapse). In the 3 months following delivery, the number of relapses increased dramatically to 68 of 222 women (=31%; annual mean relapse rate: 1.2, $P < 0.001$ versus relapse rate during the year preceding pregnancy). A high frequency of relapses during pregnancy and a high level of physical disability before pregnancy were identified as predictors of postpartum attacks [17]. A similar pattern of lack of active inflammation during pregnancy and an increase in signs of inflammation during the postpartum phase has been observed in studies using serial magnetic resonance imaging (MRI) [18,19]. In addition, Saraste et al. [20] described a patient with a record number of 200 gadolinium-enhancing lesions in a brain MRI scan performed only 4 weeks after delivery.

MRI Activity During and After Pregnancy

MRI is widely used during pregnancy, either for fetal or maternal diagnostics. In most cases, because of theoretical concerns, MRIs are not performed during the first trimester. Rise in body temperature especially locally in the uterus and acoustic noise exposure have been mentioned as potential risks. In animals, gadolinium has not been shown to be teratogenic but safety data in humans concerning gadolinium administration during pregnancy are lacking. Hence, use of gadolinium should be avoided during pregnancy.

Paavilainen et al. [19] reported the first MRI study of a larger MS cohort (28 patients), which addressed disease activity during pregnancy and the postpartum period. There was a significant increase in the number of T2-lesions ($P = 0.0009$) and diffusion-weighted imaging (DWI)-positive lesions ($P = 0.0098$) as well as, in the total lesion load measured on FLAIR-images ($P = 0.0126$) in scans performed after delivery when compared to the scans performed during pregnancy; however, no changes were observed in the number of T1-lesions ($P = 0.375$). Fourteen of the patients (50%) showed T2-activity (i.e., the scans contained one or more new or enlarging lesions) in at least one of their postpartum scans (mean 3.7 active lesions, range 1–14). The majority of the active postpartum scans (9 of 14) were performed within 5 weeks of delivery. This indicates that MS activation commonly takes place at a very early stage after the delivery. Furthermore, active lesions also were observed in two scans performed at 35–37 gestational weeks, which suggests that alterations might already take place in patients' immune systems during very late phases of pregnancy, indicating the preparation for the delivery of the fetus. In conclusion, during the 6-month postpartum period, 21 of 28 (75%) patients demonstrated MS disease activity either by a clinical MS relapse or T2-activity in the MRI scans [19].

Interestingly, blood estriol concentration begins to decline after 35 gestational weeks, reflecting the dysfunction of the aging placenta. Consequently, the loss of high estriol concentrations might lead to an increase in the disease activity in certain patients.

Pregnancy Outcome Among MS Mothers

Two large, retrospective register-based studies and a few prospective studies with smaller sample size have addressed the question of pregnancy outcome among MS patients [10–13,21]. Presently, there is no concrete evidence that MS patients are more susceptible to pregnancy or delivery complications, such as ectopic pregnancy, preeclampsia, gestational diabetes mellitus, prolonged labor, or miscarriage than healthy women are, nor are their infants more likely to be delivered preterm, be of low birth weight, have malformations, or experience an early death. Fertility problems or congenital abnormalities also are uncommon in women with MS. However, in a register-based study on MS births between 1967 and 2002, the singleton children born to MS mothers had on average 123 g lower birth weight when compared to infants of healthy control mothers; a difference stated as statistically significant [11]. Based on the same report, mothers with MS needed operative delivery more often than healthy mothers, which might be due to MS-related symptoms such as neuromuscular perineal weakness and spasticity, in addition to fatigue and exhaustion.

Delivery of MS Mothers

The possibility for a need of an operational delivery should be taken into account when planning a delivery of an MS mother but overall, the decision of an elective cesarean section should be made based on current obstetrical criteria. The mothers' functional status should always be taken into account: a mother with significant functional disability will more likely encounter problems associated with fatigue and exhaustion during the second stage of delivery.

Anesthesia During Delivery

Epidural anesthesia during delivery was not associated with increased risk of postpartum flares or disability in women with MS in the PRISMS study [5]. On the other hand, concerns have been raised about spinal anesthesia. It has been suggested that spinal anesthesia may be the explanation for postoperative relapses. The hypothetical ground for the concerns is that the local anesthetic might have a direct toxic effect on the demyelinated axons [22], but there are no real clinical data to support this view.

Treatment of MS Mothers During Pregnancy and Lactation

In a recent retrospective study in Spain, 38.6% of MS mothers on interferon-beta therapy did not discontinue the treatment until the first trimester of pregnancy [23]. Hence, a significant proportion of MS mothers may be exposed to disease-modifying therapies (DMTs) during pregnancy. Interferon-beta has been associated with an increased risk of spontaneous abortion and lower birth weight of the newborn in one small prospective study [24], but other investigators have considered the drug safe in terms of pregnancy outcome [23–26]. Taken together, the information on pregnancy outcomes for babies exposed to DMTs is increasing, but the study samples are still small. Thus, the safety of these medications has not been established fully and discontinuation of DMTs before pregnancy must still be recommended. Even though these drugs do not appear to cause any major fetal malformations, it is uncertain how they might affect the developing immune system of the fetus. In addition, the natural course of MS during pregnancy, that is, the pregnancy-associated low annual relapse rate, makes the necessity of DMTs questionable during pregnancy. Despite discontinuation of the DMTs before pregnancy, the mothers rarely experience disabling relapses during the course of pregnancy. It is still advisable for the patients to discontinue DMTs 1 month before the discontinuation of contraception, in order to allow mothers' immune systems to recover from the effects of DMT before conception. If a mother would experience a disabling relapse during pregnancy, she could be treated safely with a course of Intravenous immunoglobulin (IVIG), or after the third trimester with high-dose methylprednisolone.

Breast-Feeding

The prevalence of breast-feeding was very high (90%) in a cohort of German MS mothers and in a cohort of Finnish MS mothers [27,28]. This is in stark contrast to a South European MS population, where only 28.6% of mothers chose to nurse [23]. Breast-feeding is considered beneficial for the mother–infant relationship, and it reduces the incidence of infections and allergies experienced by the infant [29]. Moreover, both in the PRISMS study and a more recent small study performed in California [30], the MS patients who breast-fed their children had a lower relapse rate than women who did not breast-feed [5]. This probably does not reflect a positive effect of breast-feeding on MS activity; it rather implies that the mothers with active disease chose DMTs instead of breast-feeding [28].

The postpartum period is a more challenging time regarding controlling the disease activity, especially in areas of high breast-feeding prevalence. Mothers with MS want to reduce the probability of experiencing postpartum relapses in order to best manage their child, but treatment with DMTs is not recommended during nursing. One therapeutic option is IVIG, which is safe to use during breast-feeding, and which has been suggested to reduce disease activity in MS [31], although in a later study no beneficial effects could be demonstrated [32]. A retrospective study, however, suggested that IVIG may be efficient in preventing postpartum relapses [33]. Recently, a large (173 patients) multicenter, randomized, double-blind clinical trial compared two different doses of IVIG treatment during the postpartum period, but no difference was observed between the two dosing regimens [34]. A randomized, placebo-controlled study on the effect of IVIG in preventing postpartum relapses is, unfortunately, still lacking. The European Federation of Neurological Societies (EFNS) task force guidelines recommend that IVIG could be used in pregnancy in Relapsing Remitting MS (RRMS), but gives no opinion about using the drug during lactation [35]. Taken together, prophylactic treatment with IVIG could be recommended in selected cases, such as for those mothers with a high pre-pregnancy disability and/or high relapse rate before and/or during pregnancy. In such cases, IVIG infusions could be recommended already in the maternity ward, for example, at a dose of 0.4 g/kg for 3 consecutive days to prevent relapses, and if the mother wishes to breast-feed, the IVIG infusions could be continued during the nursing period on monthly basis, for example, with 0.4 g/kg on a single day once a month.

Safety of MS Medication During Pregnancy and Lactation According to the FDA Risk Classification Scheme

The American Food and Drug Administration's (FDA) pregnancy risk classification scheme gives information on the risk of whether a given medication could cause fetal loss, a major malformation, low birth weight, or infant death. This classification is based mostly on animal data or short-term human studies, and conclusions are drawn rather from lack of safety data in humans rather than from evidence of safety in human trials (Table 1.1). The FDA safety scheme for drug treatment during pregnancy and lactation are shown in Tables 1.2 and 1.3.

Table 1.1 The FDA Pregnancy Risk Classification Scheme

Category	Interpretation
A	Adequate, well-controlled studies in pregnant women have not shown an increased risk of fetal abnormalities to the fetus in any trimester of pregnancy
B	Animal studies have revealed no evidence of harm to the fetus, however, there are no adequate and well-controlled studies in pregnant women OR Animal studies have shown an adverse effect, but adequate and well-controlled studies in pregnant women have failed to demonstrate a risk to the fetus in any trimester

(*Continued*)

Table 1.1 (*Continued*)

Category	Interpretation
C	Animal studies have shown an adverse effect and there are no adequate and well-controlled studies in pregnant women OR No animal studies have been conducted and there are no adequate and well-controlled studies in pregnant women
D	Adequate well-controlled or observational studies in pregnant women have demonstrated a risk to the fetus However, the benefits of therapy may outweigh the potential risk. For example, the drug may be acceptable if needed in a life-threatening situation or serious disease for which safer drugs cannot be used or are ineffective
X	Adequate well-controlled or observational studies in animals or pregnant women have demonstrated positive evidence of fetal abnormalities or risks The use of the product is contraindicated in women who are or may become pregnant

Immunologic Basis of Pregnancy-Induced Disease Remission

Pregnancy induces alterations in the maternal immune system in order to protect the semiallogeneic fetus from an immunologic attack by the mother's immune system [36]. However, the underlying pathobiologic mechanisms responsible for the MS disease-modifying effect of pregnancy are still largely elusive. The putative justification is the pregnancy-related changes in the function of the immune system, such as a shift towards T helper 2 (Th2) type immune reactivity and expansion of regulatory T-cells [37–39]. Placenta-derived hormones, estrogens, and progesterone can directly affect the function of the immune cells via acting through estrogen and progesterone receptors. During the course of pregnancy, the placenta-derived estriol (E3) levels increase manyfold (from 0.2 ng/mL before pregnancy up to 10 ng/mL during gestational weeks 35–37). Related to this, a dramatic decrease in MS relapse frequency is observed during the latter half of pregnancy. On the other hand, the abrupt decrease in estrogen levels following delivery is associated with an increase in inflammatory activity which in MS is observed both as an increase in the relapse rate and increased lesion load in the MRI [5,19].

It has been suggested that estrogens exhibit dose-dependent biphasic effects on immune cells, whereby high estrogen levels inhibit and low estrogen levels facilitate cell-mediated immunity [40]. This could explain the higher prevalence of autoimmune diseases among women (low estrogen) and for improvement of the cell-mediated autoimmune diseases such as rheumatoid arthritis and MS during pregnancy (high estrogen). Pauklin et al. [41] recently showed that, via activation-induced

Table 1.2 Safety of MS Therapies During Pregnancy According to FDA Pregnancy Risk Classification

Medication	**FDA Category**	**Adverse Events Following in Utero Exposure**
Azatioprine	D	Neonatal immunoglobulin deficiencies and immunosuppression, low birth weight, chromosomal abnormalities, preterm labor
Cyclophosphamide	D	Skeleton, palate, limb, and eye malformations
Glatiramer acetate	B	None known in humans or animals
Interferon-beta	C	Spontaneous abortions in animals
Methotrexate	X	Neural tube defects, craniofacial and limb defects, miscarriages
Methylprednisolone	C	Fetal deformities in humans; do not use in first trimester
		Neonatal immunosuppression in humans
Mitoxantrone	D	Low birth weight, preterm delivery, kidney anomalies
Natalizumab	C	Spontaneous abortions, thymic atrophy, decreased hepatic hematopoiesis, increased splenic hematopoiesis
Prednisone	C	Fetal deformities in humans, do not use in first trimester

deaminase, estrogens could induce antibody-mediated autoimmunity; this also could contribute to the female predominance of MS. It also fits well with the notion that during pregnancy, Th2-type antibody-mediated immune responses are beneficial for the outcome of pregnancy and thus prevalent [37]. The anti-inflammatory effects of estrogens are also well documented by in vitro studies, and it has been shown that estrogen delays the onset of experimental autoimmune encephalomyelitis (EAE) [42–46].

Medicinal estriol reduces the number of inflammatory lesions in brain MRIs of MS patients [47]. A small group of female MS patients was given estriol at a dose corresponding to the late pregnancy physiological concentration (8 mg/day). This led to a reduction in the number of active lesions in the brain MRI, and alterations also were measured in systemic cytokine levels. The drug was well tolerated, and hence the results from this small preliminary study were considered very promising.

Immunoregulatory factors operative during pregnancy include tolerance-promoting signaling molecules and pregnancy-specific serum proteins such as sHLA-G, CD200, Fas-ligand, alpha-fetoprotein, and indoleamine 2,3-dioxygenase [48–50]. Moreover, a decrease in NK-cell levels, and an increase in tolerogenic HLA-G-levels, in regulatory T cells and in regulatory $CD56^{Bright}$ NK-cells have been demonstrated during

Table 1.3 Safety of MS Therapies During Lactation According to FDA Pregnancy Risk Classification

Medication	FDA Category	Safety During Lactation
Azatioprine	D	Probably hazardous
Cyclophosphamide	D	Probably hazardous
Glatiramer acetate	B	Unknown so avoid
Interferon-beta	C	Unknown so avoid
Methotrexate	X	Contraindicated
Methylprednisolone	C	Pump and discard 8–24 h after each infusion
Mitoxantrone	D	Probably hazardous
Natalizumab	C	Unknown so avoid
Prednisone	C	Avoid for 2–4 h following oral dose

MS pregnancy, while all of these phenomena are reversed in the postpartum situation where there is a high relapse rate [9,38,51,52].

Conclusion

1. The frequency of MS disease-related relapses normally is reduced greatly during the latter half of pregnancy, but after the delivery, the disease often activates.
2. Discontinuation of disease-modifying treatment is recommended about 1 month before cessation of contraception.
3. Breast-feeding is considered beneficial for the infant, but disease-modifying treatment is not recommended while breast-feeding.
4. The mothers with highest disability and highest relapse rate are most likely to experience postpartum relapses, which should be taken into account when planning the treatment after the delivery.
5. The outcome of pregnancies of MS patients is usually good.

References

[1] Orton SM, Herrera BM, Yee IM, Valdar W, Ramagopalan SV, Sadovnick AD, et al. Sex ratio of multiple sclerosis in Canada: a longitudinal study. Lancet Neurol 2006;5:932–6.
[2] Korn-Lubetzki I, Kahana E, Cooper G, Abramsky O. Activity of multiple sclerosis during pregnancy and puerperium. Ann Neurol 1984;16:229–31.
[3] Roullet E, Verdier-Taillefer MH, Amarenco P, Gharbi G, Alperovitch A, Marteau R. Pregnancy and multiple sclerosis: a longitudinal study of 125 remittent patients. J Neurol Neurosurg Psychiatry 1993;56:1062–5.
[4] Birk K, Ford C, Smeltzer S, Ryan D, Miller R, Rudick RA. The clinical course of multiple sclerosis during pregnancy and the puerperium. Arch Neurol 1990;47:738–42.

[5] Confavreux C, Hutchinson M, Hours MM, Cortinovis-Tourniaire P, Moreau T. Rate of pregnancy-related relapse in multiple sclerosis. Pregnancy in Multiple Sclerosis Group. N Engl J Med 1998;339:285–91.
[6] Saraste M, Vaisanen S, Alanen A, Airas L. Clinical and immunologic evaluation of women with multiple sclerosis during and after pregnancy. Gend Med 2007;4:45–55.
[7] Whitacre CC, Reingold SC, O'Looney PA. A gender gap in autoimmunity. Science 1999;283:1277–8.
[8] Airas L, Nikula T, Huang YH, Lahesmaa R, Wiendl H. Postpartum-activation of multiple sclerosis is associated with down-regulation of tolerogenic HLA-G. J Neuroimmunol 2007;187:205–11.
[9] Airas L, Saraste M, Rinta S, Elovaara I, Huang YH, Wiendl H. Immunoregulatory factors in multiple sclerosis patients during and after pregnancy: relevance of natural killer cells. Clin Exp Immunol 2008;151:235–43.
[10] Mueller BA, Zhang J, Critchlow CW. Birth outcomes and need for hospitalization after delivery among women with multiple sclerosis. Am J Obstet Gynecol 2002;186:446–52.
[11] Dahl J, Myhr KM, Daltveit AK, Hoff JM, Gilhus NE. Pregnancy, delivery, and birth outcome in women with multiple sclerosis. Neurology 2005;65:1961–3.
[12] Sadovnick AD, Eisen K, Hashimoto SA, Farquhar R, Yee IM, Hooge J, et al. Pregnancy and multiple sclerosis. A prospective study. Arch Neurol 1994;51:1120–4.
[13] Worthington J, Jones R, Crawford M, Forti A. Pregnancy and multiple sclerosis—a 3-year prospective study. J Neurol 1994;241:228–33.
[14] Millar JH, Allison RS, Cheeseman EA, Merrett JD. Pregnancy as a factor influencing relapse in disseminated sclerosis. Brain 1959;82:417–26.
[15] Ghezzi A, Caputo D. Pregnancy: a factor influencing the course of multiple sclerosis? Eur Neurol 1981;20:115–7.
[16] Frith JA, McLeod JG. Pregnancy and multiple sclerosis. J Neurol Neurosurg Psychiatry 1988;51:495–8.
[17] Vukusic S, Hutchinson M, Hours M, Moreau T, Cortinovis-Tourniaire P, Adeleine P, et al. Pregnancy and multiple sclerosis (the PRIMS study): clinical predictors of post-partum relapse. Brain 2004;127:1353–60.
[18] van Walderveen MA, Tas MW, Barkhof F, Polman CH, Frequin ST, Hommes OR, et al. Magnetic resonance evaluation of disease activity during pregnancy in multiple sclerosis. Neurology 1994;44:327–9.
[19] Paavilainen T, Kurki T, Parkkola R, Färkkilä M, Salonen O, Dastidar P, et al. Magnetic resonance imaging of the brain used to detect early post-partum activation of multiple sclerosis. Eur J Neurol 2007;14:1216–21.
[20] Saraste MH, Kurki T, Airas LM. Postpartum activation of multiple sclerosis: MRI imaging and immunological characterization of a case. Eur J Neurol 2006;13:98–9.
[21] Jalkanen A, Alanen A, Airas L and the Finnish Multiple Sclerosis and Pregnancy Study Group. Pregnancy outcome in women with multiple sclerosis—results from a prospective nationwide study in Finland. Mult Scler 2010;16(8):950–5.
[22] Bamford C, Sibley W, Laguna J. Anesthesia in multiple sclerosis. Can J Neurol Sci 1978;5:41–4.
[23] De Las Heras V, De Andres C, Tellez N, Tintore M. Pregnancy in multiple sclerosis patients treated with immunomodulators prior to or during part of the pregnancy: a descriptive study in the Spanish population. Mult Scler 2007;13:981–4.
[24] Boskovic R, Wide R, Wolpin J, Bauer DJ, Koren G. The reproductive effects of beta interferon therapy in pregnancy: a longitudinal cohort. Neurology 2005;65:807–11.

[25] Sandberg-Wollheim M, Frank D, Goodwin TM, Giesser B, Lopez-Bresnahan M, Stam-Morago M, et al. Pregnancy outcomes during treatment with interferon beta-1a in patients with multiple sclerosis. Neurology 2005;65:802–6.

[26] Patti F, Cavallaro T, Lo Fermo S, Nicoletti A, Cimino V, Vecchio R, et al. Is in utero early-exposure to interferon beta a risk factor for pregnancy outcomes in multiple sclerosis? J Neurol 2008;255:1250–3.

[27] Hellwig K, Brune N, Haghikia A, Müller T, Schimrigk S, Schwödiauer V, et al. Reproductive counselling, treatment and course of pregnancy in 73 German MS patients. Acta Neurol Scand 2008;118:24–8.

[28] Airas L, Jalkanen A, Alanen A, Pirttilä T, Marttila RJ. Breast-feeding, postpartum and prepregnancy disease activity in multiple sclerosis. Neurology 2010;3;75(5):474–6.

[29] Oddy WH. A review of the effects of breastfeeding on respiratory infections, atopy, and childhood asthma. J Asthma 2004;41:605–21.

[30] Langer-Gould A, Huang SM, Gupta R, Leimpeter AD, Greenwood E, Albers KB, et al. Exclusive breastfeeding and the risk of postpartum relapses in women with multiple sclerosis. Arch Neurol 2009;66(8):958–63.

[31] Fazekas F, Deisenhammer F, Strasser-Fuchs S, Nahler G, Mamoli B. Randomised placebo-controlled trial of monthly intravenous immunoglobulin therapy in relapsing–remitting multiple sclerosis. Austrian Immunoglobulin in Multiple Sclerosis Study Group. Lancet 1997;349:589–93.

[32] Fazekas F, Lublin FD, Li D, Freedman MS, Hartung HP, Rieckmann P, et al. Intravenous immunoglobulin in relapsing-remitting multiple sclerosis: a dose-finding trial. Neurology 2008;71:265–71.

[33] Achiron A, Kishner I, Dolev M, Stern Y, Dulitzky M, Schiff E, et al. Effect of intravenous immunoglobulin treatment on pregnancy and postpartum-related relapses in multiple sclerosis. J Neurol 2004;251:1133–7.

[34] Haas J, Hommes OR. A dose comparison study of IVIG in postpartum relapsing–remitting multiple sclerosis. Mult Scler 2007;13(7):900–8.

[35] Elovaara I, Apostolski S, van Doorn P, Gilhus NE, Hietaharju A, Honkaniemi J, et al. EFNS guidelines for the use of intravenous immunoglobulin in treatment of neurological diseases: EFNS task force on the use of intravenous immunoglobulin in treatment of neurological diseases. Eur J Neurol 2008;15:893–908.

[36] Chaouat G, Ledee-Bataille N, Dubanchet S, Zourbas S, Sandra O, Martal J. Reproductive immunology 2003: reassessing the Th1/Th2 paradigm? Immunol Lett 2004;92:207–14.

[37] Wegmann TG, Lin H, Guilbert L, Mosmann TR. Bidirectional cytokine interactions in the maternal–fetal relationship: is successful pregnancy a TH2 phenomenon? Immunol Today 1993;14:353–6.

[38] Sánchez-Ramón S, Navarro AJ, Aristimuño C, Rodríguez-Mahou M, Bellón JM, Fernández-Cruz E, et al. Pregnancy-induced expansion of regulatory T-lymphocytes may mediate protection to multiple sclerosis activity. Immunol Lett 2005;96:195–201.

[39] Polanczyk MJ, Hopke C, Huan J, Vandenbark AA, Offner H. Enhanced FoxP3 expression and Treg cell function in pregnant and estrogen-treated mice. J Neuroimmunol 2005;170:85–92.

[40] Gilmore W, Weiner LP, Correale J. Effect of estradiol on cytokine secretion by proteolipid protein-specific T cell clones isolated from multiple sclerosis patients and normal control subjects. J Immunol 1997;158:446–51.

[41] Pauklin S, Sernandez IV, Bachmann G, Ramiro AR, Petersen-Mahrt SK. Estrogen directly activates AID transcription and function. J Exp Med 2009;206:99–111.

[42] Liu HB, Loo KK, Palaszynski K, Ashouri J, Lubahn DB, Voskuhl RR. Estrogen receptor alpha mediates estrogen's immune protection in autoimmune disease. J Immunol 2003;171:6936–40.

[43] Polanczyk M, Zamora A, Subramanian S, Matejuk A, Hess DL, Blankenhorn EP, et al. The protective effect of 17beta-estradiol on experimental autoimmune encephalomyelitis is mediated through estrogen receptor-alpha. Am J Pathol 2003;163:1599–605.

[44] Vegeto E, Belcredito S, Etteri S, Ghisletti S, Brusadelli A, Meda C, et al. Estrogen receptor-alpha mediates the brain antiinflammatory activity of estradiol. Proc Natl Acad Sci USA 2003;100:9614–9.

[45] Kim S, Liva SM, Dalal MA, Verity MA, Voskuhl RR. Estriol ameliorates autoimmune demyelinating disease: implications for multiple sclerosis. Neurology 1999;52:1230–8.

[46] Polanczyk MJ, Jones RE, Subramanian S, Afentoulis M, Rich C, Zakroczymski M, et al. T lymphocytes do not directly mediate the protective effect of estrogen on experimental autoimmune encephalomyelitis. Am J Pathol 2004;165:2069–77.

[47] Sicotte NL, Liva SM, Klutch R, Pfeiffer P, Bouvier S, Odesa S, et al. Treatment of multiple sclerosis with the pregnancy hormone estriol. Ann Neurol 2002;52:421–8.

[48] Irony-Tur-Sinai M, Grigoriadis N, Lourbopoulos A, Pinto-Maaravi F, Abramsky O, Brenner T. Amelioration of autoimmune neuroinflammation by recombinant human alpha-fetoprotein. Exp Neurol 2006;198:136–44.

[49] Clark DA. Tolerance signaling molecules. Chem Immunol Allergy 2005;89:36–48.

[50] Bebo Jr. BF, Dveksler GS. Evidence that pregnancy specific glycoproteins regulate T-cell function and inflammatory autoimmune disease during pregnancy. Curr Drug Targets Inflamm Allergy 2005;4:231–7.

[51] Gilmore W, Arias M, Stroud N, Stek A, McCarthy KA, Correale J. Preliminary studies of cytokine secretion patterns associated with pregnancy in MS patients. J Neurol Sci 2004;224:69–76.

[52] Saraste M, Ryynänen J, Alanen A, Multanen J, Färkkilä M, Kaaja R, et al. Cerebrospinal fluid findings in multiple sclerosis patients before, during and after pregnancy. J Neurol Neurosurg Psychiatry 2006;77:1195–6.

2 Headache in Pregnancy

Debra Elliott, Xiangping Li, Peimin Zhu, Emil Gaitour

Louisiana State University Health Sciences Center, Shreveport, LA, USA

Introduction

Headache is a frequent complaint among women of childbearing age. Years ago, patients with severe chronic migraine were told by their physicians that they should not endeavor to get pregnant because they would not be able to take drugs while carrying a child. One can imagine the heartache involved in such advice! The truth is that most patients experience an improvement in headache during pregnancy. For others who have persistent severe symptoms that may cause suffering or dehydration, or represent a more sinister health problem, there are treatments that can help. Management of headaches in pregnancy poses challenges for the health care team that can be overcome with proper guidance and attention to the special needs of the fetus and gravid mother.

Epidemiology of Headache in Pregnancy

Headache is a common symptom, reported by more than 80% of women of childbearing age [1]. The majority of pregnant patients with headaches suffer from migraine or tension-type headache (TTH). A retrospective study of over 400 pregnant women reported that 30% met the International Headache Society (IHS) criteria for recurrent primary headaches. Among these women, migraine without aura (MO) was the most common headache type (64%) followed by TTH (26%) [2]. In patients who present with new onset of severe headache, with or without neurologic symptoms, more serious or life-threatening neurologic conditions need to be ruled out. This chapter discusses the epidemiology, pathophysiology, differential diagnosis, and management of major headache disorders during pregnancy.

Prevalence and Clinical Features of Migraine

Migraine is an episodic headache disorder with a 1-year prevalence of approximately 18% in women, 6% in men, and 4% in children. Three methodologically identical studies were conducted during a 15-year period with samples of more than 20,000 in the American Migraine Study I (AMS-I); 30,000 in the American Migraine Study II (AMS-II); and 160,000 in the American Migraine Prevalence and Prevention Study

Neurological Disorders and Pregnancy. DOI: 10.1016/B978-0-12-384911-3.00002-6

Table 2.1 ICHD-2 Diagnostic Criteria for Migraine Without Aura

A. At least 5 attacks fulfilling criteria B–D
B. Headache attacks lasting 4–72 h (untreated or unsuccessfully treated)
C. Headache has at least two of the following characteristics: 1. unilateral location 2. pulsating quality 3. moderate or severe pain intensity 4. aggravation by or causing avoidance of routine physical activity (e.g., walking or climbing stairs)
D. During headache at least one of the following: 1. nausea and/or vomiting 2. photophobia and phonophobia
C. Not attributed to another disorder

Source: From [6].

(AMPPS) [3–5]. They demonstrated that migraine prevalence has been stable in the United States over more than a decade. In all three studies, the average female-to-male migraine prevalence ratio was around 2.8, with a peak of 3.3 between 40 and 45 years. The ratio remained above 2.0 even after the age of menopause.

Migraine attacks occur in 6% of women and 4% of men in their teenage years, but reach the peak between ages 30 and 39 with 24% women and 7% men affected. The prevalence remains high in people in their 40s and 50s, but gradually decreases to 5% in women and 2% in men when people enter their 60s [5]. Clearly, migraine is most common in the childbearing and child-rearing years (ages of 25–55), so pre-pregnancy, pregnancy, and postpartum issues are important considerations for health care providers.

The Ad Hoc Committee on the Classification of Headache [6] described headache of migraine type as recurrent attacks of headache, widely varied in intensity, frequency, and duration. The attacks are commonly unilateral in onset; are usually associated with anorexia and sometimes with nausea and vomiting; some are preceded by, or associated with, conspicuous sensory, motor, and mood disturbances; and are often familial [6]. Migraines can be divided into two major subtypes: migraine with aura (MA) and migraine without aura (MO). MO is the most common type, accounting for approximately 80% of cases. The diagnosis of MO requires at least five lifetime attacks, lasting 4–72 h, with at least two of four pain features and at least one of two sets of associated symptoms (Table 2.1). MA is characterized by the presence of reversible focal neurologic symptoms that usually develop over 5–20 min and last for <60 min. Visual aura is overwhelmingly the most common (Table 2.2) [6]. The aura usually precedes the headache, although in many instances the aura can occur during or after the headache. More than in any other headache disorder, migraine sufferers identify triggers. Stress is the trigger most commonly listed by patients. Dietary factors also are frequently reported, although few have been scientifically validated. Oversleeping and sleep deprivation are commonly recognized triggers. Hormonal

Table 2.2 ICHD-2 Criteria for Typical Aura with Migraine Headache

A. At least 2 attacks fulfilling criteria B–D
B. Aura consisting of at least one of the following, but no motor weakness: 1. fully reversible visual symptoms including positive features (e.g., flickering lights, spots, or lines) and/or negative features (i.e., loss of vision) 2. fully reversible sensory symptoms including positive features (i.e., pins and needles) and/or negative features (i.e., numbness) 3. fully reversible dysphasic speech disturbance
C. At least two of the following: 1. homonymous visual symptoms and/or unilateral sensory symptoms 2. at least one aura symptom develops gradually ⩾5 and/or different aura symptoms occur in succession over ⩾5 minutes 3. each symptom lasts ⩾5 and ⩽60 minutes
D. Headache fulfilling criteria B–D for 1.1 *Migraine without aura* begins during the aura or follows aura within 60 min
E. Not attributed to another disorder

Source: From Headache Classification Subcommittee of the IHS [6].

headaches are triggered by variations in female estrogen levels and possibly other hormonal factors. Noise, bright lights, and fumes are commonly identified migraine triggers. Physical exertion can cause exercise-induced migraine [7].

Effect of Pregnancy on Migraine

There are a number of important issues to be addressed by the physician when a woman with migraine becomes pregnant. Below are some common questions that migraine patients might raise.

- I'm pregnant … what's going to happen to my migraine?
- I'm pregnant … is migraine going to harm my baby?
- What's going to happen to my migraine after I have the baby?

In answer to the first question, migraine in women is influenced by hormonal changes throughout the life cycle: menarche, menstruation, oral contraceptive use, pregnancy, menopause, and hormonal replacement therapy. Somerville's work in the early 1970s suggested that falling estrogen levels were the provocative factor in menstrual migraine [8]. Studies examining the natural history of migraines in pregnancy have suggested that migraine generally improves during pregnancy. Studies conducted after 1988 all used the IHS classification of migraine, improving the standardization of headache diagnosis. However, the majority of these studies is retrospective, the patients having been evaluated several years after pregnancy or, at best, in the postpartum period [9–20]. For example, in the Collaborative Perinatal Project, Chen and Leviton [15] retrospectively reviewed 55,000 pregnancies in the United States. Only 2% of these women had self-reported migraine. Of the 484 cases analyzed, 17% had a complete remission and another 62% showed some improvement with pregnancy. Granella et al. found that headache improvement during pregnancy occurred in only 43% of patients who had MA, compared with 72% of patients who had MO [18]. A large Norwegian population-based study examined the effect of pregnancy and parity on headache prevalence [19]. This study found that although the headache prevalence was lower among pregnant than among nonpregnant women, the association between headache and pregnancy was significant for nulliparous (one who has never given birth; OR = 0.5, 95% CI = 0.4–0.7), but not for primiparous (one child only) and multiparous (several children) women (OR = 0.8, 95% CI = 0.7–1.0). This was evident for both migraine and nonmigrainous headache.

A limited number of prospective studies has been conducted on the pattern of migraine during pregnancy [21–25]. Sances et al. [23] prospectively investigated the course of migraine during pregnancy and postpartum in pregnant women attending an obstetrics and gynecology department for a routine first trimester antenatal checkup. Forty-nine migraineurs (2 with MA and 47 with MO) who had experienced at least one attack during the 3 months preceding pregnancy were identified, enrolled in the study, and given a headache diary. Examinations were performed at the end of the second and third trimesters and 1 month after delivery. Migraine improved in 46.8% of the 47 MO sufferers during the first trimester, in 83.0% during the second and in 87.2% during the third, while complete remission was attained by 10.6%, 53.2%, and 78.7% of the women, respectively. Although the headache of migraine is frequently better with the stable, high estrogen levels of pregnancy, aura may occur more frequently or for the first time during pregnancy [18,24].

Recurrence during the postpartum period is common [21–23,26]. Sances et al. [23] found that migraine recurred during the first week after childbirth in 34.0% of the women and during the first month in 55.3%. Recurrence during the postpartum period is significantly less frequent in women who breast-feed [23,27]. The mechanism underlying this finding is unknown. Rather than bottle feeding representing a risk factor, it could be hypothesized that breast-feeding exerts a protective action, as breast-feeding increases the levels of the antinociceptive hormones vasopressin and oxytocin and contributes to successful natural bonding [23]. Women with menstrual migraine are most likely to experience postpartum headaches. Falling estrogen levels after delivery are blamed for this phenomenon, although lactation may delay or decrease the rate of estrogen lowering, thus decreasing the postpartum headache.

Effect of Migraine on Pregnancy

Migraine does not seem to directly affect the outcome of pregnancy [24]. Wainscott and Volans et al. [28] found that the incidence of miscarriage, toxemia, congenital anomalies, and stillbirth was not increased in a sample of 777 migraine sufferers compared with the national averages or controls. A retrospective case–control study of over 38,000 deliveries showed that mean gestational age and birth weight in babies born to women with migraine did not differ from the general population, and the proportions of low birth weight and preterm births were the same [29]. However, migraine appears to be associated with several maternal pregnancy complications.

Women with migraine during pregnancy may be at increased risk of gestational hypertension and pre-eclampsia that may appear earlier and be more severe [30–33]. A large population-based study found that migraineurs, particularly those with aura, have a higher cardiovascular risk profile than individuals without migraine. Women with migraine were more likely to have been diagnosed with gestational hypertension, even after taking into account age and number of pregnancies [34]. In a case–controlled study of pregnancy discharges, inpatient coding for peripartum migraine was associated with ischemic stroke. The results from this study also indicated associations between peripartum migraine and heart disease, venous thromboembolism, and cardiovascular risk factors such as hypertension, diabetes, and smoking [35]. However, due to the confounding presence of gestational hypertension, pre-eclampsia, and eclampsia, this study could not determine the independent effect of migraine on vascular disorders. A recent 3-year nationwide population-based study in Taiwan [36] revealed that women with migraines were at increased risk of having low birth weight infants, preterm birth, pre-eclampsia, and delivery by cesarean section, compared with unaffected mothers; however, given the large size of the sample used in this study, overpower might be a concern, giving small differences statistical significance which may not actually be clinically significant. In addition, the database did not include complete information regarding medications taken during pregnancy, the confounding role of medications in the relationship between migraines, and adverse birth outcomes were not assessed.

Tension-Type Headaches

Tension-type headache (TTH) is the most common type of primary headache, with 1-year prevalence of approximately 40% in the United States [37]. In contrast to migraine, the main pain features of TTH are bilateral location, nonpulsating quality, mild-to-moderate intensity, and lack of aggravation by routine physical activity. The pain is not accompanied by nausea, although just one of photo- or phonophobia does not exclude the diagnosis.

The International Classification of Headache Disorders-2 (ICHD-2) [6] distinguishes three main subtypes of TTH (Table 2.3):

1. Infrequent episodic TTH, with headache episodes less than 1 day a month
2. Frequent episodic TTH, with headache episodes 1–14 days a month
3. Chronic TTH, with headaches 15 or more days a month

In a recent population-based study using the ICHD-2 criteria to classify TTH subtypes, a Danish twin registry found that the 1-year-period prevalences of infrequent episodic TTH, frequent episodic TTH, and chronic TTH were 63.5%, 21.6%, and 0.9%, respectively [38].

TTH affects women slightly more often than men. The age of onset is usually between 20 and 30 years, and peak prevalence is between the ages of 30 and 39 for both sexes [37]. Clinical experience would suggest that TTH is less likely to improve during pregnancy because it is not hormonally mediated. However, TTH has not been extensively studied in pregnant women. One study noted that 48% of migraine patients improved during pregnancy compared with only 28% of patients with TTH [39].

Table 2.3 ICHD-2 Criteria for Tension-Type Headaches

2.1 Infrequent Episodic TTH	A. At least 10 episodes occurring on 1 day per month on average (12 days per year) and fulfilling criteria B–D B. Headache lasting from 30 min to 7 days C. Headache has at least two of the following characteristics: 1. bilateral location 2. pressing/tightening (nonpulsating) quality 3. mild or moderate intensity 4. not aggravated by routine physical activity such as walking or climbing stairs D. Both of the following: 1. no nausea or vomiting (anorexia may occur) 2. no more than one of photophobia or phonophobia E. Not attributed to another disorder
2.2 Frequent Episodic TTH	A. At least 10 episodes occurring on ≥1 but <15 per month for at least 3 months (≥12 and <180 days per year) and fulfilling criteria B–E for 2.1 Infrequent Episodic TTH
2.3 Chronic Tension-type Headache	A. Headaches happening on ≥15 days per month on average ≥3 months (≥180 days per year) B. Headache lasts hours or may be continuous C. Headache has at least two of the following characteristics: 1. bilateral location 2. pressing/tightening (nonpulsating) quality 3. mild or moderate intensity 4. not aggravated by routine physical activity such as walking or climbing stairs D. Both of the following: 1. no more than one of photophobia, phonophobia, or mild nausea 2. neither moderate or severe nausea nor vomiting E. Not attributed to another disorder

Source: From Headache Classification Subcommittee of the IHS [6].

Cluster Headache

The prevalence of cluster headache (CH) in reproductive-aged women is 7.5 of 100,000 women with a male to female ratio 7.5 to 1–2.5 to 1 [40]. A rise in female prevalence of cluster headache may perhaps be due to changes in women's lifestyles as they have entered the workforce. We are now slowly starting to see pregnant patients with CH. It has been shown to have a close association with both smoking and alcohol ingestion and sleep apnea, and because comorbidities can affect the outcome of pregnancy, these should be addressed [41,42].

Pathophysiology of Primary Headache During Pregnancy

The interpretation of the pathogenesis of headache during pregnancy in this chapter will focus on the influence of the gonadal female hormones on migraine. Although the true mechanism of migraine development still seems mysterious, our understanding of this common symptom has been improving over the last 50 years. The vascular theory of Wolff, an initial cerebral vasoconstriction followed by an extracranial vasodilatation, was based on the finding of the parallel decrease of temporal pulsations and headache after intravenous injection of ergotamine. This earlier hypothesis gave way to one centered on brain stem dysfunction. Compared to other hypotheses on migraine neurobiology, dysfunction of brain stem structures such as the trigeminal nucleus caudalis (TNC), locus coeruleus (LC), the periaqueductal gray matter (PAG), and such networks not only account for headache (the somatosensory component), but also for the auditory, olfactory, and visual components of migraine. Moreover, LC dysfunction could also explain distractibility and anxiety, which is often observed in migraineurs [43–46]. Migraine attacks often start with a typical premonitory phase when patients complain of tiredness, reduced concentration, irritability, yawning, and other nonheadache symptoms hours to days before the onset of aura and headache. These reports suggest that brain stem dysfunction may precede cortical spreading depression (CSD) [47,48]. Tonabersat, a possible gap-junction blocker and inhibitor of CSD that is currently being tested in humans, does not prevent migraine headache but can prevent migraine aura [43,49–51]. Although no changes are known to occur in CSD during pregnancy, researchers have suggested a role for modulation of CSD by gonadal hormones in female mice by demonstrating differences in susceptibility to CSD following ovariectomy [52].

Hormonal Influences on the Central Nervous System and Migraine During Pregnancy

During pregnancy, hormonal changes occur that affect the nervous system. The placenta becomes the primary site of production of gonadal steroids. Other minor sources of steroids include the ovary, adrenal gland, and brain. Serum levels of estradiol/estriol and progesterone begin to rise in the mother during the sixth to eighth weeks of pregnancy as the placenta begins to produce steroids. They continue to increase to their highest levels gradually, representing a 30- to 40-fold increase of estradiol and a 20-fold increase of progesterone during the third trimester [53].

Estradiol/estriol and progesterone directly affect the central nervous system (CNS). Pregnancy hormones passively diffuse across the blood–brain barrier (BBB) and act on the neurons and glia. Estrogen receptors (ER) and progesterone receptors (PR) are expressed in various regions of the brain and implicated in many different neuronal functions. As listed in Table 2.4, researchers demonstrated ERα and ERβ receptors in the TNC, brain stem nuclei, and many other regions of the brain [53].

The action of estrogen at the molecular level is carried out via nongenomic and genomic mechanisms. Through the nongenomic mechanism, estrogen uncouples μ-opioid and γ-aminobutyric acid type B ($GABA_B$) receptors from their effector systems, whereas allopregnanolone increases the opening time of $GABA_A$ receptors [54,55]. Through the genomic mechanism, gene expression levels can be changed and thus neuron function is modulated.

Table 2.4 ER in Brain Tissue

Brain Region	Rat		Monkey		Human	
	ERα	ERβ	ERα	ERβ	ERα	ERβ
Prefrontal cortex	+	+	+	+	+	+
Frontal cortex	+	+	+	−	+	+
Hippocampus	+	+	+	+	−	+
Amygdala	+	+	+	+	+	−
Paraventricular nucleus	−	+	+	+	?	?
Preoptic area	+	+	+	+	?	?
Mediobasal hypothalamus	+	+	+	+	+	−
Lateral tegmentum/pons	+	+	+	+	?	?
Dorsal raphe	+	+	+	+	+*	+*
Locus coeruleus	+	+	+	+	+	+
Spinal trigeminal nucleus	+	+	+	?	?	?
PAG	+	+	+	?	?	?
Cerebellum	+	+	+	−	?	?

Source: Modified from [53].
*Indicates the expression is studied at mRNA level.

In other studies, PR, including PRA, PRB, and 7-transmembrane progesterone receptor β isoform (7-TMPR), were expressed at different levels in many regions throughout the brain [56–58,59]. Their levels may vary between regions and change in response to stimulation and different hormonal states, such as the phases of the menstrual cycle, pregnancy, and postpartum period. Estrogen induces PRA isoform expression, whereas progesterone does not affect the expression of any PR isoforms [60,61].

The fact that migraine improves during pregnancy is at least partially attributed to the lack of fluctuation of estrogen levels during pregnancy. Numerous clinical and animal studies support the generally accepted concept that fluctuating estrogen levels may trigger migraine. Either a sharp increase or a drop in estrogen level was shown to be associated with migraine attacks, while little evidence suggests that progesterone can independently modulate or trigger migraine [4,23,62–64].

In human genetic studies, there are controversial reports on the ER and PR linkage to migraine. One study reported PR linkage with migraine-associated vertigo [65]. Another study found that PROGINS allele, PR marker, interacted synergistically with the ESR 1 594A allele, which alone was reported to be linked to migraine, to increase the risk of migraine by a factor of three [66,67]. A recent study investigated the role of common polymorphisms in the ER and PR genes in the risk for migraine in a Spanish population. Surprisingly, it did not support a major contribution of ER1 and PR to the pathogenesis of migraine [68]. However, many other physiologic and pharmacologic studies on animals and humans do suggest at least a modulatory effect of these neurohormones on migraine, through interactions with almost all of the major neurotransmitter systems, including serotonin, opioid, glutamatergic, and GABAergic as well as the sympathetic and nonsympathetic systems [53].

The serotonergic system modulates the functions of many regions in CNS. The dysfunction of this system leads to many disorders including mood disorders, neurodegenerative disease, and neurodevelopment disorders [69]. Migraineurs have been demonstrated to have low plasma serotonin interictally, with a 60% surge during attacks [70]. In the brain, serotonin is synthesized by tryptophan hydroxylase type 2 (TPH2) [71]. Levels of serotonin at the synapse are primarily determined by the serotonin reuptake transporter (SERT), which was linked to migraine in recent genetic studies [72,73]. Estrogen was also found to increase TPH expression in the monkey, whereas the addition of progesterone had no significant effect on this enzyme [74]. Estrogen and/or progesterone also modulate levels of SERT, and monoamine oxidases A and B likely through ER , PR, and NF-KappaB [74,75].

Following the earlier studies, a functional study of dorsal raphe neurons showed that during pregnancy a graded augmentation and diminution in 5-HT neuron firing rate occurs. This mirrors that of circulating progesterone concentrations. Such firing rate change in dorsal raphe neurons seems to be independent of LC activity during pregnancy [76]. These studies suggest that estrogen and progesterone may modulate the serotonin system through distinct mechanisms and participate in different physiologic functions. Regardless of the estrogen/progesterone-related 5-HT changes in raphe neurons, higher serotonin levels during pregnancy have been noted for years. This might explain the pleasant emotion and fewer headaches often observed during pregnancy.

Both estrogen and progesterone are implicated as the major gonadal hormones that modulate migraine severity during pregnancy. Increased levels of progesterone may cause changes in nervous system function important to pain-related mechanisms. These include increased release of endorphins [76,77], altered neuropeptide expression level and vascular sensitivity to them [78], decreased sensitization to glutamate or decreased α-amino-3-hydroxy-5-methyl-4-isoxazolepropionic acid (AMPA) receptor binding [79,80], and increased activity of GABAergic neurons [81,82].

ER and neuropeptides, including pituitary adenylate cyclase-activating polypeptide (PACAP), substance P (SP), calcitonin-gene-related-peptide (CGRP), have been found in human TNC and brain stem nuclei, including the LC, PAG, and raphe magnus (NRM) [83,84]. CGRP is the most studied among them. It is the most potent peptide vasodilator known and can function in the transmission of pain. 5-HT1B/D agonists, such as sumatriptan, increase intracellular calcium, which causes decrease in CGRP promoter activity [85]. 17β-estradiol and progesterone cause vasorelaxation at high nonphysiologic concentrations via rapid nongenomic pathways, but they may also manifest their actions via slow genomic pathways [86].

The expression of CGRP receptors is augmented during pregnancy, probably through ER [87,88]. In rats, pregnancy had a trophic effect on trigeminal perivascular innervation. The increase of CGRP in trigeminal innervation during pregnancy may be more related to nociception than in control of resting cerebral blood flow [88]. Receptor antagonists such as telcagepant, which is currently in phase III trials, have promise in limiting the effects of CGRP [89]. Although it is hoped that this new drug will be effective in migraine, its safety and availability for use in pregnancy will not be known for years.

There are few studies in the literature that can explain why some women experience new onset of migraine or exacerbation of migraine during pregnancy. Perhaps the imbalance between estrogen and progesterone is associated with such headache, as animal studies found that estrogen may facilitate neuronal excitation while progesterone apposes it [53]. Future studies on the linkage between PR allele or neuropeptide allele and pregnancy onset of migraine might prove worth the effort.

Tension-Type Headache and Cluster Headache

TTH is less studied than migraine. Clinical studies showed less improvement of TTH during pregnancy than migraine [39,90]. The hypothetical pathophysiologic mechanism of tension headache shares some common features with migraine, including involvement of the trigeminal system and central sensitization. Chronic TTH (CTTH) can be associated with referred pain from active trigger points (TrPs) in the posterior cervical, head, and shoulder muscles mediated through the spinal cord and the brain stem TNC. TrPs may represent the primary hyperalgesic zones responsible for the development of central sensitization in CTTH [91]. Pregnancy-related changes in endorphins and GABAergic neurotransmitter systems may apply to the attenuation of headache observed in pregnant patients with CTTH.

CH is rare in pregnancy. The acute attack of pain may be regarded as a manifestation of the trigeminal-autonomic reflex. The clinical feature of circannual and circadian periodicity, the neuroendocrine changes, and the functional imaging studies implicate the hypothalamic region as fundamental to CH [92]. A population-based questionnaire study was performed among 224 female CH patients, and the possible effect of hormonal influences on CH attacks studied. It was found that menstruation, use of oral contraceptives, pregnancy, and menopause had a much smaller influence on CH attacks than in migraine [93].

Management of Primary Headache in Pregnancy

Nonpharmacologic Treatments

Because of the uncertain safety of fetal exposure to most pharmaceuticals, many women with problematic headaches and migraine turn to nonpharmacologic treatments in pregnancy. For many acute attacks, rest, reassurance, and ice packs will be sufficient [94]. The American Academy of Neurology guidelines [95] list pregnancy, planned pregnancy, or nursing as some of the characteristics in which nonpharmacologic treatment options may be chosen, among others. These therapies can also be adjunctive to medication to improve outcome. They are categorized as physical therapies and behavioral treatments. Although some behavioral therapies are recommended with Grade A evidence to support their efficacy, evidence-based recommendations are not available for hypnosis, acupuncture, transcutaneous electrical nerve stimulation, chiropractic or osteopathic cervical manipulation, occlusal adjustment, and hyperbaric oxygen as preventive or acute therapy for migraine [1,96]. It is important to note that herbal remedies are not listed in this category, as they may indeed have pharmacologic effects and side effects which may or may not be known.

Complementary and Alternative Medicine in Pregnancy

In a recent survey of providers in Australia, the majority of obstetricians and midwives had a positive view of complementary and alternative medicine (CAM) including massage, acupuncture, vitamins, yoga, meditation, and hypnosis for a variety of ailments in pregnancy. However, 72% of obstetricians thought there was a need for more evidence [97]. Patients often turn to CAM independently, with or without health care provider input. A survey of pregnant women in Germany found that approximately half used CAM during pregnancy; headache was not addressed. Of those who consulted a provider, midwives were the main prescribers of CAM therapies. CAM often included herbal treatments that were not prescribed by or reported to their health care provider. Because of this reason, the authors concluded that the practice of using CAM in pregnancy and delivery should be used with caution, and providers should rely on those treatments backed by some positive evidence [98].

Physical Therapies

Physical treatments for headache include chiropractic manipulation and/or mobilization of the cervical spine (CMM), physical therapy (PT), acupuncture, massage, traction, craniosacral therapy, and TrP therapy. PT is often used in the treatment of TTH. It includes improvement of posture, relaxation, exercise programs, hot and cold packs, ultrasound, and electrical stimulation [99]. Patients are more likely to benefit from exercise and more active PT strategies than from passive techniques [100]. Numerous case reports [101], series [102], and reviews indicate high utilization of CMM (up to 12 million people annually) [103] and good results in many instances of headache [104] and neck and back pain [105]. CMM may be associated with an initial increase in headache intensity if delivered too vigorously. It is better tolerated when gentle muscle stretching and manual cervical traction precedes CMM and it is slowly advanced to include strengthening and aerobic conditioning [106]. Sometimes anesthetic blocks or neurolytic procedures also are used for temporary pain relief during therapy, but this has not been addressed in pregnancy. It is presumed that cervical techniques exert their effect on headaches by activating descending pain inhibitory systems from the brain stem/periaqueductal gray and/or activation of β-endorphin-driven endogenous anti-nociception [7], thus minimizing chronic nociceptive input into the CNS [107].

Due to the nature of these treatments, sham controls are difficult to produce in a scientific research setting, limiting conclusions about safety and efficacy, or providing contradictory results. In one study, researchers found no supporting evidence in eight randomized controlled trials for the efficacy of CMM in the treatment of headache [108]. For the treatment of TTH, another review found no rigorous evidence that manual therapies (CMM, connective tissue manipulation, soft tissue massage, traction, or craniosacral techniques) provided any positive effect [109]. Another systematic review in 2005 showed evidence of better efficacy of PT compared to CMM (which had possible minor benefit), acupuncture, or massage in frequent TTH. They found some benefit in migraine patients treated with a combination of PT, thermal biofeedback, relaxation training, and exercise, but found CMM to be probably more effective in TTH than in migraine [110]. More recent studies published in 2010 indicate that CMM is effective for migraine and cervicogenic headache, but inconclusive for TTH; and for neck pain, massage was most effective [111], and that cervicogenic headache patients seem to fare slightly better with CMM than they do with light massage [112].

A meta-analysis of eight studies involving acupuncture in the treatment of TTH concluded that it had limited efficacy when compared to sham controls [113], whereas a recent Cochrane review of eleven trials including over 2300 patients with episodic and/or chronic TTH revealed there may be relevant short-term benefits of adding acupuncture to routine care, and they found significant efficacy over sham interventions [114]. Acupuncture was effective for pregnancy-associated nausea and for dental pain in a review of this modality in pregnancy, but the data were equivocal or contradictory as pertains to chronic pain, back pain, and headache, despite activation of endogenous opioid mechanisms [115]. A randomized controlled trial (unblinded and with no sham procedure) looking at medical management versus medical management plus acupuncture for chronic daily headache revealed that the latter resulted in improvements in health-related quality of life and less suffering due to headaches [116]. More recent reviews of acupuncture in pregnancy corroborate the benefit in treating nausea, with some effectiveness in managing back and pelvic pain and assisting in labor. Headache was not mentioned [117,118]. Reflexology, on the other hand, has not demonstrated effectiveness in treating any medical condition including headache [119]. A controlled trial of craniosacral therapy for migraine is currently underway [120].

Most chiropractors agree that CMM is safe for pregnant patients with neck or back pain, although a majority avoids manipulation in the presence of comorbidity such as pre-eclampsia, hypertension, blood-clotting disorder, or ectopic pregnancy; and some feel it may be inappropriate in patients with gestational diabetes or in the case of multiple pregnancy [121]. Patients undergoing spinal manipulation do need to have adequate informed consent as to possible adverse events which, although are rare (5–10 per one million CMMs) can be catastrophic. Carotid and/or vertebral artery dissection [122,123], spinal cord injury, cervical nerve root damage, phrenic nerve injury, epidural hematoma, ruptured disk, and vertebral fractures can follow cervical manipulation. Patients with a known connective tissue disorder such as Ehlers–Danlos and Marfan syndrome may be more susceptible to arterial dissection; manipulation-induced vertebral fractures can occur more commonly in patients with underlying weakened vertebral bodies due to angiomata or osteoporosis. Because screening cervical radiologic tests are contraindicated in pregnancy, these patients may be at higher risk for spinal complications [124]. Fortunately, most pregnant women are young with relatively healthy bones.

Behavioral Therapies

Pregnancy is an ideal time for the patient with problematic headaches to explore behavioral therapies such as cognitive behavioral therapy, relaxation training, biofeedback, and hypnosis. This is also a time when discussions about lifestyle changes in the patient's diet, sleep, and exercise habits is especially appropriate. Trigger factors should be re-analyzed and avoided when possible. Bed rest or reduced work and home responsibilities may be helpful for some [125]. For the few that suffer from lactation headache, simply putting the baby to the breast, resulting in triggering the milk-ejection reflex, may relieve the symptoms [126].

Cognitive behavioral therapy can teach patients to identify thoughts and beliefs that generate stress and aggravate headache, and address coping strategies. It is probably most effective in patients with psychologic issues or problems such as chronic work stress, mood disorders, or adjustment disorders [127]. The exact efficacy of this modality is difficult to estimate, but is associated with very little harm if the patient is open to it. In addition, it can open the door for more intimate psychotherapy if appropriate.

Biofeedback is a method for learned control of physiologic responses of the body. These include both the voluntary system and the involuntary or autonomic system. The patient can thus learn to influence the skeletal muscles, heart rate, vascular responses (frequently indirectly measured as temperature), and sympathetic discharges (measured by the electrical galvanic skin response) to emotional or physical stimuli. With practice, biofeedback training and relaxation training results in a less excitable basal state, which may result in fewer headaches [128]. In pregnant women with recurring headache, stress management and biofeedback have been shown to decrease headache frequency by 50–79%, with lasting benefit for a year [129,130]. There are no recent studies proving benefit of hypnosis in headache treatment due to a lack of available sham procedures [131], but some patients may respond to this as a form of relaxation therapy.

Pharmacologic Treatments

Pregnancy-related health care should start before pregnancy. Because approximately 50% of pregnancies are unplanned, such an approach may serve to protect the fetus from inadvertent medication exposure. The female headache patient's reproductive status, family planning goals, and methods of contraception should be discussed on first evaluation [132]. Ethical and legal concerns would suggest including the woman's spouse or partner in any discussion which might affect the fetus [94], and communication with the obstetrician also is helpful. All women of childbearing age should be advised to take a multivitamin containing at least 0.4 mg folate daily to help decrease the risk of neural tube defects associated with some medication.

Before planned conception, medication discontinuation should be attempted and nonpharmacologic measures should be introduced. Long medication-free intervals before pregnancy are not necessary; the patient can attempt pregnancy right away [133].

Table 2.5 FDA Risk Categories

Category	Definition
A	Controlled human studies show no risk
B	No evidence of risk in humans, but there are no controlled human studies
C	Risk to humans has not been ruled out
D	Positive evidence of risk to humans from human or animal studies
X	Contraindicated in pregnancy

Source: From http://depts.washington.edu/druginfo/Formulary/Pregnancy.pdf

If medication elimination is not possible, consider changing to a more appropriate drug at the lowest effective dose.

As noted earlier, a significant minority of women will experience continued or worsened headaches during their pregnancy. In those whose headaches are severe, disabling, or associated with vomiting and possible dehydration, the benefits of pharmacologic treatment may outweigh the risks. Indeed, failure to treat chronic headache in pregnancy can lead to negative consequences such as poor nutrition, dehydration, depression, exacerbation of comorbid disease such as epilepsy or hypertension, or addiction to opioid analgesics, and/or overuse of simple analgesics compounding the chronic headache problem [132]. Decisions concerning when and what treatment is appropriate must be made on a case-by-case basis, which unfortunately will be based on inadequate information, due to a dearth of controlled studies on the subject [125].

The pharmacologic treatments include supplements and herbs, other "over-the-counter" or "off-the-shelf" medications, and prescription drugs. There are two pregnancy rating scales that are used to estimate the safety of medications in pregnancy: the Federal Drug Administration (FDA) pregnancy rating scale [134] and the Teratogen Information Service (TERIS) risk rating scale [135]. The FDA scale was devised to balance benefit versus risk, is free and readily available, and is considered an authoritative source. Some find it confusing and oversimplified, however, and 40% of drugs do not have a pregnancy rating. TERIS is based on teratogenicity only, and is a consensus of expert opinion and literature. Oddly enough, agreement between TERIS and FDA ratings is no greater than would be expected by chance alone [125]. Tables 2.5 and 2.6 include the FDA and TERIS ratings. In addition to these two sources, the American Academy of Pediatrics (AAP) Committee on Drugs provides a rating scale referable to safety during lactation, and available on the AAP website (Table 2.7) [125,133,136]. Finally, there is a compilation of drug monographs concerning prescription medications and alternative therapies and their appropriate use in breast-feeding women by Thomas Hale [137]. Comments are based on observational accounts, controlled studies, and pharmacologic data (Table 2.8). Generally speaking, drugs that are highly protein bound in the plasma are not

Table 2.6 TERIS Risk Rating

Rating	Definition	FDA-Equivalent Rating
N	None	A
N-Min	None-minimal	A
Min	Minimal	B
Min-S	Minimal-small	D
S	Small	
S-Mod	Small-moderate	
Mod	Moderate	
H	High	X
U	Undetermined	C

Source: From http://depts.washington.edu/terisweb/teris/.

Table 2.7 AAP Breast-Feeding Compatibility Ratings

Rating	Definition
1	Contraindicated
2	Requires temporary cessation of breast-feeding
3	Effects unknown but may be of concern
4	Usually compatible

Source: From [133].

Table 2.8 Hale's Lactation Risk Ratings

Rating	Definition
L1	Safest
L2	Safer
L3	Moderately safe
L4	Possibly hazardous
L5	Contraindicated

Source: From [137].

readily transferred into breast milk [133]. Other factors that impact drug levels in breast milk include the frequency the baby nurses, and the time from drug ingestion to nursing; one can minimize infant exposure by taking the medication directly after nursing or pumping and discarding breast milk following each dose [125].

Supplements and Herbs

Supplements and herbs are often misunderstood by the lay public, and the possible risks associated with them are underestimated. Therefore, patients should be adequately informed, especially those who are planning pregnancy. During patient encounters, health care providers should ask if patients are taking any of these treatments that may have not been prescribed. It is not unusual for patients to seek alternative advice. One recent observational study found that 82% of health food store clerks asked to recommend a treatment for migraine and nausea in pregnancy did so readily. Their investigation revealed that 5% of the recommended products were specifically contraindicated in pregnancy; for most others the safety was unknown [138].

Most supplements and herbs should be avoided in pregnancy. The exceptions are oral magnesium and riboflavin (vitamin B2). Magnesium is approved by the FDA for migraine prophylaxis during pregnancy. Riboflavin has shown efficacy in decreasing frequency of migraine [139]. There is no danger of toxicity associated with large doses of riboflavin. It is readily excreted in the urine and absorption by the digestive tract is relatively low. Pregnant patients should avoid butterbur root (*Petasites hybridus*) which can contain pyrrolizidine alkaloid metabolites that are toxic and carcinogenic and have been associated with Budd–Chiari syndrome (occlusion of the hepatic veins) [140]. Feverfew may be oxytocic [141] and may be teratogenic, based on rat studies [125]. Co-Q 10 is not recommended in pregnancy or lactation [142]. Caffeine may be used safely if overuse is avoided [143].

Off-the-Shelf Analgesics and Pharmaceuticals

The safest simple off-the-shelf analgesic for acute headache treatment in pregnancy and the postpartum period is acetaminophen, despite transient effects on the uterus and platelet function [132,144]. The nonsteroidal anti-inflammatory drugs (NSAIDs), ibuprofen and naproxen, should be avoided while the patient is attempting to conceive due to interference with implantation of the embryo. NSAIDs also may cause premature closure of the ductus arteriosus and fetal pulmonary hypertension and so are contraindicated in the third trimester, although they are compatible with breast-feeding [144]. Aspirin should be avoided in the third trimester as it may inhibit uterine contractions, increase bleeding of mother or baby, and also cause narrowing of the ductus arteriosus [145]. Phosphorylated carbohydrate solution (Emetrol), doxylamine (Unisom), or pyridoxine (Vitamin B6) can safely be used for nausea [94].

Prescription Medications for Acute Treatment

The goal of pharmacotherapy in pregnancy is to use the fewest and safest drugs at the lowest dose possible to achieve improvement in comfort and function, and avoid dehydration. Often the first line of treatment in a patient with a severe headache with vomiting is intravenous fluids and an intravenous antiemetic [146]. For the acute headache, prescription medications may be necessary for severe headache attacks. Most opioid analgesics are safe when used judiciously; they are rated as B unless use is prolonged or at term, in which case they have a D rating due to neonatal dependence [94]. Propoxyphene and codeine are category C drugs. Propoxyphene has been loosely associated with various malformations in early case reports [147–150]. Codeine has been associated with cleft palate and other midline malformations, such as inguinal hernias [132,144]. The sedating phenothiazines (category C) chlorpromazine, prochlorperazine, and promethazine, or metaclopromide (category B) may also be used. For a prolonged attack, prednisone (category B) or dexamethasone (category C) can break the headache cycle [133]. Barbiturates and benzodiazepines should be limited or avoided altogether due to their association with medication overuse headache, neonatal withdrawal syndromes, and possible fetal neurodevelopmental problems in the case of barbiturates [125].

Ergotamine and dihydroergotamine are to be strictly avoided, as they are oxytocic and teratogenic. Increased uterine tone and impaired placental blood flow can result in spontaneous abortion or fetal distress. Congenital defects have been reported including intestinal atresia, neurodevelopmental disorders, and Mobius syndrome [144].

The use of triptans has been studied extensively mainly through pregnancy registries organized and run by the pharmaceutical industry. The GlaxoSmithKline (GSK) registry is the longest and largest database to date, listing 829 pregnancies exposed to sumatriptan as of October 2008 [151]. The total number of major birth defects (MBDs) associated with sumatriptan exposure in the first trimester in this registry was 4.6%, excluding spontaneous abortion, induced abortion, and fetal deaths in which no defects were reported. Similarly, 4.8% of those fetuses exposed during the second trimester were born with MBDs, and none of 12 exposed in the third trimester, with an average of 4.7% across all trimesters. For comparison, data from general population studies report the incidence of MBDs as 1.6–2.2% (without versus with genetic defects) in a study in 1989, 2.1–2.7% (at 1 week versus 6 years) in 2007, and 3.4% in migraineurs in 1978. This suggests there is no substantial increase in MBD risk (when defined as greater than a two- to threefold increase) following exposure to sumatriptan thus far. Of all the MBDs recorded, ventricular septal defects were noted somewhat more commonly, comprising 0.9% of all first trimester exposures in the GSK registry, and 1.1% among pregnancy outcomes in the Swedish Medical Birth Register.

Researchers of the Norwegian Mother and Child Cohort Study, a major database of almost 70,000 primaparous women, found MBDs in 3.0% of the triptan-exposed group, 5.9% of the migraine control group, and 5.0% in the nonmigraine control group [152]. Further, they found that medical and obstetric complications were somewhat higher in the triptan-exposed group. Compared to nonmigraine controls, women who took triptan medication during pregnancy were more likely to experience emesis, fever, hypertension in the first trimester, pre-eclampsia/eclampsia, folate-deficiency anemia, hospitalization, and vaginal bleeding. Compared to migraine controls they suffered more often from folate-deficiency anemia and vaginal bleeding.

Triptan use late in pregnancy was associated with a slight increase in risk of atonic uterus and hemorrhage during labor. This could be due to serotonin effects. Serotonin stimulates myometrial contractions via 5-HT2B receptors suggesting a possible link between severe migraine and impaired uterine contractility. It is also known that serotonin has relaxant effect on porcine myometrial muscles via 5-HT7 receptors, at which triptans have an agonistic effect. At the conclusion of the Norwegian publication it was stated: "While it is important to exert caution when using any medication during pregnancy, this study indicates that migraineurs can continue an already established triptan therapy or start using triptans during pregnancy without any major risk of adverse pregnancy outcomes [152]." However, most experts agree at this time that the total reported number of exposures to triptans in pregnancy is still too low to definitively discern the safety of these medications or to recommend their use.

Prescription Medications for Preventive Treatment

If migraine headaches become excessively frequent (3–4 prolonged, severe attacks per month) or disabling, preventive treatment may rarely be indicated, for the reasons already stated earlier. None of the medications commonly used for migraine prevention have a category A or B rating for use in pregnancy. Propranolol (C) is the most commonly used β-blocker, but there are reports of intrauterine growth retardation, hypoglycemia, bradycardia, and respiratory depression associated with this drug [94,133,144]. It is probably safe to use in lactation [133,136]. Pindolol is a nonselective β-blocker which has a category B rating [144], but unfortunately, perhaps due to its intrinsic sympathetic activity, it has no demonstrated efficacy in migraine prophylaxis [153]. Labetalol (C) has also been proposed for use during pregnancy due to its unique selective α-1 and nonselective β1 and 2 adrenergic antagonist effects. It is the most commonly used medication for treating hypertension in pregnancy, as it decreases systemic vascular resistance with little change in cardiac output. Therefore, it does not impair placental blood flow, and is associated with good fetal outcome [154]. It has not been associated with any problems in lactation [136].

Selective serotonin reuptake inhibitors (SSRIs) may be considered with caution in a pregnant migraineur, especially with comorbid depression, as most are category B or C [144]. The exception is paroxetine (D), which has been linked to an increased risk of congenital heart defects [133]. Fluoxetine has both an FDA rating of B and a TERIS rating of N [94]. Its safety in lactation is unknown, but is associated with no significant levels in breast-fed infants and is rated as L2 by Hale [133]. The tricyclic antidepressants amitriptyline and nortriptyline are both category D; doxepin, desipramine, and protriptyline are category C [94] and are probably safe in lactation [133]. The anticonvulsants may be considered with comorbid migraine and epilepsy. Gabapentin and topiramate are most often suggested for use in pregnancy with an FDA category C rating [132]. There are reports of craniofacial abnormalities and hypospadias associated with topiramate exposure, and gabapentin may cause bone malformations [144]. These drugs have unknown safety in lactation [94] with L2 and L3 Hale ratings, respectively [133]. Valproic acid (D) is associated with significant fetal defects, especially neural tube defects, and is to be avoided before and during pregnancy. Ironically, it is not associated with any problems in lactation [136].

In order to minimize infant exposure to drugs during breast-feeding, the patient can be educated as to the timing of administration (take directly after feeding) and to pump and discard the first milk after administration of their medication [125]. Medications that may be used safely while breast-feeding include acetaminophen, moderate amounts of caffeine, opioid analgesics, and most NSAIDs. Those that should be avoided include bromocriptine, ergotamine, and lithium. Eletriptan has a Hale L2 rating whilst the other triptans are L3 [133] and may be used with caution. The benzodiazepines, phenobarbital, most antidepressants, neuroleptics, aspirin, and ketarolac also may be used with caution [125].

Treatment of Nonmigraine Primary Headache Types in Pregnancy

The management of TTH in pregnancy is very similar to migraine treatment. Acetaminophen and NSAIDs with nonpharmacologic strategies are used most often. Preventive treatment with prescription medication is rarely required.

For CH in pregnancy, 100% high-flow oxygen via facemask is safe and can abort up to 70% of attacks. As discussed earlier, there is limited data concerning the use of triptans in pregnancy. Prednisone is safe to use in pregnancy and lactation and can stop or attenuate the cluster bout. Verapamil, a long-standing preventive for CH, has an FDA category C rating, but is compatible with breast-feeding [125]. Intranasal lidocaine (4% solution) may be tried as well as intranasal capsaicin: no fetotoxic properties known in animals but there is no human data. Greater occipital nerve blockade can also be used in pregnancy. Lithium, methysergide, and valproic acid are contraindicated [155,156].

Trigeminal neuralgia frequently responds to carbamazepine. Recently, the rate of MBDs of infants born to patients with epilepsy and carbamazepine monotherapy (3.0%) was reported to be close to that of controls (2.1%) [157], and general IQ scores of exposed children of epileptic mothers were not reduced compared to controls in a systematic review and meta-analysis [158]. However, the FDA category for this drug is category D and many malformations have been seen in mice pups when exposed during organogenesis [159]. The potential risks probably usually outweigh the benefit for nonepileptic pregnant patients, but it is safe for lactating mothers to use postnatally.

Inadvertent Exposure

In the event of an inadvertent drug exposure during pregnancy, the health care provider should document all details of the exposure (drug, dosage, duration, and gestational age), the FDA and TERIS rating of the drug, the patient's health and family history of congenital or genetic disorders. In the case of the triptans, the appropriate pregnancy registry should be contacted before delivery of the baby. The obstetrician should be notified, and if the fetus was exposed during embryogenesis, high-resolution ultrasound may be performed to assess particular organ systems. The patient and her significant other should be educated as to the risks, including cognitive or neurodevelopmental delay that may not be predicted prenatally [94].

Secondary Headaches and Their Management

Introduction

The nervous system can be affected before, during, and after pregnancy leading to a multifaceted constellation of symptoms that challenge every neurologist encountering a pregnant woman complaining of headache. The neurologist should take into consideration not only the mother's symptoms and diseases but also any treatment of the mother and fetus during pregnancy and postpartum period. It is well known that headache affects women more often than men and more often during their childbearing years. The changes in hormonal status that accompany menarche, childbirth years, pregnancy, and the postpartum period influence the severity and intensity of primary headache and create conditions that may facilitate the occurrence of secondary headache. Even though the majority of headaches in pregnant women are primary, secondary headache must not be missed as it can represent serious and life-threatening disease requiring immediate intervention. We will discuss in this section the approach to the pregnant patient with headache and summarize current recommendation for diagnosis, workup, and treatment.

Classification

The IHS published The International Classification of Headache Disorders (ICHD) in 2004 that introduces a standardized approach to secondary headache with clear-cut characteristics whenever possible. Secondary headaches in this classification are attributed to another disorder and classified on etiologic basis. In a patient with a new onset of headache in close temporal relation to onset of another disorder known to cause headache, the headache are categorized as "attributed to" that disorder. In a patient with pre-existing primary headache, the situation is more complicated, as the headache could represent an exacerbation of existing primary headache or a new superimposed onset of secondary headache. According to the ICHD, secondary headache in a patient with pre-existing primary headache is more likely if (1) there is a close temporal relation to the potential cause; (2) the headache differs in pattern from the pre-existing disorder; (3) there is additional evidence that support a secondary cause; and (4) the disappearance of the offending cause leads to improvement of the headache [6].

It is imperative to approach the pregnant headache patient in the way that helps to differentiate the potentially dangerous secondary types of headache from primary headaches that are relatively benign. A pregnant woman with known primary headache may continue to have them during pregnancy. Often primary headache improves or resolves after the first trimester but this is not the case in all women. If the pattern of her headache has not changed during pregnancy, it is not necessary to start an extensive diagnostic workup. Women with a new onset of headache during pregnancy or a substantially altered pattern of the typical headache (different in localization, frequency, intensity, duration, or quality) should be evaluated with appropriate testing to rule out secondary causes of headache [144]. Only when all secondary causes of headache have been ruled out should headache be classified as migraine, TTH, or CH when faced with a significant change in the headache pattern.

Generalities

Headaches are common among women in their reproductive years. Over 80% of women suffer from headache in their reproductive years and consequently headaches are often encountered in pregnant women. Changes in hormonal status before pregnancy, during the pregnancy, and in the postpartum period can be a major source of headache during gestation. The vast majority of headaches during pregnancy are primary types of headache. In contrast, secondary types of headache represent a small fraction of pregnant patients who complain of headache [25].

The most common causes of secondary headache during pregnancy includes head trauma, cerebral venous thrombosis (CVT), pre-eclampsia, intracranial hypertension (ICH), or subarachnoid hemorrhage (SAH), ischemic stroke, vasculitis and vasculopathies, dehydration, brain tumors, benign ICH, other causes of increased intracranial pressure (ICP), intracranial hypotension, meningitis/encephalitis, sinusitis, cranial neuralgias, and pituitary apoplexy (PA) [144]. Pregnancy can increase the risk of bleeding from an existing arteriovenous malformation (AVM), causing SAH. In addition, the headache could occur in the setting of CVT secondary to gestational hypercoagulability. Rapid growth of some intracranial tumors such as pituitary adenoma and meningioma can lead to secondary headache during pregnancy. Changes in ICP in any direction could lead to headache in pregnant patients and may represent idiopathic intracranial hypertension (IIH) or hypotension [160].

Approach to a Patient with Headache During Pregnancy

A detailed history and physical examination that points to red flags such as altered level of consciousness, focal neurologic abnormalities, papilledema, and seizures could represent a secondary cause and warrant further extensive diagnostic evaluation. Routine investigations usually include urinalysis, complete blood count, chemistries, liver function tests, and a coagulation profile. If appropriate indications are present, computed tomography (CT) can be performed during pregnancy. The odds of having an intracranial pathologic finding on brain CT and magnetic resonance imaging (MRI) is 2.7 times higher in pregnant headache patients with an abnormal neurologic examination. However, there are no clinical features that are specifically predictive of a pathologic lesion on acute neuroimaging studies [161].

With the proper use of lead shielding, a standard CT scan of the head exposes the uterus to less than 0.01 mGy, which is much lower than the dose required to produce fetal damage [94]. Because the goal is to expose the fetus to the least risk of harm, however, CT of the head is mostly used for serious conditions like SAH and ICH in pregnant patients when quick imaging is necessary.

MRI without gadolinium is the imaging procedure of choice during pregnancy and is safe during the entire pregnancy period. It is recommended by American College of Radiology as a preferred technique as it does not expose the fetus to ionizing radiation. MRI is much more informative in conditions associated with edema and infections. MRI is also more sensitive in detecting rare disorders that may occur during pregnancy, including PA, cerebral venous sinus thrombosis, and metastatic choriocarcinoma. Another advantage of MRI is that arteriography and venography can be performed without contrast, thus detecting vascular lesions (AVM, aneurysm, and CVT). Gadolinium increases the specificity and sensitivity of MRI, but because it crosses the placenta, its use is not recommended during pregnancy, despite the fact that there is no known teratogenic effect. It is prudent to restrict the use of maternal MRI to procedures with clear medical indications, especially during the early stages of development of the fetus [162].

A spinal tap (lumbar puncture [LP]) is easily performed during pregnancy and is designed to detect many pathologic conditions. The interpretation of the CSF examination is similar to nonpregnant patients in regard to opening pressure, cell count, and protein levels [162]. As a rule, LP is performed after the possibilities of cerebral mass lesions are excluded by neuroimaging. In pregnant patients with fever, elevated white blood cell count, and/or neck rigidity, it can help to rule out infection. In those who present with the worst headache of their life or thunderclap headache, LP helps to exclude SAH. In pregnant patients with papilledema with nonfocal examination and negative imaging study, LP helps to rule out increased ICP [163].

Headache Attributed to Eclamptic Encephalopathy

Pre-eclampsia (toxemia gravidarum) and eclampsia are the main causes of perinatal morbidity and death in women. Studies have shown that 7.5% of pregnancies are complicated by pre-eclampsia. Gestational hypertension is defined as consistently elevation of systemic blood pressure above or equal to 140/90 mmHg in a previously normotensive woman after 20 weeks of pregnancy, without proteinuria. Twenty-five percent of patients who have gestational hypertension will develop pre-eclampsia/eclampsia [164]. Pre-eclampsia is a multisystem disorder that is characterized by widespread endothelial dysfunction and vasospasm causing hypertension, proteinuria, and edema. It usually develops after the twentieth week of pregnancy but can also arise in the postpartum period. If a patient with pre-eclampsia develops epileptic seizures, the syndrome is called eclampsia.

One of the most common presentations of severe pre-eclampsia and a precursor of eclampsia is headache [165]. The headache is usually mild to severe in intensity, diffuse and constant, and is often associated with scotoma, blurred vision, double vision, photophobia, amaurosis, or hemianopsia. Otherwise the neurologic examination is usually negative in pre-eclampsia, and the presence of other focal neurologic deficits should imply other pathology.

Loss of cerebral autoregulation secondary to systemic hypertension or generalized cerebral vasospasm secondary to endothelial dysfunction may explain pathogenesis of cerebral lesions in pre-eclampsia and eclampsia. Pathologic findings include cerebral edema, hypertensive encephalopathy; subarachnoid, subcortical, and petechial hemorrhages; and infarction of multiple areas of the brain and brain stem. The most affected regions are the occipital and parietal lobes within the watershed areas. The most common changes on MRI are hyperintensities in the white matter on FLAIR images in the posterior part of the cerebral hemispheres sparing the calcarine and paramedian occipital lobes. The posterior frontal white matter may also be involved, but brain stem, cerebellum, and basal ganglia rarely are [166]. Diffusion-weighted MRI allows differentiation of reversible vasogenic edema from cytotoxic edema occurring in the context of ischemic infarction [167].

The pathogenesis of headache in pre-eclampsia/eclampsia is poorly understood. It may be related to increased cerebral perfusion pressure as in hypertensive encephalopathy, cerebral ischemia from vasoconstriction, posterior leukoencephalopathy, cerebral edema, or microhemorrhages. Molecular hypotheses include the alteration of the angiotensinogen gene or circulation of vasoconstrictor endothelial toxic substances from the placenta secondary to damage of the fetal–placental barrier. Researchers have found that a substance called placental soluble fms-like tyrosine kinase 1 (sFlt1) is upregulated in pre-eclampsia and this may contribute to vascular changes [168].

There is no good explanation of why pre-eclampsia/eclampsia affects primarily the young and primigravid woman and why a shortened interval between pregnancies decreases the risk of pre-eclampsia/eclampsia. It has been hypothesized that the ischemia that complicates pre-eclampsia/eclampsia may be mediated by genetic factors that predispose to both endothelial dysfunction and to a thrombophilic state. Eclampsia-associated hemorrhagic stroke may be secondary to disturbance of cerebral autoregulation, which probably has genetic causes. The risk of pre-eclampsia increases if the patient has twin pregnancies, diabetes mellitus, hypercoagulable state, advanced age, dyslipidemia, antiphospholipid antibody syndrome, obesity, chronic hypertension, or a history of pre-eclampsia. Interestingly, smoking decreases the risk of eclampsia and hypertension during pregnancy [169]. Many cases where a diagnosis of eclampsia and pre-eclampsia was made had in reality other diseases like cerebral arterial infarction, hypertensive encephalopathy, and CVT. That suggests the need for consideration of a careful differential diagnosis in patients with eclampsia/pre-eclampsia, as well as the numerous causes of stroke in young patients that could have their onset during pregnancy.

Severe pre-eclampsia in a woman with pre-eclampsia is defined as a systolic pressure of 160 mmHg or a diastolic pressure of 110 mmHg on two occasions at least 6 h apart while the patient is resting in bed; proteinuria (500 mg of protein per 24 h or 3+ in random urine samples taken at least 4 h apart); and symptoms of end-organ damage (headache, right upper quadrant pain, visual disturbance, or altered sensorium). A percentage of women with pre-eclampsia (approximately 4–14%) could progress to HELLP syndrome, an acronym for *h*emolysis (abnormal peripheral blood smear, a bilirubin level of 1.2 mg/dL, or a lactate dehydrogenase level of 600 IU/L); *e*levated *l*iver enzyme levels (aspartate aminotransferase is 2 times normal); and *l*ow *p*latelets (platelet count of less than 100×10^3/mL). HELLP syndrome has a high rate of maternal and fetal morbidity.

The treatment for pre-eclampsia is rapid delivery of the baby, prophylactic treatment against seizures, and management of blood pressure. Magnesium sulfate, antihypertensive drugs, and antiepileptic drugs are used to prevent stroke and eclamptic seizures. Methyldopa and labetalol are appropriate first-line therapies in pre-eclampsia;

hydralazine is used as well. If severe pre-eclampsia, eclampsia, or HELLP syndrome exists, there is only one possible option: removal of the baby irrespective of the gestational age within 24–48 h of presentation via vaginal or cesarean delivery. Sometimes it is possible to delay this if the woman is able to tolerate additional time without severe consequences to allow fetal stabilization before delivery [170].

The most extensively used medication to treat the symptoms of severe pre-eclampsia and eclampsia while the woman awaits delivery is magnesium sulfate. Magnesium sulfate is better than phenytoin with or without diazepam in the prevention of seizures, not because of its anticonvulsant effect, but because it prevents the cerebrovascular complication of eclampsia. When thrombocytopenic purpura and hemolytic-uremic syndrome complicate toxemia and HELLP syndrome, severe neurologic morbidity and death is common. Plasma transfusion and plasmapheresis may be used to decrease mortality in these patients. Low-dose aspirin was successfully used in preventing eclampsia in a small trial. Another trial stated that 100 mg of aspirin daily after 17 weeks of pregnancy is effective; however, others have shown that there is no benefit if the dose is 60 mg/day. An increase in bleeding time predicts a better effect of aspirin in pregnant women [171]. The use of ketanserin, a selective serotonin-2 receptor blocker, with or without aspirin may prevent pre-eclampsia in women with hypertension diagnosed before 20 weeks of pregnancy, but this practice needs further study before it can be recommended [172]. Women with pre-eclampsia/eclampsia have a higher risk of developing stroke postpartum and need to be closely monitored not only during pregnancy but also in the puerperium, and all stroke risk factors should be monitored [173].

Headache Attributed to Ischemic Stroke

The frequency of headache in the setting of acute ischemic stroke ranges from 7% to 65%. There is a strong association of headache at stroke onset with younger age and/or a history of migraine. Women have a higher incidence of headache at stroke onset than men. Headache occurs more often in patients with cerebellar stroke. There is no significant association between vascular risk factors (hypertension, smoking, time of day), severity of stroke, and headache at stroke onset [174]. The reported incidence of stroke during pregnancy and the puerperium varies widely, ranging from 5 to 67 per 100,000 deliveries or pregnancies [175]; but probably lies between 11 and 26 per 100,000. The rates of ischemic and hemorrhagic stroke are approximately equal. Arterial stroke has a tendency to occur in the third trimester of pregnancy and postpartum period, whereas venous events occur mainly in the puerperium. Both ischemic and hemorrhagic cerebral events have the greatest risk to occur 2 days before and 1 day after delivery with an increased but declining risk over the subsequent 6-week postpartum period [176]. The estimated mortality following pregnancy-related stroke is 10–13% and it is significantly higher in Afro-American women, older women, and women who did not have prenatal care [177]. The risk of stroke during pregnancy increases with age, and is higher among Afro-American women. It is strongly associated with medical conditions like migraine headache, thrombophilia, systemic lupus erythematosus, heart disease, sickle cell disease, hypertension, and thrombocytopenia, as well as with specific complications of pregnancy such as postpartum hemorrhage, pre-eclampsia and gestational hypertension, transfusion, and postpartum infection. Eclampsia and pre-eclampsia are major causes of ischemic and hemorrhagic stroke in pregnancy and account for 25–45% of pregnancy-associated stroke [178]. Pre-eclampsia was found to be associated with an increased likelihood of ischemic stroke after multivariable adjustment for age, race, education, and number of pregnancies [173] with a respective adjusted relative risk of pre-eclampsia/eclampsia for ischemic stroke of 41 within 3 months before delivery and 35 in the first 3 days postpartum [179]. After excluding pre-eclampsia/eclampsia as causes of stroke, diagnoses such as premature atherosclerosis, hypertension, cardiac disease, hyperlipidemia, diabetes, arterial dissection, Takayasu disease, vasculitis, antiphospholipid antibody syndrome, systemic lupus erythematosis, sickle cell disease, thrombotic thrombocytopenic purpura, CVT, coagulopathies, and drugs (cocaine and other drugs) should be ruled out. Diagnoses specific to pregnancy include postpartum cerebral angiopathy, postpartum cardiomyopathy, and amniotic fluid embolus. Sometimes cerebral autosomal dominant arteriopathy with subcortical infarcts and leukoencephalopathy (CADASIL) can manifest during pregnancy. The cause of stroke remains unknown in a minority of cases.

Diagnostic workup of stroke in pregnancy is based on the same principles as in the nonpregnant patient, keeping in mind that certain procedures could be harmful for the mother or fetus. MRI without contrast, which does not have ionizing radiation, can be used to assess the brain as well as venous and arterial circulation. Two-dimensional echocardiography may be useful in gestational stroke evaluation especially to exclude cardiac thrombus or severe congestive heart failure.

Antiplatelet therapy with low-dose aspirin decreases the incidence of perinatal death and pre-eclampsia in women with risk factors for pre-eclampsia; however, the safety of other antiplatelet drugs during pregnancy is not well known. Therefore, caution is advised in administration of these medications. Anticoagulation therapy during pregnancy has limited indications and is used for current arterial or venous thromboembolism, after a prior venous thromboembolism event as a long-term anticoagulation, in antiphospholipid antibody syndrome with prior venous thromboembolism, and in patients with a mechanical heart valve. Because heparin does not cross the placenta, but warfarin does, heparin is therefore safer during pregnancy. Thrombolytic therapy in pregnancy has been used for acute ischemic stroke, but the data are limited and it is important to weigh the risks and benefits of this therapy cautiously for pregnant women and fetuses in each clinical situation [180].

Cerebrovascular Events Unique to Pregnancy

Some headaches associated with stroke during pregnancy are unique to pregnancy and deserve special attention. These are peripartum/postpartum cerebral angiopathy, cerebral autosomal dominant arteriopathy with subcortical infarcts, and leukoencephalopathy and peripartum/postpartum cardiomyopathy.

Severe excruciating headache in a pregnant patient that peaks in less than 1 min, like a "clap of thunder" could be a presentation of thunderclap headache in peripartum/postpartum cerebral angiopathy, also known as delayed peripartum vasculopathy or reversible cerebral vasoconstriction syndrome (RCVS). This is characterized by severe headaches with or without seizures and focal neurologic deficits. It affects large- and medium-sized brain arteries and may lead to SAH (22%); parenchymal ischemic or hemorrhagic strokes (7%); and permanent sequelae. The use of vasoactive drugs and migraine are risk factors in the development RCVS. Diagnosis is made by the demonstration of transient vasoconstriction in the form of "string of beads" appearance on cerebral angiography. Complete resolution occurs in 12 weeks. White matter changes that accompany the syndrome have a posterior predominance, but are not as extensive as in eclampsia. Nimodipine is used to treat the thunderclap headaches within 48 h; however, it does not prevent hemorrhagic and ischemic complications in the majority of cases [181]. Vasoconstriction is persistent and may present after headache resolution. Constriction of the middle cerebral artery at the M1 segment and the posterior cerebral artery at the P2 segment can be used as a predictor for developing posterior reversible encephalopathy syndromes and ischemic stroke [182].

Women with cerebral autosomal dominant arteriopathy with subcortical infarcts and leukoencephalopathy (CADASIL) commonly develop pre-eclampsia and neurologic symptoms while pregnant and during the postpartum period. In a recent study, 12 of 25 mothers with CADASIL confirmed by R133C NOTCH3 mutation developed neurologic symptoms in their pregnancies. In 82%, the first symptoms of disease were during pregnancy [183]. CADASIL is associated with a history of migraine, and should be taken into consideration as a possible cause of headache during pregnancy, especially if there are focal neurologic symptoms. Pregnant mothers with suspected or established diagnosis of CADASIL should be monitored carefully.

Peripartum cardiac myopathy is a dilated cardiomyopathy with left ventricular dysfunction and symptoms of heart failure, with onset in the last trimester of pregnancy or up to 5 months postpartum. It is of unknown or multifactorial etiology. It has been estimated that it occurs 1 in every 2289 live births in the United States with a mortality rate of up to 5%. The usual presentation includes symptoms of cardiac failure, but stroke and other thromboembolic phenomena may also occur. Anticoagulation is indicated when there is evidence of systemic embolism, the patient has a low ejection fraction, or there is a thrombus in the heart. Anticoagulation is continued until left ventricular function returns to normal. According to the American College of Cardiology and the American Heart Association, warfarin is probably safe up to the sixth week of pregnancy, is teratogenic with risk of embriopathy between 6 and 12 weeks of pregnancy, is relatively safe during the second and third trimesters (but can cause spontaneous fetal hemorrhages), and needs to be stopped and switched to heparin several weeks before delivery. On the other hand, unfractionated heparin or low-molecular-weight heparin is safe throughout pregnancy [184].

Headache Attributed to ICH and SAH

Headaches develop more often and are more severe in hemorrhagic stroke compared with ischemic stroke. SAH is the most common cause of severe and incapacitating headaches that have abrupt onset (thunderclap headache). This headache is often described as the worst headache of life. Headache accompanies all subarachnoidal hemorrhages and 58% of intraparenchymal hemorrhages. It is diffuse in 52% and incapacitating in 70%. The duration of headache in hemorrhagic stroke is 64.5 ± 36.5 h [185]. Headaches develop more commonly in cerebellar and lobar hemorrhages than in deep localized hemorrhages (thalamic, caudate, capsuloputaminal, brain stem). Factors associated with headache are age younger than 70, female gender, vomiting, positive meningeal signs, Glasgow coma scale less than 10, hematoma volume more than 10 mL, CT evidence of intraventricular or subarachnoidal bleed, hydrocephalus, tentorial herniation, or midline shift. In multiple logistic regression analysis, however, only meningeal signs, cerebellar or lobar location, transtentorial herniation, and female gender were significant predictors of headache at the onset of ICH. Headache pain associated with ICH is more likely secondary to concomitant subarachnoidal blood and local compression rather than the effects of ICH [186].

ICH represents 2–7% of the total cases of neurologic disorders in pregnancy, and is often due to uncontrolled hypertension [176]. The cause of hemorrhage in the majority of cases is rupture of a saccular aneurysm or AVM. Of 402 young female stroke patients, 19 had ICH and 3 had SAH. Eclampsia (37%) and AVM (26%) were the most important etiologies of hemorrhages [187]. ICH also occurs in women secondary to systemic diseases such as bleeding diatheses, cocaine toxicity, bacterial endocarditis, sickle cell disease, and moyamoya disease. However, during pregnancy we should also consider rare disorders such as PA (if physical examination reveals a field defect, reduction of visual acuity or complex ophthalmoplegia), hemorrhagic infarction of a pre-existing (unknown or known) pituitary tumor or metastases from choriocarcinoma (malignant tumor of gestational trophoblasts) [188]. In about one-third of cases the cause of ICH remains unknown. SAH that account for 3% of all stroke is secondary to a saccular aneurysm in approximately 85% of cases. Rare causes of SAH include septic aneurysm, arterial dissection, cerebral AVM, dural arteriovenous fistula, and vascular lesions around the spinal cord.

Ruptured AVM and saccular aneurysm during pregnancy should be treated with endovascular interventions before delivery [189]. Unruptured saccular aneurysm and AVM should be monitored during pregnancy with definitive treatment after pregnancy if possible. In the absence of definitive guidelines and conflicting data about the risk of rupture of saccular aneurysm and AVM during pregnancy, the approach should be tailored by a neurosurgeon and obstetrician individually. Management depends on the localization, size, and shape of the malformation, comorbidities, and other variables. The avoidance of a strenuous and painful labor is reasonable with either elective cesarean section or vaginal delivery and the use of epidural anesthesia to reduce pain and straining. The same is true in the case if an endovascular treatment fails.

Headache Attributed to CVT

Headache is the most common symptom of CVT. It is present in up to 90% of cases and it is the most frequent, and can be the only initial symptom of CVT [190].

The headache is not specific, but tends to be diffuse, progressive, and associated with papilledema, nausea, and vomiting. Other presenting features include disturbance of consciousness, focal neurologic signs, and seizures. A stroke-like presentation is possible, and has been described as a manifestation of cortical vein thrombosis [191]. Risk of CVT is higher in the postpartum period but is increased in pregnancy also. Mortality rate ranges from 4% to 36% [192]. In the United States, the incidence is 9 per 100,000 births. CVT associated with pregnancy has a more indolent course and is more benign than CVT in the general population. In the United States, there are no deaths reported among pregnant patients with peripartum CVT. Cesarean section and age greater than 25 represent risk factors for CVT. According to a large nationwide Swedish cohort with 654,957 women (1,003,489 deliveries), CVT was the most common cerebrovascular disorder affecting women between 2 days before and 1 day after delivery [193].

Magnetic resonance venogram (MRV) without contrast is the diagnostic procedure of choice in the evaluation of CVT [194]. Even though it is not as effective as conventional angiography in visualization of small veins, thrombosis of major sinuses is very well detected and it does not require contrast or ionizing radiation. In CVT, MRI shows multiple small infarcts in the gray and white matter with and without hemorrhage. If MRV fails to detect thrombosis of major sinuses, conventional angiogram or digital subtraction angiography may be used to demonstrate small vein thrombosis. This does confer a risk of ionizing radiation for the fetus, and should be considered only in an exceptional situation. CT imaging of the brain is avoided when possible, but if done may show venous infarctions that are not in an arterial distribution and a "delta sign" may be seen (hyperdensity in the sagittal sinus due to occlusion from fresh thrombus). CT is diagnostic in only one-third of the patients with CVT [195].

In pregnancy, there is increased level of C4b-binding protein and other factors that create a hypercoagulable state. Genetic thrombophilias like Factor V Leiden mutation, or protein C or S deficiency increase the risk of CVT during pregnancy. Decreased activity of protein S and the presence of antiphospholipid antibodies can be found in pregnancy-related CVT, on rare occasions there could be multiple defects of coagulation in one person. The risk of CVT is also increased by homocystinuria (hyperhomocysteinemia). Thrombophilia screening should be carried out 4 weeks after stopping anticoagulant treatment and no earlier than 6 weeks postnatally because of the effects of pregnancy on coagulation factors [196]. Infection, sickle cell disease, dehydration, and ulcerative colitis are also associated with an increased risk of development of CVT in association with pregnancy.

The treatment of CVT remains a challenging task especially in the pregnant patient. Anticoagulation with heparin is used in the treatment for the pregnant patient with CVT; however, some authorities recommend using it only in cases with a poor prognosis or associated with thromboses in other parts of the body. The duration of anticoagulation after the acute phase is unclear. Oral anticoagulation may be given after birth. Both heparin and warfarin are safe to use during breast-feeding. Local thrombolytic agents (tPA) have been used via selective venography in CVT, but this is associated with an increased risk of cerebral hemorrhage. When CVT is associated with hemorrhagic infarcts the usage of anticoagulation and thrombolytic therapy may become uncertain and mechanical removal of the thrombus together with systemic anticoagulation would be an option [197].

Headache Attributed to PA

PA is a rare acute, life-threatening condition secondary to hemorrhage or ischemia of the pituitary gland. The most frequent symptom is headache that does not respond to analgesics [198]. Headache can be retro-orbital, unilateral, bifrontal, suboccipital, or generalized and develop in 95% of apoplexy cases. Stretching of the dura mater in the walls of the sella and direct irritation of the nerve may contribute to headache. Additional symptoms include visual loss, ophthalmoplegia, nausea and vomiting, altered consciousness, and impaired pituitary function [199].

The exact pathogenesis of PA is not completely understood but ischemia and necrosis of both the anterior pituitary gland and tumor is the main possibility. In most cases, the bleeding occurs in a pre-existing adenoma. Macroadenomas are at a much higher risk of hemorrhaging than microadenomas. Rarely PA can occur in a normal pituitary gland. Mechanical compression of the pituitary stalk or vasculature or both, rather than destruction of the pituitary gland itself, results in acute pituitary failure. Serum hormone levels confirm the pituitary failure. T2-weighted gradient-echo MRI will detect intracranial hemorrhage and diffusion-weighted MRI will show high signal intensity in PA, but alone cannot distinguish apoplexy from cystic macroadenoma or craniopharyngioma [200].

Emergent stabilization is the first-line treatment and includes intravenous fluids, blood transfusions, and high-dose corticosteroids. Urgent transsphenoidal surgical decompression is reserved for patients who remain unstable after initial stabilization [201].

Headache Attributed to High ICP

Headache attributed to high ICP may cause severe daily headaches that usually awaken the patient in the morning, are pulsatile, and last for hours; and are often associated with transient obscuration of vision, intracranial noises, sustained visual loss, photopsia, diplopia, retrobulbar pain, papilledema, VI cranial nerve palsy, and peripheral visual field dysfunction [202]. During pregnancy, high ICP is usually a sign of IIH. Pregnancy is associated with IIH presentation or worsening. IIH is a disease of obese women of reproductive age and occasionally is present exclusively during pregnancy. The rate of pregnancy is the same in IIH patients and in the general population, and the visual outcome is similar in pregnant and nonpregnant women with IIH [203]. IIH of new onset usually occurs around fourteenth gestational week and persists for several months or until after delivery or longer. These women are obese and gain weight during pregnancy rapidly. Images of the brain fail to detect mass lesions or sinus thrombosis but may show slit-like ventricles. LP shows normal CSF with slightly decreased or normal protein. CSF opening pressure is elevated. Termination of pregnancy is not necessary in the majority of the cases and the baby is not affected by the disease. Visual acuity, visual fields, and the optic fundi should be monitored during the pregnancy and in the postpartum period.

Weight reduction is the mainstream of the treatment and includes diet and moderate physical activity. Acetaminophen with or without codeine could be used in the treatment of headache in these patients. More aggressive treatment is necessary for vision loss. Acetazolamide is a common agent that is used in nonpregnant patients, but its usage in pregnant patients remains controversial. There are not adequate human studies to determine its teratogenic effect. Despite of this fact it has been used without reported harm to the fetus; therefore some experts recommend it after 20 weeks of gestation. According to one study, a dosage of 1000 mg acetazolamide per day in pregnant patients with IIH resulted in healthy and normal children [204]. In severe IIH with visual loss despite of using weight reduction therapy and acetazolamide, a short 2-week course of steroids with dexamethasone or prednisone may be necessary to preserve vision. Alternatively, serial LPs can be done weekly until optic nerve sheath fenestration or lumboperitoneal shunt can be performed. Increased ICP-related headache needs adequate pain control during the delivery. IIH is not a contraindication for vaginal delivery. Epidural anesthesia can be used to avoid dramatic increases in ICP during delivery [205].

Headache Attributed to Low ICP

Headache that typically develops in the upright position and is relieved by recumbency represents orthostatic or positional headache. This type of headache is a hallmark of CSF volume depletion. The headache is usually bilateral in the fronto-occipital distribution and may be throbbing. Headache is often associated with neck stiffness, nausea, diplopia, dizziness, change in hearing, blurry vision, photophobia, interscapular pain, facial numbness or weakness, radicular upper-limb symptoms, a superior binasal visual field cut, or galactorrhea. The headache in CSF volume depletion is caused by descent of the brain and stretching of the pain-sensitive veins, meninges, and cranial nerves. This is caused by gravitational changes that occur with shifts in body position from the supine to the upright position [206]. Such a positional headache secondary to low ICP could be encountered in pregnancy as a result of leakage of CSF after LP or other cause. CSF might escape through a hole in the arachnoid and dural layers because of cranial trauma or spinal trauma (lifting, coughing, chest injury), tumor erosion, or it may occur spontaneously.

Spontaneous intracranial hypotension has specific changes on MRI that include brain sagging, cerebellar tonsil descent, decrease in size and change in shape of prepontine, perichiasmatic cisterns, basal subarachoid cisterns, displacement of optic chiasm and opening of cerebral aqueduct inferiorly, dilatation of veins and dural sinuses, subdural fluid collections, and post-contrast enhancement of the thickened dura. In severe cases, the brain sagging continues through the tentorial notch and swelling of the diencephalic and mesencephalic structures occurs secondary to impaired flow through the deformed vein of Galen [207]. If the MRI study is normal or gadolinium is contraindicated, measurement of opening CSF pressure could be tried. However, only half of the patients with intracranial hypotension have an opening pressure less than 40 mm H_2O, suggesting CSF volume depletion as a core of the problem, and not intracranial hypotension. Therefore, the LP might not be diagnostic. Variable pleocytosis with mononuclear cells and a mild-to-modest increase in CSF protein may be present in these patients.

Treatment can be administered after the confirmation of CSF volume depletion or empirically. Conservative treatment includes bed rest and hydration for several weeks. It is suggested that CSF pressure is normalized in the supine position and this may allow healing of the meningeal defect. Usage of caffeine, theophylline, and steroids all have been advocated as specific treatment; however, their efficacy remains limited. If the initial conservative treatment is not effective and the source of leakage is evident (such as in post-LP headache) a blood patch could be an effective option. If there is no obvious source of CSF leakage, further studies to identify the site of the leak are indicated. A spontaneous CSF leak is usually localized in the upper thoracic or lower cervical spine and can be localized with CT myelography of the spine, MRI, or radioisotope cisternography in nonpregnant patients. In pregnancy, the workup depends on many factors and needs to be tailored individually. Several blood patches or surgical repair of dural tear may be necessary if conservative treatment is ineffective and the exact localization of the leakage is known [208].

Headache Attributed to Lymphocytic Hypophysitis

Headache associated with a visual field cut during pregnancy may be an indication of lymphocytic hypophysitis (LH). This is an inflammation that affects the adenohypophysis characterized by diffuse infiltration of the anterior pituitary with lymphocytes and plasma cells. Epidemiologically, LH shows a strong relationship with pregnancy, especially in the last month or in the first 2 months after delivery. Prompt diagnosis and treatment are necessary for fetal and maternal safety. Hormone replacement therapy and surgery are the mainstream treatments. Most patients require long-term hormone replacement therapy; some become free from hormone replacement after mass reduction surgery [209]. When inflammation affects not only the anterior pituitary gland but also the neurohypophysis, the term "lymphocytic panhypophysitis" applies. The pathogenesis remains to be elucidated. The involvement of the neurohypophysis could be a cause of central diabetes insipidus and need treatment also [210].

Headache Attributed to Intracranial Neoplasms

The headaches that accompany brain tumors are often associated with nausea and vomiting that gradually increases during pregnancy. This is in contrast with nausea and vomiting that is of gestational origin that tends to start in the beginning of pregnancy and subsequently improves. Seizures could also be associated with intracranial neoplasms, but at the same time could represent eclampsia. Because CNS tumors are usually localized, the seizure focus is also local; however, in eclampsia the seizures are generalized, reflecting an encephalopathic origin.

The incidence of brain tumors in pregnancy represents 15 per 100,000 [211]. Many intracranial tumors that occur in women of childbearing age have the onset during pregnancy. This could be explained by gestational fluid retention, vascular engorgement, changes in hormonal status, and hormone-related tumor growth. This is especially recognized in meningiomas, schwannomas, and pituitary tumors [212]. The increasing volume may exacerbate existing tumor symptoms, or could lead to new symptoms from a tumor that was never been diagnosed.

There are no significant differences in metastatic brain tumors that affect pregnant women compared to nonpregnant women, except in the case of choriocarcinoma. This tumor metastasizes to the brain earlier in the course of disease and by the time of diagnosis up to 20% of patients have brain metastases [213]. Choriocarcinoma represents a nongerminomatous trophoblastic neoplasm that presents with cerebral and lung metastases in the pregnant patient. This tumor could present during a normal pregnancy or months after a molar pregnancy or spontaneous abortion. Patients present with headache, seizures, intracranial hemorrhages, infarctions, or gradually progressive focal deficits. The tumor may spread locally destroying the sacral plexus, cauda equine, or invade the spinal canal with symptoms specific to these sites. High serum beta chorionic gonadotropin together with a uterine sonogram usually confirms the diagnosis. A ratio of serum to CSF chorionic gonadotropin of less than 60 will suggest the presence of brain metastases. If diagnosis is made early, chemotherapy coupled with radiation and surgery will provide the best outcome [188].

Conclusion

Health care providers should begin discussing headache management before pregnancy, and help pregnant couples to choose proper treatment based on appropriate risk–benefit assessment. The CNS is responsive to hormonal changes and headaches often change during pregnancy. Most patients experience an improvement in their headache symptoms, but for those whose headaches persist, nonpharmacologic approaches are preferred when possible. Pharmacotherapy is cautiously used utilizing guidance from various risk classifications, when the patient is at risk for dehydration or untoward pain and suffering. If there is a definite change in the headache pattern or the patient experiences new headaches in pregnancy, exploration for a secondary cause is necessary. Of primary concern are pre-eclampsia/eclampsia, vascular disorders and stroke, neoplasms, PA, and causes of abnormal intracerebral pressure. The postpartum period and lactation present unique situations that may require alterations in the patient's management. Overall, a team approach involving the patient, significant other, headache specialist, and obstetrician will provide the most satisfying and safest outcome.

References

[1] Waters WE, O'Connor PJ. Epidemiology of headache and migraine in women. J Neurol Neurosurg Psychiatry 1971;34:148–53.

[2] Maggioni F, Alessi C, Maggino T, Zanchin G. Headache during pregnancy. Cephalalgia 1997;17:765–9.

[3] Lipton RB, Stewart WF, Simon D. Medical consultation for migraine: results from the American Migraine Study. *Headache* 1998;38:87–96.
[4] Lipton RB, Stewart WF, Diamond S, Diamond ML, Reed M. Prevalence and burden of migraine in the United States: data from the American Migraine Study II. Headache 2001;41:646–57.
[5] Lipton RB, Bigal ME, Diamond M, Freitag F, Reed ML, Stewart WF. On behalf of the AMPP Advisory Group Migraine prevalence, disease burden, and the need for preventive therapy. Neurology 2007;68:343–9.
[6] Headache Classification Subcommittee of the International Headache Society. The International Classification of Headache Disorders: 2nd edition. Cephalalgia 2004;24(Suppl):9–160.
[7] Silberstein SD, Saper JR, Freitag FG. Migraine diagnosis and treatment. In: Silberstein SD, Lipton RB, Dalessio DE, editors. Wolff's headache and other head pain (7th ed.). Oxford, England: Oxford University Press; 2001. p. 121–237.
[8] Somerville BW. The role of estradiol withdrawal in the etiology of menstrual migraine. Neurology 1972;22:355–65.
[9] Lance JW, Anthony M. Some clinical aspects of migraine. A prospective survey of 500 patients. Arch Neurol 1966;15:356–61.
[10] Callaghan N. The migraine syndrome in pregnancy. Neurology 1968;18:197–201.
[11] Somerville BW. A study of migraine in pregnancy. Neurology 1972;22:824–8.
[12] Granella F, Sances G, Zanferrari C, Costa A, Martignoni E, Manzoni GC. Migraine without aura and reproductive life events: a clinical epidemiological study in 1300 women. Headache 1993;33:385–9.
[13] Ratinahirana H, Darbois Y, Bousser MG. Migraine and pregnancy: a prospective study in 703 women after delivery. Neurology 1990;40(Suppl. 1):437.
[14] Rasmussen BK. Migraine and tension-type headache in a general population. Precipitating factors, female hormones, sleep pattern, and relation to lifestyle. Pain 1993;53:65–72.
[15] Chen T-C, Leviton A. Headache recurrence in pregnant women with migraine. Headache 1994;34:107–10.
[16] Cupini LM, Matteis M, Troisi E, Calabresi P, Bernardi G, Silvestrini M. Sex-hormone-related events in migrainous females. A clinical comparative study between migraine with aura and migraine without aura. Cephalalgia 1995;15:140–4.
[17] Maggioni F, Alessi C, Maggino T, Zanchin G. Headache during pregnancy. Cephalalgia 1997;17:765–9.
[18] Granella F, Sances G, Pucci E, Nappi RE, Ghiotto N, Nappi G. Migraine with aura and reproductive life events: a case–control study. Cephalalgia 2000;20:701–7.
[19] Karen A, John-Anker Z, Knut H, Lars S. The effect of pregnancy and parity on headache prevalence: the Head-HUNT study. Headache 2009;49:851–9.
[20] Kelman L. Women's issues of migraine in tertiary care. Headache 2004;44:2–7.
[21] Scharff L, Marcus DA, Turk DC. Headache during pregnancy and in the postpartum: a prospective study. Headache 1997;37:203–10.
[22] Marcus DA, Scharff L, Turk DC. Longitudinal prospective study of headache during pregnancy and postpartum. Headache 1999;39:625–32.
[23] Sances G, Granella F, Nappi RE, Fignon A, Ghiotto N, Polatti F, et al. Course of migraine during pregnancy and postpartum: a prospective study. Cephalalgia 2003;23:197–205.
[24] Ertresvåg JM, Zwart JA, Helde G, Johnsen HJ, Bovim G. Headache and transient focal neurological symptoms during pregnancy, a prospective cohort. Acta Neurol Scand 2005;111:233–7.

[25] Melhado EM, Maciel Jr. JA, Guerreiro CAM. Headache during gestation: evaluation of 1101 women. Can J Neurol Sci 2007;34:187–92.
[26] Stein G, Morton J, Marsh A, Collins W, Branch C, Desaga U, et al. Headaches after childbirth. Acta Neurol Scand 1984;69:74–9.
[27] Wall VR. Breastfeeding and migraine headaches. J Hum Lact 1992;8:209.
[28] Wainscott G, Volans G, Sullivan F, Wilkinson M. The outcome of pregnancy in women suffering from migraine. Postgrad Med J 1978;54:98–102.
[29] Banhidy F, Acs N, Horváth-Puhó E, Czeizel A. Pregnancy complications and delivery outcomes in pregnant women with severe migraine. Eur J Obstet Gynecol Reprod Biol 2006;134:157–63.
[30] Facchinetti F, Allais G, D'Amico R, Benedetto C, Volpe A. The relationship between headache and preeclampsia: a case–control study. Eur J Obstet Gynecol Reprod Biol 2005;121:143–8.
[31] Adeney KL, Williams MA, Miller RS, Frederick IO, Sorensen TK, Luthy DA. Risk of preeclampsia in relation to maternal history of migraine headaches. J Matern Fetal Neonatal Med 2005;18:167–72.
[32] Adeney KL, Williams MA. Migraine headaches and preeclampsia: an epidemiologic review. Headache 2006;46:794–803.
[33] Facchinetti F, Allais G, Nappi R, D'Amico R, Marozio L, Bertozzi L, et al. Migraine is a risk factor for hypertensive disorders in pregnancy: a prospective cohort study. Cephalalgia 2009;29:286–92.
[34] Scher AI, Terwindt GM, Picavet HS, Verschuren WMM, Ferrari MD, Launer LJ. Cardiovascular risk factors and migraine: the GEM population-based study. Neurology 2005;64:614–20.
[35] Bushnell CD, Jamison MG, James A. Migraines during pregnancy linked to stroke and vascular diseases: US population based case–control study. BMJ 2009;338:b664.
[36] Chen H-M, Chen S-F, Chen Y-H, Lin H-C. Increased risk of adverse pregnancy outcomes for women with migraines: a nationwide population-based study. Cephalalgia 2010;30:433–8.
[37] Schwartz BS, Stewart WF, Simon D, Lipton RB. The epidemiology of tension-type headache. JAMA 1998;279:381–3.
[38] Russell MB, Levi N, Saltyte-Benth J, Fenger K. Tension-type headache in adolescents and adults: a population based study of 33,764 twins. Eur J Epidemiol 2006;21:153–60.
[39] Rasmussen BK. Migraine and tension-type headache in a general population: precipitating factors, female hormones, sleep pattern and relation to lifestyle. Pain 1993;53:65–72.
[40] Calhoun AH, Peterlin BL. Treatment of cluster headache in pregnancy and lactation. Curr Pain Headache Rep 2010;14:164–73.
[41] Graff-Radford SB, Newman A. Obstructive sleep apnea and cluster headache. Headache 2004;44:607–10.
[42] Sahota PK, Jain SS, Dhand R. Sleep disorders in pregnancy. Curr Opin Pulm Med 2003;9:477–83.
[43] Sprenger T, Goadsby PJ. Migraine pathogenesis and state of pharmacological treatment options. BMC Med 2009;7:71–6.
[44] Aston-Jones G, Cohen JD. An integrative theory of locus coeruleus-norepinephrine function: adaptive gain and optimal performance. Annu Rev Neurosci 2005;28:403–50.
[45] Weiller C, May A, Limmroth V, Juptner M, Kaube H, Schayck RV, et al. Brain stem activation in spontaneous human migraine attacks. Nat Med 1995;1:658–60.
[46] Afridi SK, Matharu MS, Lee L, Kaube H, Friston KJ, Frackowiak RS, et al. A PET study exploring the laterality of brainstem activation in migraine using glyceryl trinitrate. Brain 2005;128:932–9.

[47] Kelman L. The premonitory symptoms (prodrome): a tertiary care study of 893 migraineurs. Headache 2004;44:865–72.

[48] Giffin NJ, Kowacs F, Libri V, Williams P, Goadsby PJ, Kaube H. Effect of the adenosine A1 receptor agonist GR79236 on trigeminal nociception with blink reflex recordings in healthy human subjects. Cephalalgia 2003;23:287–92.

[49] Goadsby PJ, Ferrari MD, Csanyi A, Olesen J, Mills JG. Randomized, double-blind, placebo-controlled, proof-of-concept study of the cortical spreading depression inhibiting agent tonabersat in migraine prophylaxis. Cephalalgia 2009;29:742–50.

[50] Hauge AW, Asghar MS, Schytz HW, Christensen K, Olesen J. Effects of tonabersat on migraine with aura: a randomised, doubleblind, placebo-controlled crossover study. Lancet Neurol 2009;8:718–23.

[51] Wolthausen J, Sternberg S, Gerloff C, May A. Are cortical spreading depression and headache in migraine causally linked? Cephalalgia 2009;29:244–9.

[52] Eikermann-Haerter K, Kudo C, Moskowitz MA. Cortical spreading depression and estrogen. Headache 2007;47(Suppl. 2):S79–85.

[53] Martin VT, Behbehani M. Ovarian hormones and migraine headache: understanding mechanisms and pathogenesis—part I. Headache 2006;46:3–23.

[54] Kelly MJ, Qiu J, Wagner EJ, Ronnekleiv OK. Rapid effects of estrogen on G protein-coupled receptor activation of potassium channels in the central nervous system (CNS). J Steroid Biochem Mol Biol 2002;83:187–93.

[55] Twyman RE, Macdonald RL. Neurosteroid regulation of GABAA receptor single-channel kinetic properties of mouse spinal cord neurons in culture. J Physiol 1992;456:215–45.

[56] Zhu Y, Rice CD, Pang Y, Pace M, Thomas P. Cloning, expression, and characterization of a membrane progestin receptor and evidence it is an intermediary in meiotic maturation of fish oocytes. Proc Natl Acad Sci USA 2003;100:2231–6.

[57] Zhu Y, Bond J, Thomas P. Identification, classification, and partial characterization of genes in humans and other vertebrates homologous to a fish membrane progestin receptor. Proc Nat Aca Sci USA 2003;100:2237–42.

[58] Curran-Rauhut MA, Petersen SL. The distribution of progestin receptor mRNA in rat brainstem. Brain Res Gene Expr Patterns 2002;1:151–7.

[59] Brinton RD, Thompson RF, Foy MR, Baudry M, Wang J, Finch CE, et al. Progesterone receptors: form and function in brain. Front Neuroendocrinol 2008;29:313–39.

[60] Guerra-Araiza C, Villamar-Cruz O, González-Arenas A, Chavira R, Camacho-Arroyo I. Changes in progesterone receptor isoforms content in the rat brain during the oestrous cycle and after oestradiol and progesterone treatments. J Neuroendocrinol 2003;15:984–90.

[61] Guerra-Araiza C, Coyoy-Salgado A, Camacho-Arroyo I. Sex differences in the regulation of progesterone receptor isoforms expression in the rat brain. Brain Res Bull 2002;59:105–9.

[62] Somerville BW. The role of progesterone in menstrual migraine. Neurology 1971; 21:853–9.

[63] Amir BY, Yaacov B, Guy B, Gad P, Itzhak W, Gal I. Headaches in women undergoing in vitro fertilization and embryo-transfer treatment. Headache 2005;45:215–9.

[64] Gupta S, Villalón CM, Mehrotra S, de Vries R, Garrelds IM, Saxena PR, et al. Female sex hormones and rat dural vasodilatation to CGRP, periarterial electrical stimulation and capsaicin. Headache 2007;47:225–35.

[65] Lee H, Sininger L, Jen JC, Cha YH, Baloh RW, Nelson SF. Association of progesterone receptor with migraine-associated vertigo. Neurogenetics 2007;8:195–200.

[66] Colson NJ, Lea RA, Quinlan S, MacMillan J, Griffiths LR. The estrogen receptor 1 G594A polymorphism is associated with migraine susceptibility in two independent case/control groups. Neurogenetics 2004;5:129–33.

[67] Colson NJ, Lea RA, Quinlan S, MacMillan J, Griffiths LR. Investigation of hormone receptor genes in migraine. Neurogenetics 2005;6:17–23.
[68] Corominas R, Ribasés M, Cuenca-León E, Cormand B, Macaya A. Lack of association of hormone receptor polymorphisms with migraine. Eur J Neurol 2009;16:413–5.
[69] Daubert EA, Condron BG. Serotonin: a regulator of neuronal morphology and circuitry. Trends Neurosci Sep. 2010;33(9):424–34.
[70] Peterlin BL, Rapoport AM. Clinical pharmacology of the serotonin receptor agonist, zolmitriptan. Expert Opin Drug Metab Toxicol 2007;3:899–911.
[71] Walther DJ, Peter JU, Bashammakh S, Hortnagl H, Voits M, Fink H, et al. Synthesis of serotonin by a second tryptophan hydroxylase isoform. Science 2003;299:76.
[72] Marziniak M, Mössner R, Schmitt A, Lesch KP, Sommer C. A functional serotonin transporter gene polymorphism is associated with migraine with aura. Neurology 2005;64:157–9.
[73] Bayerer B, Engelbergs J, Savidou I, Boes T, Küper M, Schorn CF, et al. Single nucleotide polymorphisms of the serotonin transporter gene in migraine—an association study. Headache 2010;50:319–22.
[74] Pecins-Thompson M, Brown NA, Kohama SG, Bethea CL. Ovarian steroid regulation of tryptophanhydroxylase mRNA expression in rhesus macaques. J Neurosci 1996;16:7021–9.
[75] Bethea CL, Lu NZ, Gundlah C, Streicher JM. Diverse actions of ovarian steroids in the serotonin neural system. Front Neuroendocrinol 2002;23:41–100.
[76] Genazzani AR, Facchinetti F, Parrini D. Beta-lipotrophin and beta-endorphin plasma levels during pregnancy. Clin Endocrinol (Oxf) 1981;14:409–18.
[77] Dawson-Basoa MB, Gintzler AR. 17-Beta-estradiol and progesterone modulate an intrinsic opioid analgesic system. Brain Res 1993;601:241–5.
[78] Sarajari S, Oblinger MM. Estrogen effects on pain sensitivity and neuropeptide expression in rat sensory neurons. Exp Neurol 2010;224:163–9.
[79] Cyr M, Ghribi O, Di Paolo TJ. Regional and selective effects of oestradiol and progesterone on NMDA and AMPA receptors in the rat brain. Neuroendocrinol 2002;12:445–52.
[80] Nilsen J, Brinton RD. Impact of progestins on estradiol potentiation of the glutamate calcium response. Neuroreport 2002;13:825–30.
[81] Twyman RE, Macdonald RL. Neurosteroid regulation of GABAA receptor single-channel kinetic properties of mouse spinal cord neurons in culture. J Physiol 1992;456:215–45.
[82] Shughrue PJ, Merchenthaler I. Estrogen is more than just a "sex hormone": novel sites for estrogen action in the hippocampus and cerebral cortex. Front Neuroendocrinol 2000;21:95–101.
[83] Uddman R, Tajti J, Hou M, Sundler F, Edvinsson L. Neuropeptide expression in the human trigeminal nucleus caudalis and in the cervical spinal cord C1 and C2. Cephalalgia 2002;22:112–6.
[84] Tajti J, Uddman R, Edvinsson L. Neuropeptide localization in the "migraine generator" region of the human brainstem. Cephalalgia 2001;21:96–101.
[85] Durham PL, Russo AF. Stimulation of the calcitonin gene-related peptide enhancer by mitogen-activated protein kinases and repression by an antimigraine drug in trigeminal ganglia neurons. J Neurosci 2003;23:807–15.
[86] Suzuki T, Nakamura Y, Moriya T, Sasano H. Effects of steroid hormones on vascular functions. Microsc Res Tech 2003;60:76–84.
[87] Aukes AM, Bishop N, Godfrey J, Cipolla MJ. The influence of pregnancy and gender on perivascular innervation of rat posterior cerebral arteries. Reprod Sci 2008;15:411–9.

[88] Mowa CN, Usip S, Collins J, Storey-Workley M, Hargreaves KM, Papka RE. The effects of pregnancy and estrogen on the expression of calcitonin gene-related peptide (CGRP) in the uterine cervix, dorsal root ganglia and spinal cord. Peptides 2003;24:1163–74.

[89] Tepper SJ, Stillman MJ. Clinical and preclinical rationale for CGRP-receptor antagonists in the treatment of migraine. Headache 2008;48:1259–68.

[90] Marcus DA, Scharff L, Turk DC. Longitudinal prospective study of headache during pregnancy and postpartum. Headache 1999;39:625–32.

[91] Fernández-de-las-Peñas C, Cuadrado ML, Arendt-Nielsen L, Simons D, Pareja JA. Myofascial trigger points and sensitization: a updated pain model for tension-type headache. Cephalalgia 2007;27:383–93.

[92] Goadsby PJ. Pathophysiology of cluster headache: a trigeminal autonomic cephalgia. Lancet Neurol 2002;1:251–7.

[93] Van Vliet JA, Favier. I, Helmerhorst FM, Haan J, Ferrari MD. Cluster headache in women: relation with menstruation, use of oral contraceptives, pregnancy, and menopause. J Neurol Neurosurg Psychiatry 2006;77:690–2.

[94] Silberstein SD. Headaches in pregnancy. Neurol Clin 2004;22:727–56.

[95] Silberstein SD. Practice parameter: evidence-based guidelines for migraine headache (an evidence-based review): report of the Quality Standards Subcommittee of the American Academy of Neurology. Neurology 2000;55:754–62.

[96] Sándor PS, Áfra J. Nonpharmacologic treatment of migraine. Curr Pain Headache Rep 2005;9:202–5.

[97] Gaffney L, Smith CA. Use of complementary therapies in pregnancy: the perceptions of obstetricians and midwives in South Australia. Aust N Z J Obstet Gynacol 2004;44:24–9.

[98] Kalder M, Knoblauch K, Hrgovic I, Münstedt K. Use of complementary and alternative medicine during pregnancy and delivery. Arch Gynecol Obstet Feb. 23, 2010 E pub ahead of print.

[99] Bendtsen L, Jensen R. Tension-type headache. Neurol Clin 2009;27:525–35.

[100] Sun-Edelstein C, Mauskap A. Complementary and alternative approaches to the treatment of tension-type headache. Curr Pain Headache Rep 2008;12:447–50.

[101] Alcantara J, Cossette M. Intractable migraine headaches during pregnancy under chiropractic care. Complement Ther Clin Pract 2009;15:192–7.

[102] Schoensee SK, Jensen G, Nicholson G, Gossman M, Katholi C. The effect of mobilization on cervical headaches. J Orthop Sports Phys Ther 1995;21:184–96.

[103] Heiner JD. Cervical epidural hematorma after chiropractic spinal manipulation. Am J Emerg Med 2009;27:1023.e1–1023.e2.

[104] Gaul C, Eismann R, Schmidt T, May A, Leinisch E, Wieser T, et al. Use of complementary and alternative medicine in patients suffering from primary headache disorders. Cephalalgia 2009;29:1069–78.

[105] Bronfort G, Haas M, Evans RL, Bouter LM. Efficacy of spinal manipulation and mobilization for low back pain and neck pain: a systematic review and best evidence synthesis. Spine 2004;4:335–56.

[106] Biondi DM. Cervicogenic headache: a review of diagnostic and treatment strategies. J Am Osteopath Assoc 2005;105(Suppl. 2):S16–22.

[107] Jensen R, Roth JM. Physiotherapy of tension-type headaches. In: Olesen J, Tfelt-Hansen P, Welch KMA, editors. The headaches. 3rd ed. Philadelphia, PA: Lippincott Williams & Wilkins; 2006. p. 721–5.

[108] Astin JA, Ernst E. The effectiveness of spinal manipulation for the treatment of headache disorders: a systematic review of randomized clinical trials. Cephalalgia 2002;22:617–23.

[109] Fernández-de-Las-Peñas C, Alonso-Blanco C, Cuadrado ML, Miangolarra JC, Barriga FJ, Pareja JA. Are manual therapies effective in reducing pain from tension-type headache? A systemic review. Clin J Pain 2006;22:278–85.
[110] Biondi DM. Physical treatments for headache: a structured review. Headache 2005;45:738–46.
[111] Bronfort G, Haas M, Evans R, Leininger B, Triano J. Effectiveness of manual therapies: the UK evidence report. Chiropr Osteopat 2010;18:1–33.
[112] Haas M, Spegman A, Peterson D, Aickin M, Vavrek D. Dose response and efficacy of spinal manipulation for chronic cervicogenic headache: a pilot randomized controlled trial. Spine 2010;10:169–71.
[113] Davis MD, Kononowech RW, Rolin SA, Spierings EL. Acupuncture for tension-type headache: a meta-analysis of randomized, controlled trials. J Pain 2008;8:667–77.
[114] Granato A, Grandi FC, Stokelj D, Musho S, Pizzolato G. Acupuncture in tension-type headache. Neuroepidemiology 2010;35:160–2.
[115] Kaptchuk TJ. Acupuncture: theory, efficacy, and practice. Ann Intern Med 2002;136:374–83.
[116] Remy RC, Kaufman JS, Kaptchuk TJ, Chen W, Miller WC, Callahan LF, et al. A randomized, controlled trial of acupuncture for chronic daily headache. Headache 2005;45:1113–23.
[117] Smith CA, Cochrane S. Does acupuncture have a place as an adjunct treatment during pregnancy? A review of randomized controlled trials and systematic reviews. Birth 2009;36:246–53.
[118] Smith C, Dahlen H. Caring for the pregnant woman and her baby in a changing maternity service environment: the role of acupuncture. Acupunct Med 2009;27:123–5.
[119] Ernst E. Is reflexology an effective intervention? A systemic review of randomised controlled trials. Med J Aust 2009;191:263–6.
[120] Mann JD, Faurot KR, Wilkinson L, Curtis P, Coeytaux RR, Suchindran C, et al. Craniosacral therapy for migraine: protocol development for an exploratory controlled clinical trial. BMC Complement Altern Med 2008;8:28–40.
[121] Stuber K. The safety of chiropractic during pregnancy: a pilot e-mail survey of chiropractors' opinions. Clin Chiropract 2007;10:24–35.
[122] Nadgir RN, Loevner LA, Ahmed T, Moonis G, Chalela J, Slawek K, et al. Simultaneous bilateral internal carotid and vertebral artery dissection following chiropractic manipulation: case report and review of the literature. Neuroradiology 2003;45:311–4.
[123] Khan AM, Ahmad N, Li X, Korsten MA, Rosman A. Chiropractic sympathectomy: carotid artery dissection with oculosympathetic palsy after chiropractic manipulation of the neck. Mt Sinai J Med 2005;72:207–10.
[124] Schmitz A, Lutterbey G, von Engelhardt L, von Falkenhausen M, Stoffel M. Pathological cervical fracture after spinal manipulation in a pregnant patient. J Manipulative Physiol Ther 2005;28:633–6.
[125] Loder E. Migraine in pregnancy. Semin Neurol 2007;27:425–33.
[126] Thorley V. Lactational headache: a lactation consultant's diary. J Hum Lact 1997;13:51–3.
[127] Sun-Edelstein C, Mauskap A. Complementary and alternative approaches to the treatment of tension-type headache. Curr Pain Headache Rep 2008;12:447–50.
[128] Holroyd KA, Martin PR, Nash JM. Psychological treatments for tension-type headache. In: Olesen J, Tfelt-Hansen P, Welch KMA, editors. The headaches. 3rd ed. Philadelphia, PA: Lippincott Williams & Wilkins; 2006. p. 711–9.
[129] Marcus DA, Scharff L, Turk DC. Nonpharmacological management of headaches during pregnancy. Psychosom Med 1995;57:527–35.

[130] Scharff L, Marcus DA, Turk DC. Maintenance of effects in the nonmedical treatment of headaches during pregnancy. Headache 1996;36:285–90.
[131] Sándor PS, Áfra J. Nonpharmacologic treatment of migraine. Curr Pain Headache Rep 2005;9:202–5.
[132] Brandes JL. Headache related to pregnancy: management of migraine and migraine headache in pregnancy. Curr Treat Options Neurol 2008;10:12–19.
[133] Lucas S. Medication use in the treatment of migraine during pregnancy and lactation. Curr Pain Headache Rep 2009;13:392–8.
[134] http://depts.washington.edu/druginfo/Formulary/Pregnancy.pdf
[135] http://depts.washington.edu/terisweb/teris/.
[136] American Academy of Pediatrics Committee on Drugs. Transfer of drugs and other chemicals into human milk. Pediatrics 2001;108:776–89.
[137] Hale TW. Medications and mothers' milk. Amarillo, TX: Hale Publishing; 2008.
[138] Buckner KD, Chavez MD, Raney EC, Stoehr JD. Health food stores recommendations for nausea and migraines during pregnancy. Ann Pharmacother 2005;39:274–9.
[139] Schoenen J, Jacquy J, Lenaerts M. Effectiveness of high-dose riboflavin in migraine prophylaxis. A randomized controlled trial. Neurology 1998;50:466–70.
[140] National Toxicology Program, National Institute of Environmental Health Sciences, National Institutes of Health. Supporting nomination for toxicological evaluation by the National Toxicology Program. Accessed at http://ntp.niehs.nih.gov/NTP/Noms/Support_Docs/Butterbur_Nov2009.pdf; 2009.
[141] National Institute of Health, National Center for Complementary and Alternative Medicine. Herbs at a Glance, NCCAM Publication No. D342 accessed at http://nccam.nih.gov/health/feverfew/; 2008.
[142] U.S. National Library of Medicine and the National Institute of Health, Medline Plus. Coenzyme Q-10, accessed at http://www.nlm.nih.gov/medlineplus/druginfo/natural/patient-coenzymeq10.html; 2009.
[143] Nehlig A, Debry G. Potential teratogenic and neurodevelopmental consequences of coffee and caffeine exposure: a review of human and animal data. Neurotoxicol Teratol 1994;**16**:5311–543.
[144] Menon R, Bushnell CD. Headache and pregnancy. Neurologist 2008;14:108–19.
[145] Briggs G, Freeman R, Yaffe S. Drugs in pregnancy and lactation. 3rd ed. Baltimore, MD: Williams and Wilkins; 1990.
[146] Lay CL, Broner SW. Migraine in women. *Neurol* Clin 2009;27:503–11.
[147] Barrow MV, Souder DE. Propoxyphene and congenital malformations. JAMA 1971;217:1551–2.
[148] Ringrose CAD. The hazard of neurotrophic drugs in the fertile years. Can Med Assoc J 1972;106:1058.
[149] Golden NL, King KC, Sokol RJ. Propoxyphene and acetaminophen: possible effects on the fetus. Clin Pediatr 1982;21:7524.
[150] Golden SM, Perman KI. Bilateral clinical anophthalmia: drugs as potential factors. South Med J 1980;73:14047.
[151] Cunnington M, Ephross S, Churchill P. The safety of sumatriptan and naratriptan in pregnancy: what have we learned? Headache 2009;49:1414–22.
[152] Nezvalová-Henriksen K, Spigset O, Nordeng H. Triptan exposure during pregnancy and the risk of major congenital malformations and adverse pregnancy outcomes: results from the Norwegian Mother and Child Cohort Study. Headache 2010;50:563–75.
[153] Shimzu T. Beta blockers in migraine prophylaxis. Brain Nerve 2009;61:1125–30.

[154] Dey R, Khan S, Akhouri V, Wootton J, Bajwa ZH. Labetalol for prophylactic treatment of intractable migraine during pregnancy. Headache 2002;42:642–5.

[155] Giraud P, Chavet S. Cluster headache during pregnancy: case report and literature review. Headache 2009;49:136–9.

[156] Jurgens TP, Schaefer C, May A. Treatment of cluster headache in pregnancy and lactation. Cephalalgia 2009;29:391–400.

[157] Mawer G, Briggs M, Baker GA, Bromley R, Coyle H, Eatock J, et al. Pregnancy with epilepsy: obstetric and neonatal outcome of a controlled study. Seizure 2010;19:112–19.

[158] Banach R, Boskovic R, Einarson T, Koran G. Long-term developmental outcome of children of women with epilepsy, unexposed or exposed prenatally to antiepilepic drugs: a meta-analysis of cohort studies. Drug Safety 2010;33:73–9.

[159] Afshar M, Moallem SA, Houshang Mohammadpour A, Sheravi A, Majid JS, Jafar Golalipour M. Teratogenic effects of carbamazepine on embryonic eye development in pregnant mice. Cutan Ocul Toxicol 2010;29:10–15.

[160] Marcus D. Headache in pregnancy. Curr Treat Options Neurol 2007;9:23–30.

[161] Ramchandren S, Cross B, Liebeskind D. Emergent headaches during pregnancy: correlation between neurologic examination and neuroimaging. Am J Neuroradiol 2007;28:1085–7.

[162] Kanal E, Barkovich J, Bell C, Borgstede J, Bradley W, Froelich J, et al. ACR guidance document for safe MR practices: 2007. AJR Am J Roentgenol 2007;188:1447–74.

[163] De Luca GC, Bartleson JD. When and how to investigate the patient with headache. Semin Neurol 2010;30:131–44.

[164] Hauth JC, Ewell MG, Levine RJ, Esterlitz JR, Sibai B, Curet LB, et al. Pregnancy outcomes in healthy nulliparas who developed hypertension. Calcium for Preeclampsia Prevention Study Group. Obstet Gynecol 2000;95:24–8.

[165] Report of the National High Blood Pressure Education Program Working Group on High Blood Pressure in Pregnancy. Am J Obstet Gynecol 2000;183(Suppl):1–22.

[166] Bartynski WS, Boardman JF. Distinct imaging patterns and lesion distribution in posterior reversible encephalopathy syndrome. Am J Neuroradiol 2007;28:1320–7.

[167] Schaefer PW, Buonanno FS, Gonzalez GG, Schwamm LH. Diffusion-weighted imaging discriminates between cytotoxic oedema and vasogenic oedema in a patient with eclampsia. Stroke 1997;28:1082–5.

[168] Jim B, Sharma S, Kebede T, Acharya A. Hypertension in pregnancy. Cardiol Rev 2010;18:178–89.

[169] Yang Q, Wen SW, Smith GN, Chen Y, Krewski D, Chen XK, et al. Maternal cigarette smoking and the risk of pregnancy-induced hypertension and eclampsia. Int J Epidemiol 2006;35:288–93.

[170] Haddad B, Sibai BM. Expectant management of severe preeclampsia: proper candidates and pregnancy outcome. Clin Obstet Gynecol 2005;48:430–40.

[171] Jim B, Sharma S, Kebede T, Acharya A. Hypertension in pregnancy. Cardiol Rev 2010;18:178–89.

[172] Lidwien M, Hanff LM, Visser W, Roofthooft DWE, Vermes A, Hop WCJ, et al. Insufficient efficacy of intravenous ketanserin in severe early-onset pre-eclampsia. Eur J Obstet Gynecol Reprod Biol 2006;128:199–203.

[173] Brown DW, Dueker N, Jamieson DJ, Cole JW, Wozniak MA, Stern BJ, et al. Pre-eclampsia and the risk of ischemic stroke among young women: results from the stroke prevention in young women study. Stroke 2006;37:1055–9.

[174] Tentschert S, Wimmer R, Greisenegger S, Lang W, Lalouschek W. Headache at stroke onset in 2196 patients with ischemic stroke or transient ischemic attack. Stroke 2005;36:e1–3.

[175] Tang SC, Jeng JS. Management of stroke in pregnancy and the puerperium. Expert Rev Neurother 2010;10:205–15.
[176] Davie CA, O'Brien P. Stroke and pregnancy. J Neurol Neurosurg Psychiatry 2008;79:240–5.
[177] Chang J, Elam-Evans LD, Berg CJ, Herndon J, Flowers L, Seed KA, et al. Pregnancy-related mortality surveillance United States, 1991–1999. MMWR Surveill Summ 2003;52:1–8.
[178] James AH, Bushnell CD, Jamison MG, Myers ER. Incidence and risk factors for stroke in pregnancy and the puerperium. Obstet Gynecol 2005;106:509–16.
[179] Tang C, Wu C, Lee T, Hung S, Yang CC, Lee C, et al. Preeclampsia–eclampsia and the risk of stroke among peripartum in Taiwan. Stroke 2009;40:1162–8.
[180] Tang SC, Jeng JS. Management of stroke in pregnancy and the puerperium. Expert Rev Neurother 2010;10:205–15.
[181] Ducros A, Bousser M. Reversible cerebral vasoconstriction syndrome. Pract Neurol 2009;9:256–67.
[182] Chen S, Fuh J, Wang S, Chang F, Lirng J, Fang Y, et al. Magnetic resonance angiography in reversible cerebral vasoconstriction syndromes. Ann Neurol 2010;67:648–56.
[183] Roine S, Poyhonen M, Timonen S, Tuisku S, Marttila R, Sulkava R, et al. Neurologic symptoms are common during gestation and puerperium in CADASIL. Neurology 2005;64:1441–3.
[184] Ramaraj R, Sorrell VL. Peripartum cardiomyopathy: causes, diagnosis, and treatment. Cleve Clin J Med 2009;76:289–96.
[185] Arboix A, Massons J, Oliveres M, Arribas MP, Titus F. Headache in acute cerebrovascular disease: a prospective clinical study in 240 patients. Cephalalgia 1994;14: 37–40.
[186] Melo TP, Pinto AN, Ferro JM. Headache in intracerebral hematomas. Neurology 1996;47:494–500.
[187] Jeng J, Tang S, Yip P. Incidence and etiologies of stroke during pregnancy and puerperium as evidenced in Taiwanese women. Cerebrovasc Dis 2004;18:290–5.
[188] Huang CY, Chen CA, Hsieh CY, Cheng WF. ICH as initial presentation of gestational choriocarcinoma: a case report and literature review. Int J Gynecol Cancer 2007;17:1166–71.
[189] Piotin M, de ouza Filho C, Kothimbakam R, Moret J. Endovascular treatment of acutely ruptured intracranial aneurysms in pregnancy. Case reports. Am J Obstet Gynecol 2001;185:1261–2.
[190] Ravishankar K. Incidence and pattern of headache in cerebral venous thrombosis. J Pak Med Assoc 2006;56:561–4.
[191] Jacobs K, Moulin T, Bogousslavsky J, Woimant F, Dehaene I, Tatu L, et al. The stroke syndrome of cortical vein thrombosis. Neurology 1996;47:376–82.
[192] Canhao P, Ferro JM, Lindgren AG, Bousser M, Stam J, Barinagarrementeria F. Causes and predictors of death in cerebral venous thrombosis. Stroke 2005;36:1720–5.
[193] Salonen RH, Lictenstein P, Bellocco R, Petersson G, Cnattingius S. Increased risks of circulatory disease in late pregnancy and puerperium. Epidemiology 2001;12:456–60.
[194] Lockhart EM, Baysinger CL. Intracranial venous thrombosis in the parturient. Anesthesiology 2007;107:652–8.
[195] Bousser MG. Cerebral venous thrombosis: diagnosis and management. J Neurol 2000;247:252–8.
[196] Cakmak S, Derex L, Berruyer M, Nighoghossian N, Philippeau F, Adeleine P, et al. Cerebral venous thrombosis: clinical outcome and systematic screening of prothrombotic factors. Neurology 2003;60:1175–8.

[197] Medel R, Monteith SJ, Crowley RW, Dumont AS. A review of therapeutic strategies for the management of cerebral venous sinus thrombosis. Neurosurg Focus 2009;27:1–9.

[198] Dubuisson AS, Beckers A, Stevenaert A. Classical pituitary tumor apoplexy: clinical features, management and outcomes in a series of 24 patients. Clin Neurol Neurosurg 2007;109(1):63–70.

[199] Murad-Kejbou S, Eggenberger E. Pituitary apoplexy: evaluation, management, and prognosis. Curr Opin Ophthalmol 2009;20:456–61.

[200] Semple P, Jane J, Lopes B, Laws E. Pituitary apoplexy: correlation between magnetic resonance imaging and histopathological results. J Neurosurg 2008;108:909–15.

[201] Nawar RN, AbdelMannan D, Selman WR, Arafah BM. Pituitary tumor apoplexy: a review. J Intens Care Med 2008;23:75–90.

[202] Ambika S, Arjundas D, Noronha V, Anshuman Clinical profile, evaluation, management and visual outcome of idiopathic intracranial hypertension in a neuro-ophthalmology clinic of a tertiary referral ophthalmic center in India. Ann Indian Acad Neurol 2010;13:37–41.

[203] Tang RA, Dorotheo EU, Schiffman JS, Bahrani HM. Medical and surgical management of idiopathic intracranial hypertension in pregnancy. Curr Neurol Neurosci Rep 2004;4:398–409.

[204] Lee AG, Pless M, Flalardeau J, Capozzoli T, Wall M, Kardon RH. The use of acetazolamide in idiopathic intracranial hypertension during pregnancy. Am J Ophthalmol 2005;139:855–9.

[205] Bagga R, Jain V, Gupta KR, Gopalan S, Malhotra S, Das CP. Choice of therapy and mode of delivery in idiopathic intracranial hypertension during pregnancy. Med Gen Med 2005;7:42–6.

[206] Mokri B. Low cerebrospinal fluid pressure syndromes. Neurol Clin North Am 2004;22:55–74.

[207] Savoiardo M, Minati L, Farina L, De Simone T, Aquino D, Mea E, et al. Spontaneous intracranial hypotension with deep brain swelling. Brain 2007;130:1884–93.

[208] Schievink WI. Spontaneous spinal cerebrospinal fluid leaks and intracranial hypotension. JAMA 2006;295:2286–96.

[209] McGrail KM, Beyerl BD, Black PM, Klibanski A, Zervas N. Lymphocytic adenohypophysitis of pregnancy with complete recovery. Neurosurgery 1987;20:791–3.

[210] Yasuyuki A, Koichiro N, Hiroki I, Sachiko H, Yoshiharu W, Yoshiyuki H, et al. A case of lymphocytic panhypophysitis (LPH) during pregnancy. Endocrine 2007;32:117–21.

[211] Haas JF, Janisch. W, Staneczek W. Newly diagnosed primary intracranial neoplasms in pregnant women: a population-based assessment. J Neurol Neurosurg Psychiatry 1986;49:874–80.

[212] Carroll RS, Zhang J, Black PM. Expression of estrogen receptors alpha and beta in human meningiomas. J Neurooncol 1999;42:109–16.

[213] DeAngelis LM. Central nervous system neoplasms in pregnancy. Adv Neurol 1994;64:139–52.

[214] Klink R, Robichaud M, Debonnel G. Gender and gonadal status modulation of dorsal raphe nucleus serotonergic neurons. Part I: Effects of gender and pregnancy. Neuropharmacology 2002;43:1119–28.

3 Myasthenia Gravis and Pregnancy

Fernanda Campos da Silva[1,2,3], *Luciana Carneiro do Cima*[3,4], *Renato Augusto Moreira de Sá*[1,3]

[1]Universidade Federal Fluminense, Niterói, Brazil
[2]Hospital Geral de Bonsucesso, Rio de Janeiro, Brazil
[3]Grupo Perinatal, Rio de Janeiro, Brazil
[4]Instituto Fernandes Figueira, Rio de Janeiro, Brazil

Introduction

Myasthenia gravis (MG) is a chronic autoimmune disorder in which autoantibodies against the acetylcholine receptor (AChR Abs) at the neuromuscular junction impair neuromuscular transmission, causing weakness of skeletal muscles. It is considered a rare disease in the general population and also in pregnancy. The overall incidence ranges from 50 to 125 cases per million population [1]. Women are more affected than men at a ratio of 6:4. It may occur at any age, but female incidence peaks in the third decade of life, whereas the male mean age of onset is at 42 years [2]. Thus, like other autoimmune diseases, MG occurs commonly in women in childbearing age.

Clinical Features

Main signs and symptoms include diplopia and ptosis that represent involvement of extrinsic ocular muscles. Fifteen percent of patients will only have this ocular involvement, but it may progressively affect the bulbar muscles used for swallowing. In addition, when limbs are affected, fluctuating weakness and easy fatigability of skeletal muscles are seen. Weakness has often a proximal distribution, worsens with sustained exertion, and improves after rest. The disease typically has periods of remission and exacerbations that may be triggered by certain medications, intercurrent infections, surgery, general anesthesia, emotional stress, menses, pregnancy, and puerperium [1] (Box 3.1). A myasthenic crisis occurs when there is involvement of respiratory muscles requiring mechanical ventilation. It is not unusual for patients with MG to have other autoimmune diseases such as hypothyroidism (13%), systemic lupus erythematosus, rheumatoid arthritis (5–6%), or polymiositis (1%) [3]. Box 3.2 shows clinical features of MG.

Neurological Disorders and Pregnancy. DOI: 10.1016/B978-0-12-384911-3.00003-8

Box 3.1 Factors That Increase the Weakness in MG

- Physical exertion
- Hot temperature
- Drugs—e.g., aminoglycosides, phenytoin, local anesthetics
- Emotional upsets
- Surgery
- Infections
- Menses
- Hyperthyroidism
- Pregnancy
- Hypokalemia

Box 3.2 Clinical Features of MG

- Can present at any age, typically bimodal peak, with first peak in the third decade and the second peak in sixth and seventh decades ("young women and old men").
- Weakness and fatigue of the voluntary muscles are the most important features. Symptoms worsen or appear on exertion and improve at rest or with anticholinesterases. Typically there is a diurnal variation, with worsening of symptoms in the later part of the day.
- Ocular muscle weakness is usually the initial presentation and may be the only feature through the course in about 10% of patients. The ptosis (and diplopia) is exacerbated by the prolonged upward gaze toward a fixed target for 1 min.
- In most cases, weakness progresses from ocular muscles to involve other muscles in a craniocaudal direction. The weakness of intercostal muscles and diaphragm leads to dyspnea on exertion or at rest. The orthopnea with rapid resolution on sitting up and diaphragmatic paradox are important clinical signs of neuromuscular breathlessness.
- Deep tendon reflexes are intact or may be brisk.
- There are no objective sensory deficits.
- In severe cases, respiratory failure may ensue, requiring intubation and mechanical ventilation.
- Symptoms may fluctuate and there may be remissions of variable periods, particularly in early stages.

Diagnosis

Diagnosis of MG should start with a complete history and physical examination. Other neuromuscular conditions including mitochondrial myopathy, thyroid ophthalmopathy, and Lambert–Eaton myasthenic syndrome must be excluded. Serum AChR Abs is present in 70–90% of patients with general involvement, and 50% of patients with purely ocular MG. It confirms clinical diagnosis [4]. Other antibodies may be present, such as those against the muscle-specific receptor tyrosine kinase that may be useful in seronegative patients [5]. Electronic testing is also used for diagnosis and to assess severity. Typical pattern includes an abnormal decline in the size of evoked potentials noted on repetitive supermaximal muscle motor nerve stimulation [1]. Abnormal jitter and blocking are detected virtually in all patients who have MG and a weak muscle is tested. The method is especially interesting in seronegative patients.

Approximately 75% of patients have thymic abnormalities, and 10% have thymomas [1]. Thymomas are more frequent in patients over the age of 30. Because 30% are invasive at the time of diagnosis, all thymomas should be surgically removed. Women of childbearing age who have MG have an enlarged thymus and circulating autoantibodies in most cases.

General Aspects of Preconception Care

The onset of MG can be triggered during pregnancy or postpartum. In pre-existing MG, exacerbations are frequently unpredictable and not unusual during pregnancy, labor, or the postpartum period. Although a good outcome is possible, there are some important clinical considerations for the myasthenic patient planning a pregnancy. Pregnancy is associated with important hemodynamic changes essential for fetal growth and well-being. These include a rise in blood volume and renal clearance that interfere with absorption of oral medications that may need dosage adjustments. The growing fetus many times restricts the diaphragm and compromises the respiratory function in normal pregnancy. Symptoms may be worse in MG, especially with previous respiratory involvement.

Myasthenic patients considering pregnancy should seek preconception counseling in order to improve their clinical condition, minimize the use of immunosuppressive drugs, and address the need for thymectomy. It is also important to maximize treatment to concomitant disorders, such as arterial hypertension, diabetes mellitus, and hypothyroidism, as all add risk to the future pregnancy.

All issues and risks should be made clear to patients to enable them to make a conscious decision based on the most current information available. Those with involvement of the respiratory muscles should be advised not to get pregnant until improvement of their clinical condition. They should also be aware that the effects of pregnancy in MG is often unpredictable, and so is the opposite: the effects of the disease in pregnancy cannot be predicted.

Effect of Pregnancy on MG

Pregnancy may change the course of MG, often in an unpredictable way. The clinical state at the beginning of pregnancy does not predict the occurrence of exacerbation or remission [6]. It is also interesting to notice that each pregnancy has its effect on

MG. The course of future pregnancies cannot be predicted by the ongoing pregnancy. In one review of 322 pregnancies in 225 myasthenic patients, exacerbation, remission, and no change in disease occurred in 41%, 29%, and 30%, respectively [7]. Additionally, postpartum exacerbations were noted in 30% of all patients. It seems that the first trimester and the postpartum period are the times of highest risk of exacerbation [2]. Despite these findings, the long-term outcome of MG is not altered by pregnancy [6]. The maternal mortality risk is inversely related to the duration of the disease with the highest risk being in the first year. It is thus recommended that myasthenic women postpone pregnancy for the first year or two after diagnosis [8].

Normal physiologic changes associated with pregnancy, especially the hemodynamic changes and alteration in gastrointestinal absorption, may affect the clinical course of MG. Besides, common symptoms of the first trimester, such as nausea and vomiting, can lead to subtherapeutic levels of medication, sometimes requiring parenteral therapy. Another important consideration concerns infections in the myasthenic pregnant woman. Infections should be treated aggressively because they can precipitate severe exacerbations. Special attention is required for respiratory infections. When diaphragmatic muscle weakness is present, it may become more symptomatic during pregnancy because of the respiratory restriction caused by increase in abdomen. A simple upper respiratory tract infection can lead to a life-threatening respiratory crisis in need of mechanical ventilation [9]. Complaints of cough or dyspnea should be evaluated promptly.

Alpha-fetoprotein (AFP) has been studied as a factor influencing MG in pregnancy. AFP has been identified as a factor inhibiting binding of antiacetylcholine receptor antibodies to acetylcholine receptors, with a level of 60,000 ng/mL inhibiting 93% of autoantibodies from binding [7]. Varying levels of AFP could partially explain variations in clinical course during pregnancy.

Effect of MG in Pregnancy

Preterm delivery is a major complication of pregnancy, responsible for high neonatal morbidity and mortality. It is defined by births occurring at less than 37 weeks gestation. Its etiology in the general population and a possible association with MG are not completely understood. The overall incidence of preterm delivery is 10% and reported incidence in MG is variable. In one case series evaluating clinical outcome in myasthenic patients, 36.5% of pregnancies ended before 37 weeks [7]. This group also found a high rate of perinatal death, 68 per 1000 live births. Another large series found no increase in preterm deliveries in MG [6]. However, their population had increased incidence of fetal anomalies, which were responsible for a death rate of 18 per 1000 live births, higher than the general population (2.2 deaths per 1000 live births).

Another common medical problem in obstetrics is pre-eclampsia. Pre-eclampsia is a hypertensive syndrome that complicates 5% of pregnancies, and is considered a major cause of maternal and perinatal death. Maternal complications include hypertensive crisis, cerebral events such as convulsions and hemorrhage, hepatic involvement in HELLP syndrome, and renal lesions. Because there is no treatment for pre-eclampsia, management options focus on preventing these severe complications and anticipating delivery. Damage to the central nervous system is prevented by administration of magnesium sulfate. Despite being a first-line drug in treatment of pre-eclampsia, its use is contraindicated in myasthenic patients. Excess magnesium at the neuromuscular junction causes a relative depression of muscle fiber excitability, which may further exacerbate weakness and fatigability. In one case report, an undiagnosed myasthenic patient treated with magnesium sulfate for pre-eclampsia experienced severe proximal muscle weakness approximately 15 min after magnesium administration [10]. Another report suggests that the administration of magnesium sulfate for seizure prophylaxis precipitated a myasthenic crisis [11]. Narcotics and sedatives may be used under careful supervision as anticonvulsive agents. Seizure prophylaxis may be achieved by administration of phenobarbital.

Myasthenic pregnant women who develop pre-eclampsia are also at increased risk if they use corticosteroids. High-dose corticosteroids may increase fluid retention and aggravate hypertension in patients with severe pre-eclampsia. These patients are at increased risk for developing pulmonary edema and should be monitored closely for worsening respiratory status. Decreased urine output commonly seen in severe pre-eclampsia calls for frequent need of dose adjustment of medications to avoid toxicity. In addition, cholinergic side effects can mimic symptoms of pre-eclampsia. Severe hypertension should be treated with a regime that includes hydralazine. Management of pre-eclampsia in the myasthenic pregnant woman is challenging with less therapeutic options and increased maternal risk.

Preterm birth and pre-eclampsia are not the only concerns in myasthenic pregnant women. Other life-threatening risks include respiratory failure and cholinergic crisis due to overmedication. It is of use to monitor pulmonary function as the patient progresses through gestation. In addition, an electrocardiogram is indicated for the reported risk of focal myocardial necrosis in some patients with MG [12]. Care includes evaluation of thyroid function to rule out coexisting thyroid disease.

Fetal assessment tests that rely on alterations of fetal movement or heart rate response to fetal movement are not always reliable in the myasthenic patient. This includes the patient's perception of fetal movement. During a myasthenic crisis, continuous fetal monitoring of a viable fetus is indicated because the patient and fetus may be hypoxic.

Polyhydramnios as a severe complication resulting from impaired fetal swallowing has been described in several case reports. In extreme cases, fetal arthrogryposis multiplex congenita may be observed in pregnant myasthenic patients. In these cases, lack of fetal movement causes joint contractures and paralysis of the fetal diaphragm results in the development of pulmonary hypoplasia [13]. In some studies evaluating arthrogryposis multiplex congenita, high maternal antiacetylcholine receptor autoantibody titers appear related to the occurrence of fetal/neonatal symptoms [13]. Decreased fetal breathing and total body movements were observed on ultrasound with increasing antibody titers (Table 3.1). Passive placental transfer of antiacetylcholine receptor IgG can be responsible for symptoms in the fetus prenatally and may cause transient neonatal MG after delivery.

Table 3.1 Evaluation Modalities for Pregnancy Complicated with MG

Maternal	Fetal	Neonatal
Baseline motor power survey	Ultrasound	Observation
Pulmonary function test	Biophysical profile	Pulse oximetry
Electrocardiogram	Amniotic fluid index	Respiratory rate
Thyroid function test	Kick counts	Ability to feed

Treatment

Care of a myasthenic pregnant woman has some challenging considerations, and requires a multidisciplinary approach with neurologists, obstetricians, and neonatologists. In pregnancy, treatment aims at optimizing muscle strength in the mother, minimizing the risk of exacerbations, and protecting the fetus. The therapeutic regimen for a myasthenic woman who is pregnant or planning a pregnancy should be individualized. Considerations should be made about severity and distribution of muscle weakness. When bulbar and respiratory muscles are affected, treatment needs to be more aggressive, as potentially life-threatening exacerbations may compromise mother and fetus. In general, if a woman is under treatment for MG at the diagnosis of pregnancy, her drug regimen should not change [14].

Cholinesterase Inhibitors

Principles of treatment are not different from the nonpregnant population. Treatment should include oral cholinesterase inhibitors as first-line agents, such as pyridostigmine and neostigmine. This may be sufficient to treat mild cases. Pyridostigmine is considered safe for use in pregnancy and the recommended dosage is less than 600 mg/day. There is no evidence of a teratogenic effect in rats and humans [15]. Dosage adjustments are more frequent in pregnancy not only because of changes in blood volume and renal clearance, but also because of variability in the disease course. Increments should be accomplished first by reducing medication interval. If unsuccessful, the dosage can be increased slowly to avoid side effects [14].

Immunosuppressant Drugs

Long-term management of MG frequently requires use of immunosuppressant drugs, for example, corticosteroids, azathioprine (AZA), cyclosporine (CsA), and mycophenolate mofetil (MMF). Usually, maximum benefits with steroids and AZA are achieved after 6–12 months. They all cross the placenta and reach the fetus, but most times cannot safely be excluded from treatment options.

Corticosteroids (FDA Risk—B/C)[1]

The corticosteroids most commonly used are the short-acting prednisolone and methylpredinisolone. Clinical experience with these drugs extends to many thousands of women-years. Despite concerns about teratogenic effects in animals, these drugs have not been shown to cause fetal abnormalities in the humans [16], nor have they been shown to affect the fetal hypothalamo-pituitaryadrenal axis. They also seem to be safe in lactation.

The complications associated with the use of corticosteroids in a pregnant patient are the same as in those that may occur in nonpregnant patients, including immunosuppression, avascular necrosis of bone, osteopenia, hypertension, hyperglycemia, cataracts, and striae. However, there may be pregnancy-specific complications such as premature rupture of the membranes and exacerbation of gestational diabetes and hypertension [17].

The routine use of oral calcium and vitamin D supplements is recommended to help prevent osteoporosis. The lowest possible dose needed to control disease activity should be used, and a patient who has been treated with corticosteroids during pregnancy should be given "stress doses" of hydrocortisone for any emergency surgery, cesarean section, or prolonged labor and delivery. Neonates should be monitored for evidence of adrenal insufficiency and infection. Women who choose to breast-feed while taking high doses of glucocorticoids should wait 4h after ingesting a dose to resume breast-feeding, a strategy that will decrease the amount of glucocorticoid in the milk [18].

Azathioprine (FDA Risk—D)

AZA and its metabolite 6-mercaptopurine are purine analogs that were initially developed as chemotherapeutic agents. They are now widely used in the treatment of autoimmune diseases and transplant recipients. Radioactive labeling studies in humans have revealed 64–93% of AZA administered to mothers appears in fetal blood, the majority as the inactive metabolite thiouric acid [19]. Although sporadic anomalies have been reported, no definite association between the drug and the observed abnormalities has been established. There seems to be no effect on fertility and no reported increase in abortion.

AZA crosses the placenta, but the fetal liver lacks the enzyme that converts AZA to its active metabolites. This fetal enzyme deficiency seems to protect the fetus from possible teratogenic effects of AZA early in pregnancy [20]. Women who have MG and take AZA generally are advised against pregnancy, although there has not been a definite demonstration of teratogenicity in humans at therapeutic dosages and many normal pregnancies are reported while on the drug [2]. Because of the potential for carcinogenesis and the unknown long-term effects of fetal immunosuppression,

[1]The United States Food and Drug Administration (FDA) pregnancy risk categories are as follows: A, no risk in controlled clinical studies in humans; B, human data reassuring or when absent, animal studies show no risk; C, human data are lacking; animal studies show risk or are not done; D, positive evidence of risk, benefit may outweigh; X, contraindicated during pregnancy.

use of AZA should be reserved for pregnant women whose disease is severe or life threatening. In addition, reduction of the AZA dose at 32 weeks gestation may prevent serious neonatal leukopenia and thrombocytopenia [21]. Close prenatal monitoring for growth and long-term evaluation of the offspring are essential.

Cyclosporine (FDA Risk—C)

CsA is a large molecule of fungal origin that blocks interleukin-2 and reduces the activity of T lymphocytes. It is most commonly used to prevent solid organ rejection, but has been used more recently to treat a variety of connective tissue diseases. Maternal side effects of CsA include hypertension, nephrotoxicity, hepatotoxicity, tremor, hirsutism, paresthesia, seizures, gout, and gingival hypertrophy [22]. CsA was not toxic to the exposed fetuses at the maternal dosage of 10 mg/kg/day, whereas it was embryotoxic at dosages of 25–100 mg/kg/day [23].

More than 800 pregnancies receiving CsA have been reported, mainly in transplant recipients. The observed rate of 3% of congenital malformations has not exceeded the rate reported in the general population, nor has any particular pattern of abnormalities emerged. Renal and liver functions were normal in 166 newborn infants exposed to CsA in utero [24]. A meta-analysis evaluated the risk of congenital malformations, preterm delivery, or low birth weight from CsA treatment during pregnancy [25]. The calculated odds ratio (OR) of 3.83 for malformations did not achieve statistical significance. The overall prevalence of 4.1% of malformations in the study population did not vary substantially from that reported in the general population. The OR for prematurity did not reach statistical significance, although the overall prevalence rate was 56.3%. It is not clear whether maternal therapy with CsA or the underlying maternal disease was associated with increased rates of prematurity and low birth weight (less than 2500 g).

The decision to continue treatment with the drug in a stable patient depends on the need for disease control, and it should be made jointly with the patient while weighing the potential risks and benefits. Although there was no increased risk of congenital anomalies in the exposed fetuses reported, the number of cases is small and the long-term effects of CsA exposure in utero are unknown. Of the few newborns reported with anomalies, no consistent pattern of congenital defects occurred, which makes antenatal detection difficult. Breast-feeding should be discouraged in women using CsA.

Plasmapheresis and Intravenous Immunoglobulin (IVIG)

Plasmapheresis or intravenous immunoglobulin (IVIG) can be used to manage severe MG symptoms or crisis during pregnancy or to avoid immunosuppressive agents and their side effects [8]. The frequency of the treatments should be guided by the clinical course. The potential risks related to these treatments should be weighed against the severity of myasthenic weakness [26].

With plasmapheresis, there is a theoretic risk of inducing premature labor because of the removal of circulating hormones. Fetal monitoring during the third trimester is recommended. Monitoring of fluid balance and using a left lateral decubitus position during the procedure are helpful in avoiding hypotension. The safety of IVIG use during pregnancy has not been investigated in MG, but the obstetric literature contains many reports of IVIG therapy for various conditions encountered during pregnancy, including autoimmune thrombocytopenia purpura, antiphospholipid syndrome, and neonatal alloimmune thrombocytopenia. IVIG infusions seem to be well tolerated and the occurrence of major and minor side effects is uncommon. Specific contraindications to IVIG use include a previous episode of IVIG-induced anaphylaxis and selective IgA deficiency. Serious side effects include aseptic meningitis, acute renal failure, thromboembolic events, and anaphylactic reactions. Hyperviscosity and volume overloading associated with IVIG infusion may be of greater significance in pregnancy. Less severe but more common side effects include headache, nausea, and fever [2].

Thymectomy

Thymectomy has been recommended for the treatment of MG especially if a thymoma is present. Complete remission of the disease occurs in 45% of patients several years after surgery. Due to this delayed effect, surgery may be postponed until after delivery. Whereas the prevalence of exacerbation is thought to be higher in nonthymectomized as compared with thymectomized pregnant women, there is a case series that describes severe exacerbations in patients with previous thymectomies [27].

Labor and Delivery

Obstetric complications are not very common during delivery [28]. Active labor is divided into two phases: the first stage of labor and the second stage of labor. During the first stage, uterine contractions are responsible for cervical dilation and effacement, and end when there is maximum dilation and the fetus is ready to be born. The second stage is the actual birth of the fetus. Besides uterine contractions, this phase needs maternal efforts to be completed. The first stage of labor is not affected by MG because the uterus is composed of smooth muscle and lacks the postsynaptic acetylcholine receptor. However, the second stage of labor may be affected because the voluntary striated abdominal muscles used during expulsive efforts may easily weaken [29]. Excessive maternal fatigue may result and, therefore, precipitate a myasthenic crisis. Appropriate steps should be taken to circumvent the effects of maternal muscle weakness on delivery. Operative vaginal delivery (forceps, vacuum extraction) should be considered in order to reduce maternal fatigue and weakness [2]. Myasthenic fatigue occurring during labor can be helped by cholinesterase inhibitors. These should be administered parenterally because of unpredictable gastric absorption. Neostigmine doses of 1.5 mg intramuscularly or 0.5 mg intravenously are equivalent to 60 mg of pyridostigmine taken orally.

A cesarean section is only recommended for obstetric reasons [30], as surgical procedures pose a multitude of risks to the myasthenic patient. Such procedures should be reserved for patients with myasthenic exacerbation or myasthenic crisis [8].

Anesthesia

Consultation with an anesthesiologist before labor is recommended, because patients with myasthenia who undergo general anesthesia may be at increased risk for requiring mechanical ventilation [31]. Selection of anesthetic technique is dependent on several factors. Regional anesthesia is recommended for mild to moderate disease when vaginal delivery is anticipated, allowing for adequate anesthesia if vacuum or forceps are needed. General endotracheal anesthesia is recommended for the patient with severe disease and with respiratory or bulbar involvement for better control of airway, secretions, and oxygenation [12].

Nondepolarizing muscle relaxants should be avoided as patients with MG have altered acetylcholinesterase activity. Due to the relative resistance to succinylcholine, larger doses are often required leading to a prolonged block. Some authors recommend that relaxation be provided with inhaled agents during the induction of general anesthesia. It seems that patients with MG are more sensitive to inhaled anesthetics including enflurane, halothane, and isoflurane [12].

Sedatives, opioids, and tranquilizers can potentiate respiratory depression in this population and should be administered judiciously. When using opioids or other sedatives for pain control, pulse oximetry and frequent assessment of respiratory rate is recommended. Nonsteroidal anti-inflammatory medications such as ketorolac tromethamine also may be used for postpartum or postoperative pain [32].

During labor, anticholinesterase medications should be administered parenterally to avoid erratic gastrointestinal absorption due to the impaired gastric emptying process. The parenteral dose of pyridostigmine is equivalent to one-thirtieth of the patient's oral dose [2].

Magnesium sulfate for the management of eclampsia should be used with caution in myasthenic women because it can precipitate weakness by interfering with neuromuscular transmission [2].

The maternal respiratory status (respiratory rate, pulse oximetry, arterial blood gas analysis) should be monitored carefully because stress and fatigue associated with labor and delivery may precipitate worsening of disease.

The postpartum period is also a moment of vulnerability for the myasthenic patient. Approximately one-third of patients experience exacerbation of the disease during the first 3 weeks after giving birth [8]. During this period, the patient is best managed on the medication dosage on which they were stable before pregnancy [14].

Breast-Feeding

The American Academy of Pediatrics classifies pyridostigmine, prednisone, and prednisolone as compatible with breast-feeding [33]. Large doses of anticholinesterase drugs may cause gastrointestinal symptoms in the breast-fed newborn. Some clinicians recommend that mothers wait at least 4h after taking their corticosteroid dose before nursing. The question as to whether it is safe for women receiving immunosuppressive agents (IS) other than corticosteroids to breast-feed is not answered completely. ISs are excreted in breast milk but it is not clear if such breast milk concentrations are significant biologically or have any substantial clinical effects on the infant. Breast-feeding for mothers taking AZA, CsA, or methotrexate generally is not recommended by the World Health Organization (WHO) Working Group on Drugs and Human Lactation. AZA is excreted into breast milk in small amounts. Undetectable levels of 6-mercaptopurine (the active metabolite) in the milk were found in nursing women on AZA [34]. Despite these reports, breast-feeding while receiving AZA is not recommended [18].

Estimates of neonatal exposure to CsA in breast milk indicate it is likely to be far less than the levels to which the fetus is exposed prenatally [35]. In a group of seven infants breast-fed by mothers receiving CsA, it was estimated that the infants ingested less than 300 ng/day of CsA, and all infant blood levels were below 30 ng/mL, the detection limit of the drug assay [36]. In a single case report, CsA levels were undetectable in a neonate at various times during 10.5 months of exclusive breast-feeding from a woman on CsA therapy [37].

Methotrexate is excreted in breast milk in small quantities. Although the amount of methotrexate ingested daily through milk is less than 0.5% of the pediatric therapeutic dosage of this drug (0.12 mg/kg), the American Academy of Pediatrics lists methotrexate as contraindicated during breast-feeding [18], and the WHO Working Group on Drugs and Human Lactation does not recommend breast-feeding for mothers using this drug, unless no alternative is available [38].

Because human breast milk confers many benefits to the infant, mothers should review the risk of the drugs against the disadvantages of formula feeding. Some mothers also find that loss of sleep from night feeding worsens symptoms of MG and choose not to breast-feed so they can have help with infant care.

Anticholinesterase drugs are found in breast milk in low levels and are therefore considered safe in pregnancy unless high dosages are required [1].

Effects on the Fetus and Neonate

Fetal complications of MG include arthrogryposis multiplex congenita and neonatal myasthenia. Arthrogryposis multiplex congenita is a rare condition in which the fetus develops multiple joint contractures due to the lack of movement during pregnancy. There is increased neonatal death due to pulmonary hypoplasia and polyhydramnios [2]. There is a high risk of recurrence in subsequent pregnancies, and the lack of symptoms in the mother does not relate to a smaller risk of arthrogryposis multiplex congenita in the infant [29].

Transient neonatal MG develops in 10–20% of infants born to myasthenic mothers due to transplacental passage of IgG antiacetylcholine receptor antibodies. Symptoms of respiratory distress, poor sucking and swallowing, ptosis, feeble cry, facial paresis, and flaccid tone usually appear within 48 h of birth and may persist for up to 3 months [14]. Respiratory arrest can occur, resulting in the need for ventilatory support [39]. The variable timing of neonatal MG seems at least partially due to the protective effects of AFP which inhibits the binding of antibodies to the acetylcholine receptors [29], as well as the transfer of water-soluble anticholinesterase medications from the mother to the newborn [28].

Despite the fact that the severity and duration of the disease in the mother do not correlate with the risk of developing neonatal MG, among mothers with a child affected by transient neonatal MG, the risk of recurrence with subsequent pregnancies is approximately 75% [12]. Autoantibodies are found in the colostrum and breast milk of myasthenic patients with high antibody titers, but because there is no correlation between levels of the mother's antibodies and neonatal disease, breastfeeding is considered safe for unaffected neonates [6].

All infants of myasthenic mothers should be observed in a special care nursery for the first 48–72h of life. Treatment of neonatal MG consists of supportive care, anticholinesterase medications and, when needed, plasmapheresis. The symptoms improve progressively as antibody titers gradually decrease [2].

A retrospective analysis of data from the Medical Birth Registry of Norway found that neonates of mothers with MG who had undergone thymectomy were less likely to develop neonatal MG than those born to mothers without thymectomy (9/72 [13%] versus 17/63 [27%], relative risk 0.4, 95% CI 0.16–0.94) [40]. These results suggest that thymectomy has a protective effect against neonatal MG. However, the strength of this study is limited by the retrospective design, lack of randomization and blinding, and wide confidence intervals [32].

It is important to note that the beneficial effects of thymectomy are delayed for all patients and may take years to accrue. The 1-year remission rate of myasthenia after thymectomy is <20%.

Thus, thymectomy in the year before conception is unlikely to result in clinical remission of myasthenia in the mother before pregnancy, and its impact on the risk of neonatal MG is undetermined. In the study discussed earlier, 25 of the 41 thymectomized mothers had undergone thymectomy on an average of 5 years before the first birth [40], allowing more time for the benefit of thymectomy to accumulate.

References

[1] Drachman D. Myasthenia gravis. N Engl J Med 1994;330:1797–810.

[2] Ciafaloni E, Massey J. Myasthenia gravis and pregnancy. Neurol Clin 2004;22:771–82.

[3] Uncu G, Kucukerdogan L, Ozan H, Cengiz C. Pregnancy and myasthenia gravis: a case report. Clin Exp Obstet Gynecol 1995;22:145–7.

[4] Lindstrom J. Nicotinic acetylcoline receptors in health and disease. Mol Neurobiol 1997;15:193–222.

[5] Hoch W, McConville J, Helms S, Newsom-Davis J, Melms A, Vincent A. Autoantibodies to the receptor tyrosine kinase MuSK in patients with myasthenia gravis without acetylcoline receptor antibodies. Nat Med 2001;7:365–8.

[6] Batocchi AP, Majolini L, Evoli A, Lino MM, Minisci C, Tonali P. Course and treatment of myasthenia gravis in pregnancy. Neurology 1999;52:447–52.

[7] Plauche WC. Myasthenia gravis in mothers and their newborns. Clin Obstet Gynecol 1991;34:82.

[8] Djelms J, Sustarko M, Mayer D, Ivanisec M. Myasthenia gravis in pregnancy: a report on 69 cases. Eur J Obstet Gynecol Reprod Biol 2002;104:21–5.
[9] Pijnenborg JMA, Hansen ECM, Brolman HAM, Oei SG, Andriessen P, Dellemijn PL. A severe case of myasthenia gravis during pregnancy. Gynecol Obstet Invest 2000; 50:142–3.
[10] Bashuk RG, Krendel DA. Myasthenia presenting as weakness after magnesium administration. Muscle Nerve 1990;13:708–12.
[11] Cohen BA, London RS, Goldstein PJ. Myasthenia gravis and preeclampsia. Obstet Gynecol 1976;48:35S–7S.
[12] Lu CH, Liou CM, Chen YS, Hung CJ, Tso HS. Anesthetic management in myasthenic parturient. Anaesthesiol Sin 1992;30:193–7.
[13] Verspyck E, Mandelbrot L, Dommergues M, Huon C, Woimant F, Baumann C, Vernet-Der Garabedran B. Myasthenia gravis with polyhydramnios in the fetus of an asymptomatic mother. Prenat Diagn 1993;13:539–42.
[14] Stafford IP, Dildy GA. Myasthenia gravis and pregnancy. Clin Obstet Gynecol 2004;48(1):48–56.
[15] Levine BS, Parker RM. Reproductive and developmental toxicity studies of pyridostigmine bromide in rats. Toxicology 1991;69:291–300.
[16] Briggs GG, Freeman RK, Yafe SJ. Drugs in pregnancy and lactation, 4th ed. Baltimore: Williams and Wilkins; 1994.
[17] American College of Rheumatology Ad Hoc Committee on Clinical Guidelines Guidelines for monitoring drug therapy in rheumatoid arthritis. Arthritis Rheum 1996;39:723–31.
[18] Committee on Drugs, American Academy of Pediatrics The transfer of drugs and other chemicals into human milk. Pediatrics 1994;93:137–50.
[19] Saarikoski S, Seppala M. Immunosupression during pregnancy: transmission of azathioprine and its metabolites from the mother to the fetus. Am J Obstet Gynecol 1973;115:1100–6.
[20] Polifka JE, Friedman JM. Teratogen update: azathioprine and 6-mercaptopurine. Teratology 2002;65:240–61.
[21] Davison JM, Dellagrammatikas H, Parkin JM. Maternal azathioprine therapy and depressed haemopoiesis in the babies of renal allograft patients. Br J Obstet Gynaecol 1985;92:233–9.
[22] Simms CJ. Organ transplantation and immunosuppressive. Clin Obstet Gynaecol 1991;34:100–11.
[23] Mason RJ, Thomson AW, Whiting PH, Gray ES, Brown PA, Catto GR. Cyclosporine-induced fetotoxicity in the rat. Transplantation 1985;39:9–12.
[24] Shaheen FAM, Al-Sulaiman MH, Al-Khader AA. Long-term nephrotoxicity after exposure to CsA in utero. Transplantation 1993;56:224–5.
[25] Bar Oz B, Hackman R, Einarson T, Koren G. Pregnancy outcome after CsA therapy during pregnancy: a meta-analysis. Transplantation 2001;71:1051–5.
[26] Samuels P, Pfeifer SM. Autoimmune diseases in pregnancy. The obstetrician's view. Rheum Dis Clin North Am 1989;15:307–22.
[27] Mitchell PJ, Bebbington M. Myasthenia gravis in pregnancy. Obstet Gynecol. 1992;80:178–81.
[28] Thanvi BR, Lo TCN. Update on myasthenia gravis. Postgrad Med J 2004;80:690–700.
[29] Sax TW, Rosenbaum RB. Neuromuscular disorders in pregnancy. Muscle Nerve. 2006 Nov;34(5):559–71.

[30] Shehata HA, Okosun H. Neurological disorders in pregnancy. Curr Opin Obstet Gynecol 2004;16:117–22.
[31] Leventhal SR, Orkin FK, Hirsh RA. Prediction of the need for postoperative mechanical ventilation in myasthenia gravis. Anesthesiology 1980;53:26.
[32] Bird SJ, Stafford IP, Dildy GA. Management of myasthenia gravis in pregnancy. www.uptodate.com. Review vesion January, 2010.
[33] Committee on Drugs. American Academy of Pediatrics. The transfer of drugs and other chemicals into human breast milk. Pediatrics 1994;93:137–50.
[34] Buckley LM, Bullaboy CA, Leichtman L, Marquez M. Multiple congenital anomalies associated with weekly low-dose methotrexate treatment of the mother. Arthritis Rheum 1997;40:971–3.
[35] Thiru Y, Bateman DN, Coulthard MG. Successful breast-feeding while mother was taking cyclosporine. BMJ 1997;315:463.
[36] Nyberg G, Haljamae U, Frisenette-Fish C. Wennergren M, Kjellmer I. Breast-feeding during treatment with cyclosporine. Transplantation 1998;65:253–5.
[37] Munoz-Flores-Thiagarajan KD, Easterling T, David C, Bond EF. Breast-feeding by a cyclosporine-treated mother. Obstet Gynecol 2001;97:816–8.
[38] The WHO Working Group. In: Bennet PN, editor. Drugs and human lactation; 1988 p. 286–7.
[39] Burke ME. Myasthenia gravis and pregnancy. J Perinat Neonatal Nurs 1993;7:11.
[40] Hoff JM, Daltveit AK, Gilhus NE. Myasthenia gravis in pregnancy and birth: identifying risk factors, optimising care. Eur J Neurol 2007;14:38.

4 Postpartum Angiopathy and Related Disorders

Jennifer E. Fugate, Alejandro A. Rabinstein

Department of Neurology, Mayo Clinic, Rochester, MN, USA

Background and Context

Acute stroke is a rare but potentially devastating complication during pregnancy or in the puerperium. Whether pregnancy confers an increased risk of stroke compared to age-matched nonpregnant women is not clear and has been studied with conflicting results. A large population-based study in the United States using the Nationwide Inpatient Sample found an estimated threefold increase in stroke incidence in pregnant women [1], while other studies have found the risk to be as high as 13-fold increase [2,3]. In contrast, Kittner et al. [4] found an increased risk within 6 weeks after delivery but found no increased risk during pregnancy itself.

The increased risk of stroke in the postpartum period has been a more consistent finding. Traditional cerebrovascular risk factors (e.g., hypertension, smoking, arterial vascular disease, hyperlipidemia) can contribute, but there are additional factors that pertain to the unique physiology of pregnancy. Several factors contribute to a hypercoagulable state in normal pregnancy. Concentrations of von Willebrand factor, factor VIII, and fibrinogen are increased [5,6], resistance to protein C develops, and concentrations of protein S are reduced. In addition, platelet aggregation may be increased by higher prolactin concentrations [7]. Postpartum angiopathy (PPA), peripartum cardiomyopathy, eclampsia, dural sinus thrombosis, and intracranial hemorrhage are other potential causes of stroke in this population.

Postpartum Angiopathy

Introduction

PPA, a cerebral vasculopathy, is considered comparatively rare, but may be underrecognized. The diagnosis is made based on neurologic symptoms in the postpartum setting with documented angiographic findings of multifocal segmental vasoconstriction. Our understanding of this condition is largely derived from case reports and small retrospective series, conferring a poor understanding of its true incidence, spectrum, and natural history.

Neurological Disorders and Pregnancy. DOI: 10.1016/B978-0-12-384911-3.00004-X

Clinical Features

Symptoms of PPA are usually encountered in the first 1–2 weeks after an uncomplicated pregnancy and delivery, but can be delayed for up to 6 weeks postpartum [8]. Classically patients present with abrupt, excruciating headaches (so-called "thunderclap headaches"). The pain is commonly holocephalic and may be accompanied by nausea, visual disturbances, encephalopathy, or seizures (Table 4.1). Though there have been cases reported without headache [9–13], the absence of this symptom should raise suspicion for other diagnoses, as it is a prominent and early feature in the vast majority of described cases. Headaches can be persistent or may fluctuate and manifest as recurrent thunderclap headaches over several days. Generalized seizures are the second most commonly reported neurologic symptom in PPA, followed by visual disturbances and encephalopathy [14]. A variety of visual disturbances can occur, including transient scotomas, visual field deficit, and cortical blindness.

Focal neurologic deficits (e.g., hemiparesis, sensory loss, aphasia) from ischemic stroke (caused by severe vasoconstriction) or intracranial hemorrhage may develop. In this setting, the patient often will have had several days of headache preceding the onset of hemiparesis, which may initially fluctuate in severity. Because ischemic strokes in PPA often involve the watershed zones between the anterior and middle cerebral arteries, bilateral lower extremity hyperreflexia and/or weakness can be seen.

Hypertension is commonly but not invariably present at initial clinical presentation. In our review of nearly 50 cases in the English literature, nearly half of patients (23/49, 47%) with PPA had a systolic blood pressure <160 mmHg at symptom onset (unpublished data).

Table 4.1 Frequency of Clinical and Radiologic Findings in PPA Based on a Review of 49 Cases in the English Literature (Unpublished Data)

	n (%)
Clinical Symptoms	
Headache	42 (86)
Generalized seizures	28 (57)
Focal neurologic deficits	17 (35)
Visual disturbances	15 (31)
Encephalopathy	14 (29)
Radiologic	
PRES	19 (39)
Intracranial hemorrhage	18 (37)
IPH	11 (22)
SAH	7 (14)
Ischemic stroke	13 (27)

PRES, posterior reversible encephalopathy syndrome; IPH, intraparenchymal hemorrhage; SAH, subarachnoid hemorrhage.

Radiologic Findings

Our interpretation of the frequency and severity of radiographic findings seen in PPA is confounded by a selection bias of the patients who undergo brain imaging. Neurologic symptoms late in pregnancy and in the puerperium often prompt a clinical diagnosis of eclampsia (if concomitant hypertension and proteinuria are present) or even "atypical eclampsia" in the absence of those features. Brain imaging is not always performed in these circumstances, and many patients are treated with intravenous magnesium sulfate with resolution of symptoms. If imaging is performed, computed tomography (CT) or magnetic resonance imaging (MRI) may be performed to visualize the brain parenchyma but is often performed without arteriography. Even when vascular imaging is obtained, timing could be an additional factor affecting diagnosis and estimated frequency, as in early PPA initial angiographic studies can be normal with repeat studies showing vasoconstriction [15]. Authors of a recent study of reversible cerebral vasoconstriction syndromes (which only included one patient with PPA) found that vasoconstriction reached a maximum about 2 weeks after onset of headache and often persists longer than symptoms [16].

Noninvasive techniques such as magnetic resonance angiography (MRA) and computed tomography angiography (CTA) or conventional cerebral angiography are used to evaluate the cerebral vasculature. Multifocal areas of vessel narrowing involving multiple large- and medium-sized arteries are characteristic and should raise suspicion for the diagnosis of PPA (Figure 4.1). Vessel caliber may be dilated or normal between areas of constriction. When dilated, the appearance may be that of "beads on a string." The anterior cerebral, middle cerebral, distal basilar, and superior cerebellar arteries are most commonly affected [8]. Serial transcranial Doppler (TCD) has also been used to follow blood velocity trends, indirectly assessing the degree of vasoconstriction. Caveats with this approach are that TCD can show normal blood flow velocities in some patients [17], and elevated velocities may reflect hyperemia rather than vasoconstriction.

Brain MRI or head CT findings vary and can demonstrate evidence of ischemic stroke, reversible vasogenic edema, or acute intracranial hemorrhage. Imaging may be initially normal (up to 35% of cases), but most of the time subsequent imaging reveals an abnormality. Posterior reversible encephalopathy syndrome (PRES) is the most commonly identified abnormality, seen in 40% (unpublished data) to 54% of cases [14]. Intracranial hemorrhage, often lobar intraparenchymal or small convexal subarachnoid hemorrhage occurs in nearly 40% and ischemic stroke in nearly 30% [14] (Table 4.1).

Differential Diagnosis

Other potentially life-threatening disorders can present in the postpartum setting similar to thunderclap headaches and should be excluded (Table 4.2). Aneurysmal subarachnoid hemorrhage, cerebral venous sinus thrombosis, arterial dissection, and pituitary apoplexy must be included in the differential diagnosis. Brain imaging and in most cases, cerebrospinal fluid (CSF) examination for xanthochromia, cell count,

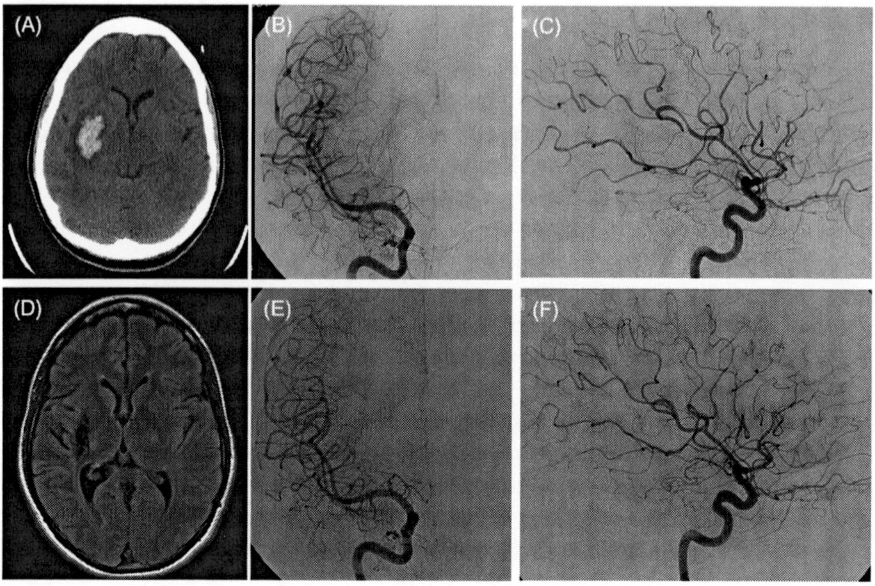

Figure 4.1 PPA A 28-year-old woman experienced thunderclap headache and left hemiparesis 1 day after an uncomplicated caesarean section. At presentation, head CT (A) revealed right basal ganglia hemorrhage. Cerebral digital subtraction angiography (right internal carotid artery injection, B and C) demonstrated multifocal smooth narrowings of middle cerebral artery branches. Follow-up imaging 3 months later (MRI, D, and cerebral angiography E and F) demonstrated evolution of hemorrhage and resolution of arterial narrowing.

Table 4.2 Differential Diagnosis of Severe Postpartum Headache

Pre-eclampsia/eclampsia
Cerebral venous sinus thrombosis
Pituitary apoplexy
PPA
Aneurysmal subarachnoid hemorrhage
Carotid artery dissection
CNS vasculitis
Intracranial hypotension (CSF leak)

CNS, central nervous system; CSF, cerebrospinal fluid; PPA, postpartum angiopathy.

total protein, and glucose should be done. Angiography can exclude ruptured cerebral aneurysms, dissection, or cerebral venous thrombosis.

Vasculitis of the central nervous system, an inflammatory disorder that warrants urgent immunosuppressive treatment, can be difficult to differentiate from vasoconstriction. This can present with headaches, but generally these are more insidious in onset. Angiographic abnormalities in vasculitis tend to involve distal intracranial arteries rather than the proximal circle of Willis arteries that are commonly involved in PPA. Still, the multifocal arterial narrowings that occur with vasculitis may be impossible to differentiate radiographically from PPA. Abnormal CSF results and laboratory tests including erythrocyte sedimentation rate, C-reactive protein, antinuclear antibodies, and antineutrophil cytoplasmic antibodies may be helpful in a vasculitis workup. Nevertheless, the two disorders might only be differentiated in retrospect, with PPA usually demonstrating more rapid clinical and radiographic resolution.

Pathophysiology

The pathophysiology underlying PPA is unknown. Because most patients recover rapidly, definitive pathologic evaluation is usually not available. Postmortem examination has been performed in three fatal cases and these have revealed no inflammatory changes or evidence of vasculitis. In one case, there was a single patch of subendothelial thickening involving a posterior cerebral artery [18], in another a slight intimal thickening and focal disruption of the elastic lamina of one vertebral artery [19], and in the third no vascular abnormality was found [20]. CSF analysis usually is normal or may reveal mild pleocytosis or elevation of protein. These features, in addition to the transitory nature of both the symptoms and angiographic findings, support a vasospastic process as the underlying pathophysiology rather than a true inflammatory vasculitis.

The use of vasoactive medications (e.g., bromocriptine, ergot alkaloids) has been implicated in the development of PPA [11,21,22], but causality is difficult to prove. It has been theorized that the neurovasculature has an enhanced susceptibility to sympathomimetic medications because of hormonal fluctuations [11,21–24]. Nevertheless, many cases have been reported in the absence of vasoactive medication administration [13,15,19,25,26]. If this theory were comprehensive, one might expect this disorder to be more commonly appreciated with the high frequency of postpartum women receiving vasoactive medications.

A second theory purports that the vasoconstriction is a response to severe hypertension. The fact that a substantial proportion of women are not hypertensive above the normal upper limits of cerebral autoregulation argues against this theory. Additionally, clinical and radiologic resolution does not seemingly correspond to prompt treatment of hypertension.

Similarities seen in PPA and eclampsia have led to speculation that they share a common pathophysiology and thus might be part of the same disease process [10,14,20,27]. Although more commonly described following an uncomplicated pregnancy and delivery, PPA has been described in association with eclampsia [28]. A recent review of the literature demonstrated the commonly overlapping clinical and radiologic features between the two [14]. For example, both often present with headache, encephalopathy, visual disturbance, or focal neurologic deficit. Both can have cytotoxic or vasogenic edema seen on brain MRI, and arterial vasoconstriction detected by angiography has been observed in both.

Several theories regarding the pathophysiology of pre-eclampsia or eclampsia have been proposed. In pre-eclampsia, there are several circulating factors that are elevated compared to normal pregnant women. These include antiangiogenic proteins, soluble fms-like tyrosine kinase 1 (sFlt1), and soluble endoglin [29–31] as well as placental proteins activin A and inhibin A [32]. Whether these are of pathogenic significance or merely markers of the disease is unknown. However, there is experimental evidence that both sFLt and endoglin cause endothelial dysfunction [33], which would argue for their direct contribution to the pathogenesis.

Management

Management of PPA is based on anecdotes; there is no established treatment that is considered the standard of care. Furthermore, no treatment has been shown to alter the natural history of the disorder. Many therapies including magnesium sulfate, calcium channel blockers, corticosteroids, and immunosuppressants have been tried. Because the differentiation between vasculitis and PPA can be difficult early, a short course of steroids may be justified but probably should be discontinued if rapid angiographic resolution is demonstrated. Generally patients are treated with the vasodilator intravenous magnesium sulfate on an empiric basis, particularly if seizures are present. After vasoconstriction has been angiographically documented, calcium channel blockers are often started. One case described improvement in angiographic spasm and clinical symptoms after administration of intra-arterial nimodipine followed by intravenous and oral nimodipine [34]. In fatal cases, hypervolemia, balloon angioplasty and stenting, intra-arterial vasodilators, and intrathecal calcium channel blockers are among the therapies that were tried, but were ultimately unsuccessful[18–20].

Optimal blood pressure management in PPA is likewise not well established. It is crucial to maintain at least normal blood pressure in patients with severe vasoconstriction, as reduced cerebral perfusion will result if systemic hypotension occurs. Hemodynamic augmentation with vasopressors has been tried in fulminant cases, but this has not been shown to be beneficial. Theoretically, one could surmise that this might exacerbate vasoconstriction, either by direct sympathomimetic effects or by furthering reactive vasoconstriction as a response to abrupt hypertension. However, patients with fulminant vasoconstriction develop massive brain infarctions, thus attempts to improve cerebral perfusion by augmentation of blood pressure appear to be justified. Intra-arterial vasodilators or angioplasty may also be reasonable therapeutic trials in these cases.

Prognosis

Most affected patients with PPA achieve full recovery or near-complete recovery, though this is not uniformly the case. Headaches may linger for weeks, and patients may be left with neurologic sequelae including mild aphasia, visual deficit, or mild hemiparesis. PPA is grouped with several disorders under the heading of "reversible cerebral vasoconstriction syndromes" (Table 4.3). This name may falsely suggest

Table 4.3 Conditions and Precipitating Factors That Have Been Associated with Reversible Cerebral Vasoconstriction Syndrome, Also Referred to as the "Call-Fleming Syndrome"

Postpartum
Postpartum alone, eclampsia, pre-eclampsia
Primary Headache Disorders
Orgasmic headache
Migraine headache
Bath-related thunderclap headache
Medications
Ergot derivatives (e.g., bromocriptine, lisuride)
Serotonergic drugs (e.g., SSRIs, triptans, trazodone)
Pseudoephedrine
Isometheptene
Oral contraceptives
Chemotherapeutic agents
Illicit Drugs
Cocaine
Marijuana
Medical Conditions
Pheochromocytoma
Hyperparathyroidism
Porphyria
Systemic lupus erythematosus
Autonomic dysreflexia with spinal cord injury
Neurosurgical Procedures
Head Trauma

SSRI, selective serotonin reuptake inhibitor.

that it is consistently a benign process. However, substantial morbidity (due to intracranial hemorrhage, cerebral infarction, and status epilepticus) and several fatalities have been well described [12,18–20].

References

[1] James AH, Bushnell CD, Jamison MG, Myers ER. Incidence and risk factors for stroke in pregnancy and the puerperium. Obstet Gynecol 2005;106:509–16.

[2] Wiebers DO, Whisnant JP. The incidence of stroke among pregnant women in Rochester, Minn, 1955 through 1979. JAMA 1985;254:3055–7.

[3] Sharshar T, Lamy C, Mas JL. Incidence and causes of strokes associated with pregnancy and puerperium. A study in public hospitals of Ile de France. Stroke in Pregnancy Study Group. Stroke 1995;26:930–6.

[4] Kittner SJ, Stern BJ, Feeser BR, Hebel R, Nagey DA, Buchholz DW, et al. Pregnancy and the risk of stroke. N Engl J Med 1996;335:768–74.

[5] Clark P, Brennand J, Conkie JA, McCall F, Greer IA, Walker ID. Activated protein C sensitivity, protein C, protein S and coagulation in normal pregnancy. Thromb Haemost 1998;79:1166–70.
[6] Treadwell SD, Thanvi B, Robinson TG. Stroke in pregnancy and the puerperium. Postgrad Med J 2008;84:238–45.
[7] Wallaschofski H, Donne M, Eigenthaler M, Hentschel B, Faber R, Stepan H, et al. PRL as a novel potent cofactor for platelet aggregation. J Clin Endocrinol Metab 2001;86:5912–9.
[8] Singhal AB, Bernstein RA. Postpartum angiopathy and other cerebral vasoconstriction syndromes. Neurocrit Care 2005;3:91–7.
[9] Will AD, Lewis KL, Hinshaw Jr. DB, Jordan K, Cousins LM, Hasso AN, et al. Cerebral vasoconstriction in toxemia. Neurology 1987;37:1555–7.
[10] Raps EC, Galetta SL, Broderick M, Atlas SW. Delayed peripartum vasculopathy: cerebral eclampsia revisited. Ann Neurol 1993;33:222–5.
[11] Janssens E, Hommel M, Mounier-Vehier F, Leclerc X, Guerin du Masgenet B, Leys D. Postpartum cerebral angiopathy possibly due to bromocriptine therapy. Stroke 1995; 26:128–30.
[12] Ursell MR, Marras CL, Farb R, Rowed DW, Black SE, Perry JR. Recurrent intracranial hemorrhage due to postpartum cerebral angiopathy: implications for management. Stroke 1998;29:1995–8.
[13] Song JK, Fisher S, Seifert TD, Cacayorin ED, Alexandrov AV, Malkoff MD, et al. Postpartum cerebral angiopathy: atypical features and treatment with intracranial balloon angioplasty. Neuroradiology 2004;46:1022–6.
[14] Fletcher JJ, Kramer AH, Bleck TP, Solenski NJ. Overlapping features of eclampsia and postpartum angiopathy. Neurocrit Care 2009;11:199–209.
[15] Singhal AB. Postpartum angiopathy with reversible posterior leukoencephalopathy. Arch Neurol 2004;61:411–6.
[16] Chen, SP, Fuh, JL, Wang, SJ, Chang, FC, Lirng, JF, Fang, YC, et al. Magnetic resonance angiography in reversible cerebral vasoconstriction syndromes. Ann Neurol 2010; 67:648–56.
[17] Konstantinopoulos PA, Mousa S, Khairallah R, Mtanos G. Postpartum cerebral angiopathy: an important diagnostic consideration in the postpartum period. Am J Obstet Gynecol 2004;191:375–7.
[18] Singhal AB, Kimberly WT, Schaefer PW, Hedley-Whyte ET. Case records of the Massachusetts General Hospital. Case 8-2009. A 36-year-old woman with headache, hypertension, and seizure 2 weeks postpartum. N Engl J Med 2009;360:1126–37.
[19] Geraghty JJ, Hoch DB, Robert ME, Vinters HV. Fatal puerperal cerebral vasospasm and stroke in a young woman. Neurology 1991;41:1145–7.
[20] Williams TL, Lukovits TG, Harris BT, Harker Rhodes C. A fatal case of postpartum cerebral angiopathy with literature review. Arch Gynecol Obstet 2007;275:67–77.
[21] Comabella M, Alvarez-Sabin J, Rovira A, Codina A. Bromocriptine and postpartum cerebral angiopathy: a causal relationship? Neurology 1996;46:1754–6.
[22] Roh JK, Park KS. Postpartum cerebral angiopathy with intracerebral hemorrhage in a patient receiving lisuride. Neurology 1998;50:1152–4.
[23] Crippa G, Sverzellati E, Pancotti D, Carrara GC. Severe postpartum hypertension and reversible cerebral angiopathy associated with ergot derivative (methergoline) administration. Ann Ital Med Int 2000;15:303–5.
[24] Raroque Jr. HG, Tesfa G, Purdy P. Postpartum cerebral angiopathy. Is there a role for sympathomimetic drugs? Stroke 1993;24:2108–10.

[25] Geocadin RG, Razumovsky AY, Wityk RJ, Bhardwaj A, Ulatowski JA. Intracerebral hemorrhage and postpartum cerebral vasculopathy. J Neurol Sci 2002;205:29–34.

[26] Kubo S, Nakata H, Tatsumi T, Yoshimine T. Headache associated with postpartum cerebral angiopathy: monitoring with transcranial color-coded sonography. Headache 2002;42:297–300.

[27] Donaldson JO. Eclampsia and postpartum cerebral angiopathy. J Neurol Sci 2000;178:1.

[28] Trommer BL, Homer D, Mikhael MA. Cerebral vasospasm and eclampsia. Stroke 1988;19:326–9.

[29] Levine RJ, Lam C, Qian C, Yu KF, Maynard SE, Sachs BP, et al. Soluble endoglin and other circulating antiangiogenic factors in preeclampsia. N Engl J Med 2006;355:992–1005.

[30] Levine RJ, Maynard SE, Qian C, Lim KH, England LJ, Yu KF, et al. Circulating angiogenic factors and the risk of preeclampsia. N Engl J Med 2004;350:672–83.

[31] Chaiworapongsa T, Romero R, Kim YM, Kim GJ, Kim MR, Espinoza J, et al. Plasma soluble vascular endothelial growth factor receptor-1 concentration is elevated prior to the clinical diagnosis of pre-eclampsia. J Matern Fetal Neonatal Med 2005;17:3–18.

[32] Reddy A, Suri S, Sargent IL, Redman CW, Muttukrishna S. Maternal circulating levels of activin A, inhibin A, sFlt-1 and endoglin at parturition in normal pregnancy and preeclampsia. PLoS One 2009;4:e4453.

[33] Venkatesha S, Toporsian M, Lam C, Hanai J, Mammoto T, Kim YM, et al. Soluble endoglin contributes to the pathogenesis of preeclampsia. Nat Med 2006;12:642–9.

[34] Klein M, Fesl G, Pfister HW, Straube A, Bruckmann H, Hoffmann LA, et al. Intra-arterial nimodipine in progressive postpartum cerebral angiopathy. Cephalalgia 2009;29:279–82.

5 Neurology of Pre-eclampsia and Eclampsia

Roger E. Kelley, Maike Tiede Blaya, Patricia Colon

Department of Neurology, Tulane University School of Medicine, New Orleans, LA, USA

Pathophysiology

There are certain risk factors for the development of hypertension and proteinuria in later stages of pregnancy. There are several identified contributing factors to an increased risk of pre-eclampsia. It is now generally acknowledged that the initial pathogenesis appears to be tied in with the placenta. As the human embryo is implanted within the uterus, there is pronounced decidualization of the endometrium while the embryo produces trophoblastic invasion of the maternal spiral arteries in order to maintain adequate placental nutrition to the developing fetus. In the normal pregnancy, the trophoblast becomes embedded in the vessel wall and the muscular and elastic components of the affected vessels become disrupted. This remodeling of the spiral arteries results in dilated, low-resistance vessels that are unable to constrict when exposed to vasoactive stimulation [1]. This ensures that there is adequate circulation for the placenta and fetus. There is impairment of this physiologic process in pre-eclampsia with the trophoblastic invasion disrupted. This is associated with retention, by the spiral arteries, of their endothelial lining and musculature. There is resultant compromise of perfusion into the intervillous space, which adversely affects blood flow to the placenta and fetus, which can lead to ischemic hypoxia and oxidative stress.

Although often self-limited, pre-eclampsia is not necessarily benign for the fetus. There is commonly intrauterine growth retardation as well as low birth weight, prematurity, and risk of perinatal stroke. Furthermore, the potential systemic manifestations of pre-eclampsia can evolve into an encephalopathy with predisposition to seizures, and even death; in the mother, this is termed eclampsia.

It is theorized that impaired perfusion of placental tissue results in toxic factors that are released into the systemic circulation with resultant damage to maternal endothelial cells [2]. Susceptibility to such an occurrence includes premorbid risk factors such as underlying hypertension, glucose intolerance, and hyperlipidemia, which constitutes much of what has been termed the metabolic syndrome [3]. Of particular note is the potential association of smoking with pre-eclampsia [4]. However, somewhat surprisingly, there is roughly a one-third reduced risk of pre-eclampsia in smokers that has been theorized to be related to a possible protective

Neurological Disorders and Pregnancy. DOI: 10.1016/B978-0-12-384911-3.00005-1

effect of either heme oxygenase, an enzyme involved in the endogenous generation of carbon monoxide, or the carbon monoxide itself which is a by-product of the cigarette smoke [4].

There appears to be a familial predisposition to pre-eclampsia [5] that may well be reflective of a genetic predisposition to risk factors associated with pre-eclampsia including components of the metabolic syndrome. However, differential gene expression also might play a role. In a study of potential placental genes that might predispose to pre-eclampsia, Hoegh et al. [6] reported what they viewed as a surprisingly low differential gene expression when comparing biopsies from 11 pre-eclamptic placentas when compared to 18 normal controls.

Neurologic Manifestations of Pre-eclampsia/Eclampsia

Spectrum of Manifestations

Pre-eclampsia and eclampsia are not distinct disorders but are differentiated according to the severity of the clinical symptoms. The mildest disorder in this continuum is pregnancy-induced hypertension (PIH). In pre-eclampsia, hypertension and proteinuria are present, and when convulsions occur in addition to these signs, the condition is referred to as eclampsia [7]. Some patients may be diagnosed with PIH and never progress to a more severe presentation. Furthermore, up to 28% of patients with a diagnosis of eclampsia do not have pre-eclampsia or PIH preceding this presentation [8]. Because pre-eclampsia and eclampsia are a continuum and possibly share the same pathophysiologic mechanisms, we will use the term pre-eclampsia/eclampsia.

By definition, the central nervous system (CNS) is commonly affected in patients with pre-eclampsia/eclampsia and is a cause of significant morbidity and possibly death in those affected [9]. Death from pre-eclampsia/eclampsia is usually attributable to cerebral hemorrhage in patients with thrombocytopenia either in isolation or as part of HELLP (hemolysis, elevated liver enzymes, and low platelets) syndrome [8]. Fortunately, the neurologic deficits often are reversible.

Incidence and Prevalence

In the United States, pre-eclampsia affects roughly 5% of women, and eclampsia occurs in 5–7 of every 10,000 births (0.05–0.07%) with international rates, overall, approximately the same as the United States. However, eclampsia occurs in 0.17–1% of pregnant women in developing countries [7]. The neurologic manifestations that may occur associated with pre-eclampsia/eclampsia syndrome are varied and are listed in Table 5.1.

Headache

Headache is the most common neurologic symptom in pre-eclampsia/eclampsia, reported in 78–83% of the patients [9]. New-onset headache may be the

Table 5.1 Neurologic Manifestations of Pre-eclampsia/Eclampsia Syndrome

Headache
Seizures
Visual disturbances
Reversible posterior leukoencephalopathy syndrome
Subarachnoid hemorrhage
Ischemic stroke
Cerebral venous thrombosis
Altered mental status
Cognitive dysfunction
Intracranial hypertension

initial complaint in a pregnant woman presenting with pre-eclampsia/eclampsia. Progressive headache always precedes seizure activity in eclampsia and does not respond to routine over-the-counter remedies [10]. The headache syndrome in pre-eclampsia/eclampsia has no typical characteristics. It has been described by patients as throbbing or pounding, pressure-like, or sharp like a knife. The location also varies. Aura usually is not seen [11]. Rapid resolution of the headache associated with pre-eclampsia/eclampsia is seen with administration of magnesium sulfate [10].

If the patient experiences sudden onset of a severe headache (thunderclap headache) associated with nausea and vomiting, the physician should have a high index of suspicion for subarachnoid hemorrhage (SAH). A possible association between migraine headaches and pre-eclampsia has been suggested [12].

Visual Disturbances

Visual symptoms may occur in 40% of pre-eclamptic women [13] and they present in a variety of ways from blurred vision, diplopia, homonymous hemianopsia, to cortical blindness [14]. Anton's and Balint syndrome have also been described in association with pre-eclampsia/eclampsia [15,16]. Initially attributed to retinal arteriolar vasospasm or thrombosis, visual disturbances are now recognized to be associated with cerebral edema demonstrated on neuroimaging techniques by low-density areas on CT brain scan and by hyperintense lesions on T2-weighted and fluid attenuation inversion recovery (FLAIR) MRI [16].

Cortical blindness, when it occurs, is usually reversible and the majority of patients recover vision over a period ranging from 2h to 21 days [14]. Cerebral edema has been attributed to endothelial dysfunction and reversible posterior leukoencephalopathy syndrome (RPLS) [17,18] (Figure 5.1). Brief episodes of positive visual symptoms, such as scintillating scotomata, chromatopsia, as well as colored and mainly circular elementary visual hallucinations, should prompt rapid investigation to evaluate for possible occipital seizures [16].

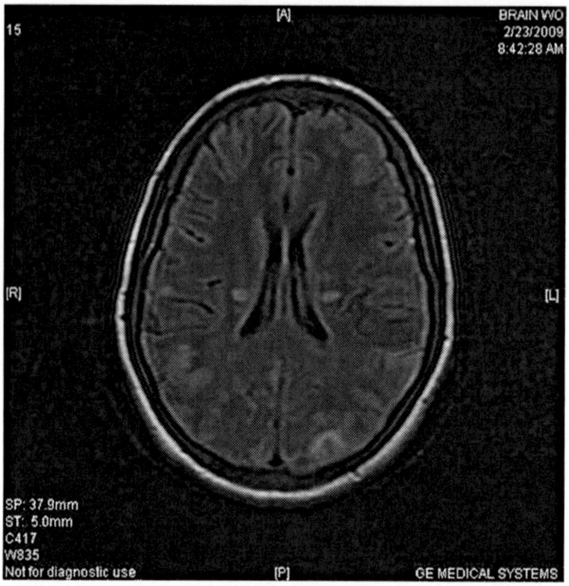

Figure 5.1 Transverse FLAIR MRI brain scan, in a 24-year-old woman in the 40th week of gestation, demonstrating the typical signal intensity changes reflective of RPLS. She presented with a seizure reflective of her eclampsia. Note the particular involvement of the parieto-occipital lobes, bilaterally, along with some subcortical hyperintensity as well.

Cerebrovascular Disease

Intracranial Bleed

Cerebral hemorrhage is reported to be the most common cause of death in patients with eclampsia [7]. SAH occasionally is reported in pre-eclampsia/eclampsia [19]. Nontraumatic SAH usually results from rupture of a berry aneurysm or arteriovenous malformation (AVM). A large case-crossover study did not find an increased risk of aneurysmal SAH or AVM during pregnancy, delivery, or puerperium [20]. SAH in pre-eclampsia/eclampsia is thought to be the result of rupture of cortical petechiae over the surface of the brain or rupture of small pial veins, as a complication of RPLS, and usually carries a favorable prognosis [18,21]. Patients usually present with sudden onset of severe headache associated with signs of increased intracranial pressure, such as nausea, vomiting, loss of consciousness, cranial nerve palsies, and other focal neurologic deficits. Signs of meningeal irritation may be present early in some patients, such as neck pain, neck stiffness, low back pain, and bilateral leg pain [20]. Mechanisms of SAH, outside of bleeding from aneurysms and AVMs, can include dissection [21], Moyamoya disease [22], and idiopathic perimesencephalic SAH [23].

Intraparenchymal bleed is more common in older women with underlying chronic hypertension. The areas most frequently affected include the striatocapsular area, thalamus, cerebellum, and brain stem. Patients with longstanding uncontrolled hypertension and atherosclerosis also tend to bleed in these same locations. The presentation and outcome is very much reflective of the size and location of the hematoma. Typically, hemispheric hematomas greater than 30 cm^3 in size have a worse prognosis, while relatively small hematomas of the pons can be devastating.

Other Situations Associated with Intracranial Bleed

Patients with cerebral venous thrombosis (CVT) may also present with intracranial bleed. Other potential etiologies that are recognized, with or without pregnancy, include bleeding into a primary or metastatic brain tumor, bleeding secondary to vasculitis, septic embolism, vessel dissection, or hemorrhagic transformation of a cerebral infarction.

Reversible Posterior Leukoencephalopathy Syndrome

RPLS is an acute cerebral illness and was described in 1996 [24]. In terms of clinico-radiologic correlation, RPLS is characterized by reversible vasogenic subcortical edema without infarction and, in the majority of cases, patients present with encephalopathy, seizures, headache, and visual abnormalities [25]. Visual changes range from loss of acuity, visual neglect, or homonymous hemianopia to complete blindness. This syndrome usually happens in patients with underlying predisposing medical conditions and oftentimes a triggering factor can be identified [18].

In RPLS, the sudden increase of the systemic blood pressure is postulated to disrupt the cerebral vascular reactivity leading to vasogenic edema similar to the mechanism associated with eclampsia. Interestingly, the neurologic manifestations of eclampsia are identical to those of hypertensive encephalopathy [26] and RPLS [7,18].

Pre-eclampsia/eclampsia is believed to be a dysfunction in placental implantation and poor placental perfusion inducing hypoxia with consequent release of vasoactive substances into the maternal circulation, causing endothelial dysfunction and systemic hypertension. The endothelial dysfunction may predispose to blood–brain barrier (BBB) disruption with increased permeability even with moderate changes in blood pressure. Both BBB disruption and endothelial dysfunction contribute to breakthrough of autoregulation, leading to extravasation of fluid and red blood cells out of the vessels and causing vasogenic edema and pericapillary hemorrhages [26, 27]. The occipital lobes are particularly more vulnerable to loss of autoregulation because the sympathetic innervations are relatively sparse in the posterior circulation [28]. In addition, the distal terminal branches are more often involved compared to proximal main vessels. These theories help to explain the radiologic findings of symmetric hyperintensities seen on FLAIR MRI, usually in the posterior white and gray matter, seen in eclampsia and hypertensive encephalopathy or RPLS (Figure 5.1). RPLS is now hypothesized to be the primary mechanism of injury in eclampsia.

Ischemic Stroke

Stroke is associated with greater than 12% of maternal deaths. Etiologic factors associated with ischemic stroke during pregnancy are varied and include hypercoagulability, cerebral sino-venous thrombosis (CVT), paradoxical cerebral embolism, postpartum cerebral angiopathy, peripartum cardiomyopathy, arrhythmias, and less specific vascular sequelae of pre-eclampsia/eclampsia [29]. Pre-eclampsia/eclampsia are the most common cause of both cerebral infarct and intracranial hemorrhage in pregnancy and puerperium [30,31]. Pre-eclampsia/eclampsia is present in 24–47% of ischemic strokes and 14–44% of intracranial hemorrhages diagnosed during pregnancy [32].

It has long been assumed that most strokes associated with pregnancy are secondary to venous infarcts because these studies were collecting retrospective data before the advent of the newer imaging techniques [28,33]. However, based on more recent information, pregnancy-related infarctions are most commonly attributable to arterial occlusion [34] (Figure 5.2). There is an increased risk of ischemic stroke in patients with pre-eclampsia/eclampsia and the risk appears to persist even beyond pregnancy and puerperium in these patients [31,35].

CVT is the occlusion of the cerebral cortical sinuses and veins resulting in venous infarction with associated focal neurologic symptoms and signs. It is more common in the third trimester of the pregnancy and postpartum period because of the hypercoagulable state during this period [28]. There is no data showing an increased risk of CVT in patients with pre-eclampsia/eclampsia compared to healthy pregnant patients, but hypertension is considered one of the risk factors for CVT especially during the peripartum period [36]. CVT may be mistaken for postpartum eclampsia especially in the absence of hypertension and proteinuria. CT scan in CVT may show characteristics of thrombosed sagittal sinus (delta sign and cord sign) and hemorrhagic infarction [10].

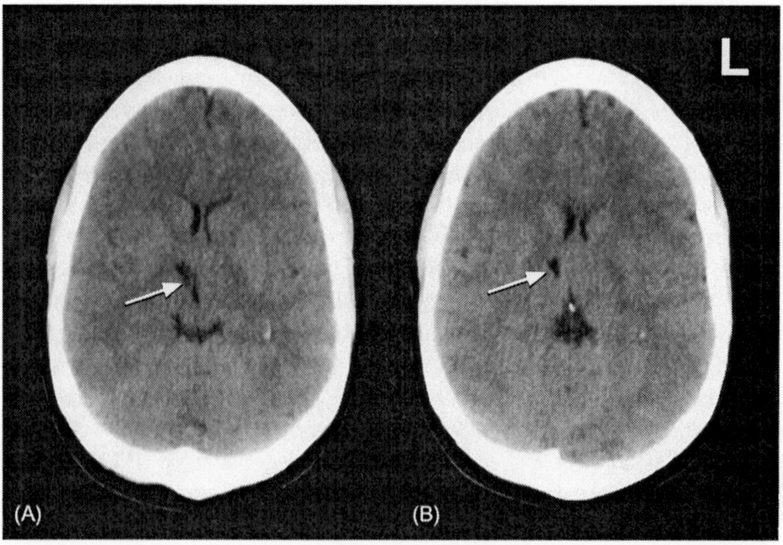

Figure 5.2 Noncontrast CT brain scan in a 26-year-old patient with pre-eclampsia who developed the sudden onset of severe headache and left-sided sensory loss. There is a subcortical small vessel ischemic stroke in the region of the thalamus (arrows) seen on two different slices (A and B).

The clinical and therapeutic approach to women with stroke during pregnancy should be similar to the approach to stroke in young adults [28]. Factors such as maternal risk versus benefit and fetal risks must be taken into account when considering a specific treatment. Thrombolytics and heparin are both category C in pregnancy. Warfarin is category X. Antiplatelets may be considered for a short period, balancing risks and benefits [37].

Epilepsy

Evaluation of Eclamptic Seizures

The term eclampsia was first described in the seventeenth century, when a group of French physicians noticed that epilepsy was a chronic condition, whereas seizures in pregnancy represented an acute process [36,38]. Eclampsia is defined as the presence of new-onset tonic–clonic seizures in a woman with pre-eclampsia. Seizures distinguish eclampsia from pre-eclampsia. It is a rare but serious complication. Seizures may appear with or without preceding hypertension, edema, or proteinuria. Other causes of seizures in the peripartum period include various vascular etiologies such as venous sinus thrombosis, stroke, or SAH due to ruptured aneurysms. Other causes of seizures during pregnancy are listed in Table 5.2.

Eclampsia can be classified according to the time of presentation. Approximately half of all reported cases of eclampsia are preterm, and about three-fourths are intrapartum or within 2 days of delivery. A significant portion of eclamptic patients develops convulsions following delivery, and this often carries a worse prognosis. Postpartum eclampsia is frequently associated with adult respiratory distress syndrome (ARDS) and disseminated intravascular coagulopathy (DIC) [39].

Table 5.2 Causes of Seizures in Pregnancy

Cause	Mechanism
Vascular	Ischemic, ICH, SAH, CVT/hypercoagulable states
Hypertension	Cerebral edema, malignant hypertension
Structural abnormalities	Brain tumors, abscesses, AVMs
Infections	Meningo-encephalitis, subdural empyema, brain abscess
Migraine	Migrainous infarction
Toxic	Amphetamines, cocaine, theophylline, tramadol, atypical antipsychotics
Metabolic	Hyponatremia, hypocalcemia, hyperglycemia, hypoglycemia, hypomagnesemia
Epilepsy	Underlying condition

Only patients with focal findings on examination or atypical presentations necessitate brain imaging. The majority of these patients are managed by obstetricians due to the urgent need for delivery. MRI brain scan may show curvilinear abnormalities at the gray–white matter junction, particularly in the parietal and occipital regions. Such findings can help differentiate eclampsia from other causes of seizures [40].

Management of Seizures

Although most eclamptic patients are treated by obstetricians intrapartum, those that return with new-onset seizures in the postpartum period are often admitted to the neurology service. Despite extensive controversy between the neurology and obstetric communities in the United States regarding the management of eclamptic seizures, magnesium sulfate has become the mainstay of treatment.

Empirical evidence supports the effectiveness of magnesium sulfate in preventing and treating eclamptic seizures. The Eclampsia Trial Collaborative Group, a multinational study involving 1687 women with eclampsia, demonstrated that magnesium sulfate effectively reduced the risk of recurrent seizures in eclamptic women by 52% when compared to diazepam, and by 67% when compared to phenytoin [41].

Therapeutic levels of magnesium can be obtained by administering a 6-g intramuscular loading dose followed by 2 g/h intravenous infusion, or alternatively with a 2- to 4-g intravenous bolus followed by a 1 g/min infusion, or a combination of both [42,43,53]. The goal serum concentration is considered to be 4–8 mg/dL (2.0–3.5 mol/L). Magnesium is excreted in the urine; thus, impaired renal function may affect serum levels. Magnesium therapy has a narrow therapeutic index and symptoms of toxicity include loss of deep tendon reflexes at blood levels of 8–12 mg/dL, respiratory depression at concentrations of >14 mg/dL, muscular paralysis and respiratory arrest at levels >15–17 mg/dL. Cardiac arrest can occur above 30 mg/dL. Recommended treatment for toxicity includes calcium gluconate.

The mechanism of action of magnesium sulfate remains unclear. Several possible theories exist including acting as a vasodilator, protecting the BBB, and action as a central anticonvulsant. This theory was reinforced by transcranial Doppler (TCD) studies that have shown that vasospasm of the middle cerebral artery can be reversed with administration of intavenous magnesium sulfate [44,45]. The increase in blood flow helps prevent ischemia and thus minimizes a major cause of cortical irritability.

Concerns have been raised that magnesium sulfate may mask the outward signs of convulsions through its dose-dependent depression of neuromuscular transmission without treating the cause of seizure [46,47]. Studies have shown that there is minimal, if any, change in the electroencephalogram (EEG) obtained during magnesium therapy [48]. The possible anticonvulsant activity of magnesium sulfate may also be related to its role as an *N*-methyl-D-aspartate (NMDA) receptor antagonist [47–49]. Seizures are thought to be mediated in part by stimulation of glutamate receptors, such as the NMDA receptor [50,51]. Magnesium levels increase in the cerebrospinal fluid (CSF) after systemic administration [52]. In animals, studies have demonstrated that magnesium crosses the intact BBB and enters the CNS in correlation with the serum level [53]. NMDA receptors can be blocked by magnesium ions, thus minimizing neuronal damage and helping prevent seizures [54].

Eclampsia continues to be a significant cause of maternal and fetal death throughout the world. Approximately 10% of eclamptic patients who fail to receive therapy will experience recurrent seizures. There is a marked reduction in morbidity and mortality with early treatment with magnesium sulfate.

Neurobehavioral Aspects of Pre-eclampsia/Eclampsia

A patient who is suffering from the encephalopathy that characterizes eclampsia will, by definition, have altered sensorium, especially if seizures develop. However, behavioral aspects probably have an impact on the predisposition to pre-eclampsia/eclampsia as well. It is generally felt that a healthy lifestyle tends to be protective against these potential complications of pregnancy. Risk factors for pre-eclampsia/eclampsia include smoking [55], obesity [56], and hypertension [57]. It is not a great stretch to draw a correlation between taking care of one's physical, and presumably mental, health and protecting against problems related to pregnancy. The patient's perspective is important as well in terms of determining whether they will be attentive to prenatal care [58]. This can be impacted not only by socioeconomic issues [59], but also by educational and cultural aspects [60]. It is not out of the realm of possibility that stress might play a role in predisposition, but promotion of physical and leisure activity does not necessarily translate into reduction in risk [61,62]. Furthermore, stress is not necessarily a major contributing factor in either human [63] or animal studies [64]. However, secondary features of stress, such as increased cigarette consumption, elevated blood pressure, dynamics of the sexual relationship [65,66], or even increased tea consumption [67] might play some role.

References

[1] van Beek E, Peeters LLH. Pathogenesis of preeclampsia: a comprehensive model. Obstet Gynecol Surv 1998;53:233–9.

[2] Bersinger NA, Smarason AK, Muttukrishna S, Groome NP, Redman CW. Women with preeclampsia have increased levels of pregnancy-associated plasma protein A (PAPP-A), inhibin A and activin A, and soluble E-selectin. Hypertens Pregnancy 2003;22:45–55.

[3] Magnussen EB, Vatten LJ, Smith GD, Romundstad PR. Hypertensive disorders in pregnancy and subsequently measured cardiovascular risk factors. Obstet Gynecol 2009;114:961–70.

[4] Bainbridge SA, Sidle EH, Smith GN. Direct placental effects of cigarette smoke protect women from pre-eclampsia: the specific roles of carbon monoxide and antioxidant systems in the placenta. Med Hypotheses 2005;64:17–27.

[5] Lie RT, Rasmussen S, Brunborg H, Gjessing HK, Lie-Nielsen E, Irgens LM. Fetal and maternal contributions to risk of pre-eclampsia: population based study. Br Med J 1998;316:1343–7.

[6] Hoegh AM, Borup R, Nielsen FC, Sorensen S, Hviid TVF. Gene expression profiling of placentas affected by pre-eclampsia. J Biomed Biotechnol 2010;2010:1–11.
[7] Shah AK, Rajamani K, Whitty JE. Eclampsia: a neurologic perspective. J Neurol Sci 2008;271:158–67.
[8] McCrae KR, Samuels P, Schreiber AD. Pregnancy-associated thrombocytopenia: pathogenesis and management. Blood 1992;80:2697–714.
[9] Thomas SV. Neurological aspects of eclampsia. J Neurol Sci 1998;155:37–43.
[10] Shah AK, Whitty JE. Characteristics of headache in women with eclamplia. Neurology 1999;52(Suppl 2):A85–86.
[11] Adeney KL, Williams MA. Migraine headaches and pre-eclampsia: an epidemiologic review. Headache 2006;46:794–802.
[12] Lipton RB, Bigal ME, Steiner TJ, Silberstein SD, Olesen J. Classification of primary headaches. Neurology 2004;63:427–35.
[13] Weiner CP. The clinical spectrum of preeclampsia. Am J Kidney Dis 1987;9:312–6.
[14] Cunningham FG, Fernandez CO, Hernandez C. Blindness associated with preeclampsia and eclampsia. Am J Obstet Gynecol 1995;172:1291–8.
[15] Zeeman GG. Neurologic Complications of Pre-eclampsia. Semin Perinatol 2009;33(Issue 3):166–72.
[16] Panayiotopoulos CP. Elementary visual hallucinations, blindness, and headache in idiopathic occipital epilepsy: differentiation from migraine. J Neurol Neurosurg Psychiatry 1999;66:536–40.
[17] Witlin AG, Friedman SA, Egerman RS, Frangieh AY, Sibai BM. Cerebrovascular disorders complicating pregnancy—beyond eclampsia. Am J Obstet Gynecol 1997;176:1139–48.
[18] Lee VH, Wijdicks EF, Manno EM, Rabinstein AA. Clinical spectrum of reversible posterior leukoencephalopathy syndrome. Arch Neurol 2008;65:205–10.
[19] Shah AK. Non-aneurysmal primary subarachnoid hemorrhage in pregnancy-induced hypertension and eclampsia. Neurology 2003;61:117–20.
[20] Groenestege AT, Rinkel GE, van der Bom JG, Algra A, Klijn CM. The risk of aneurysmal subarachnoid hemorrhage during pregnancy, delivery, and the puerperium in the ultrecht population. Stroke 2009;40:1148–51.
[21] Arnold M, Camus-Jacqmin M, Stapf C, Ducros A, Viswanathan A, Berthet K, et al. Post-partum cervicocephalic artery dissection. Stroke 2008;39:2377–9.
[22] Matsumoto Y, Asada M, Mukubou M. Postpartum subarachnoid hemorrhage due to Moyamoya disease associated with renal artery stenosis. J Obstet Gynaecol Res 2009;34:787–9.
[23] Hirsch KG, Froehler MT, Juang J, Ziai WC. Occurrence of perimesencephalic subarachnoid hemorrhage. Neurocrit Care 2009;10:339–43.
[24] Hinchey J, Chaves C, Appignani B, Breen J, Pao L, Wang A, et al. A reversible posterior leukoencephalopathy syndrome. N Engl J Med 1996;334:494–500.
[25] Garg RK. Posterior leukoencephalopathy syndrome. Postgrad Med J 2001;77:24–8.
[26] Schwartz RB, Feske SK, Polak JF, DeGirolami U, Iaia A, Beckner KM, et al. Preeclampsia–eclampsia: clinical and neuroradiographic correlates and insights into the pathogenesis of hypertensive encephalopathy. Radiology 2000;217:371–6.
[27] Edvinson L, Owman C, Sjoberg NO. Autonomic nerves, mast cells, and amine receptors in human brain vessels. A histochemical and pharmacological study. Brain Res 1976;115:377–93.
[28] Treadwell SD, Thanvi B, Robinson TG. Stroke in pregnancy and the purperium. Postgrad Med J 2008;84:238–45.

[29] Liang CC, Chang SD, Lai SL, Hsieh CC, Chueh HY, Lee TH. Stroke complicating pregnancy and the puerperium. Eur J Neurol 2006;13:1256–60.
[30] Sharshar T, Lamy C, Mas JL. Incidence and causes of strokes associated with pregnancy and puerperium. A study in public hospitals of Ile de France. Stroke in pregnancy study group. Stroke 1995;26:930–6.
[31] Waddy S, Stern BJ. Cerebrovascular disease in pregnancy. In: Washington JM, editor. Neurologic disorders in pregnancy. New York: Parthenon; 2004. p. 39–51.
[32] Jaigobin C, Silver FL. Stroke and pregnancy. Stroke 2000;31:2948–51.
[33] Brown DW, Dueker N, Jamieson DJ, Cole JW, Wozniak MA, Stern BJ, et al. Preeclampsia and the risk of ischemic stroke among young women: results of the stroke prevention and young women study. Stroke 2006;37:1055–9.
[34] Lanska DJ, Kryscio RJ. Risk factors of peripartum and postpartum stroke and intracranial venous thrombosis. Stroke 2000;31:1274–82.
[35] Askie LM, Henderson-Smart DJ, Stewart LA, for the PARIS Collaborative Group Antiplatelet agents for prevention of pre-eclampsia: a meta-analysis of individual patient data. Lancet 2007;369:1791–8.
[36] de Sauvages FBS. Pathologia methodica, seu de Cognoscendis morbis, 3rd ed. Leyden: Fratum de Tournes; 1759. p. 286
[37] de Sauvages F. Pathologia methodica, seu de Cognoscendis morbis, 1st ed. Monspelii: Martel; 1739. p.120
[38] Phelan JP. Pulmonary edema in obstetrics. Obstet Gynecol Clin North Am 1991;18:319–31.
[39] Digre KB, Varner MW, Osborn AG, Crawford S. Cranial magnetic resonance imaging in severe preeclampsia vs eclampsia. Arch Neurol 1993;50:399–406.
[40] The Eclampsia Trial Collaborative Group. Which anticonvulsant for women with eclampsia? Evidence from the collaborative eclampsia trial. Lancet 1995;345:1455–63.
[41] Pritchard JA, Cunningham FG, Pritchard SA. The Parkland Memorial Hospital protocol for treatment of eclampsia: evaluation of 235 cases. Am J Obstet Gynecol 1984;148:951–60.
[42] Belfort MA, Moise Jr. KJ. Effect of magnesium sulfate on maternal brain blood flow in preeclampsia: a randomized placebo controlled study. Am J Obstet Gynecol 1992;167:661–6.
[43] Belfort MA, Saade GR, Moise Jr. KJ. The effect of magnesium sulfate on maternal and fetal blood flow in pregnancy-induced hypertension. Acta Obstet Gynecol Scand 1993;72:526–30.
[44] Donaldson JO. Does magnesium sulfate treat eclamptic convulsions? Clin Neuropharmacol 1986;9:37–45.
[45] Kaplan PW, Lesser RP, Fisher RS, Repke JT, Hanley DF. No, magnesium sulfate should not be used in treating of eclamptic seizures. Arch Neurol 1988;45:1361–4.
[46] Sibai BM, Spinnato JA, Watson DL, Lewis JA, Anderson JD. Effect of magnesium sulfate on electroencephalographic finding in preeclampsia–eclampsia. Obstet Gynecol 1984;64:261–6.
[47] Goldman RS, Finkbeiner SM. Therapeutic use of magnesium sulfate in selected cases of cerebral ischemia and seizure. N Engl J Med 1988;319:1224–5.
[48] Hallak M, Berman RF, Irtenkauf SM, Janusz C, Cotton DB. Magnesium sulfate treatment decreases *N*-methyl-D-aspartate receptor binding in the rat brain: an autoradiographic study. J Soc Gynecol Invest 1994;1:25–30.
[49] Lipton SA, Rosenberg PA. Excitatory amino acids as a final common pathway for neurologic disorders. N Engl J Med 1994;330:613–20.

[50] Dingledine R, Hynes MA, King GL. Involvement of *N*-methyl-D-aspartate receptors in epileptiform bursting in the rat hippocampal slice. J Physiol 1986;380:175–89.

[51] Thurnau GR, Kemp DB, Jarvis A. Cerebrospinal fluid levels of magnesium in patients with preeclampsia after treatment with intravenous magnesium sulfate: a preliminary report. Am J Obstet Gynecol 1987;157:1435–8.

[52] Hallak M, Berman RF, Irtenkauf SM, Evans MI, Cotton DB. Peripheral magnesium sulfate enters the brain and increases the threshold for hippocampal seizures in rats. Am J Obstet Gynecol 1992;167:1605–16.

[53] Yang YC, LeeCH Kuo CC. Ionic flow enhances low-affinity binding: a revised mechanistic approach into Mg^{2+} block of NMDA receptors. J Physiol 2010;588:633–50.

[54] Karumanchi SA, Levine RJ. How does smoking reduce the risk of preeclampsia? Hypertension 2010;55:1100–1.

[55] Robinson SH, Teoh TG. Management of maternal obesity prior to and during pregnancy. Semin Fetal Neonatal Med 2010;15:77–82.

[56] Chandiramani M, Joash K, Shennan AH. Options and decision-making: hypertensive disorders of pregnancy. Future Cardiol 2010;6:535–46.

[57] Kalim N, Anwar I, Khan J, Blum LS, Moran AC, Botlero R, et al. Postpartum hemorrhage and eclampsia: differences in knowledge and care-seeking behavior in two districts of Bangladesh. J Health Popul Nutr 2009;27:156–69.

[58] Silva LM, Coolman M, Steegers EA, Jaddoe VW, Moll HA, Hofman A, et al. Low socioeconomic status is a risk factor for preeclampsia: the Generation R Study. J Hypertens 2008;26:1200–8.

[59] Moran AC, Winch PJ, Sultana N, Kalim N, Afzal KM, Koblinsky M, et al. Patterns of maternal care seeking behaviours in rural Bangladesh. Trop Med Int Health 2007;12:823–32.

[60] Magnus P, Trogstad L, Owe KM, Olsen SF, Nystad W. Recreational physical activity and the risk of preeclampsia: a prospective cohort of Norwegian women. Am J Epidemiol 2008;168:952–7.

[61] Tyldum EV, Romundstad PR, Slordahl SA. Pre-pregnancy physical activity and preeclampsia risk: a prospective population-based cohort study. Acta Obstet Gynecol Scand 2010;89:315–20.

[62] Vollebregt KC, van der Wal MF, Wolf H, Vrijkotte TG, Boer K, Bonsel GJ. Is psychosocial stress in first ongoing pregnancies associated with pre-eclampsia and gestational hypertension? BJOG 2008;115:607–15.

[63] Falcao S, Solomon C, Monat C, Berube J, Gutkowska J, Lavoie JL. Impact of diet and stress on development of preeclampsia-like symptoms in p57kip2 mice. Am J Physiol Heart Circ Physiol 2009;296:119–26.

[64] Kho EM, McCowan LM, North RA, Roberts CT, Chan E, Black MA, et al. Duration of sexual relationship and its effect on preeclampsia and small for gestational age perinatal outcome. J Reprod Immunol 2009;82:66–73.

[65] Roberts JM, Pearson GD, Cutler JA, Lindheimer MD, National Heart Lung and Blood Institute. Summary of the NHLBI working group on research on hypertension during pregnancy. Hypertens Pregnancy 2003;22:109–27.

[66] VanWijk MJ, Kublickiene K, Boer K, VanBavel E. Vascular function in preeclampsia. Cardiovasc Res 2000;47:38–48.

[67] Wei SQ, Xu H, Xiong X, Luo ZC, Audibert F, Fraser WD. Tea consumption during pregnancy and risk of pre-eclampsia. Int J Gynaecol Obstet 2009;105:123–6.

6 Epilepsy and Pregnancy

John W. Kevill[1], *Eduardo Gonzalez-Toledo*[1,2]

[1] Department of Neurology, Louisiana State University Health Sciences Center, Shreveport, LA, USA
[2] Department of Radiology, Louisiana State University Health Sciences Center, Shreveport, LA, USA

Introduction

A woman with epilepsy who becomes pregnant or simply wants to have a child poses many questions that are difficult for the physician to answer. The prospective mother's questions are seemingly more uncomfortable in our evidence-based medicine of today than in bygone days when much less was known about the subject. Can I conceive if I am on antiepileptic medication? What will happen to my seizures if I am pregnant? Will seizures hurt the baby? Will my seizure medication hurt the baby? Can I just stop my seizure medication? I was told I cannot have a baby if I have epilepsy, is that true? There are no simple answers. The physician faces similar, difficult-to-answer questions regarding management that are no less unsettling. What is worse for the baby, seizures or antiepileptic medication? What antiseizure medication is most effective for the mother? What antiseizure medication is safest for the baby? Can birth defects due to antiepileptic drugs be prevented? What else I do not know? In general, these questions cannot be answered by medical studies producing Class I evidence [1]. It is unlikely that such evidence will ever be available due to the ethics of controlled studies on pregnant women.

The fact is that most women with epilepsy will have perfectly healthy children so it is not unreasonable for them to try to do so. Recent evidence suggests that the risk of fetal malformations has been overstated and that the shift to newer antiepileptic drugs and the use of folic acid has reduced the incidence [2]. Medical science has greatly improved the lives of patients with epilepsy over the past 50 years. The repeal of all the eugenic marriage laws in the United States that prohibited marriage (and therefore reproduction) of epileptics is stark evidence of this change in the way society views epilepsy. The medical view of epilepsy has changed as well. Diagnosis of epilepsy is now accurate and relatively rapid. Electroencephalogram-Video (EEG-video) monitoring can clarify events that were only suspected to be seizures and demonstrate clearly those that are not. Improved imaging can identify a treatable cause for seizures in many cases. Tremendous advances in genetics have allowed the elucidation of many syndromes that involve clear molecular abnormalities that predispose a patient to seizures. Treatment has improved dramatically in the past 20 years with many new pharmacologic and nonpharmacologic options that are safer and often

Neurological Disorders and Pregnancy. DOI: 10.1016/B978-0-12-384911-3.00006-3

more effective than older treatments. However, when all these medical advances come up against the problem of epilepsy in pregnancy, our breathtaking advance slows to a crawl. As with many areas of medicine, the full array of options cannot be used due to concerns about the second patient who does not have a disorder but will be exposed to the effects of treatment. Progress has been slow but definite [3].

This chapter will examine the available evidence for treatment of epilepsy and will review the most recent guidelines. Issues regarding the patient with epilepsy (meaning the pregnant mother) will be first. The effect of epilepsy and its treatment on conception begins the discussion. The effects of pregnancy on epilepsy and epilepsy on pregnancy will follow. The special case of seizures caused by pregnancy (eclamptic seizures) will be covered separately. Largely due to pregnancy registries, there is a growing body of knowledge regarding the effects of both epilepsy and its treatment on the developing fetus. Birth defects and the fetal anticonvulsant syndrome have been the focus in this area but there is growing evidence that antiseizure medications have more subtle effects on learning and development that should impact medication choice. The chapter will conclude with most recent recommendations for managing a woman with epilepsy through the process from conception to birth and somewhat beyond. Women with epilepsy can have children safely but with higher risk of complications (to both mother and fetus) than in the general population. Minimizing this risk and the responsibility of physicians is the purpose of this chapter.

History

Children born to mothers with epilepsy have an increased risk of an adverse outcome. The risks are relatively small with proper management. It is now recognized that the vast majority of women with epilepsy can have healthy children. This has not always been the case.

Pregnancy is mentioned infrequently in ancient writings regarding epilepsy. Most writing on epilepsy before Hippocrates ascribed epilepsy to magical forces or punishment for sin. The Greek usage of the term "the sacred disease" reflects this. Hippocrates published "The Sacred Disease" in 400 BC as a statement to the general public to combat superstition. "The fact is that the cause of this affliction is in the brain" [4]. He also discussed the role of the uterus which he felt could cause seizures when displaced but little else is mentioned regarding epilepsy and pregnancy [5]. Physicians in the middle ages continued to recognize the uterus as a source of seizures in women. Guainerius in 1516 noted differences between hysterical seizures and "idiopathic" epilepsy based on clinical description of the events and the recognition that patients with hysterical seizures remembered events during the episode [6]. This is one of the earliest writings to recognize the phenomena of psychogenic seizures or pseudoseizures. Vapors arising from the uterus were felt to explain epileptic attacks but some authors felt that these vapors could cause hysterical seizures as well.

The nineteenth century brought about the beginning of our current understanding of epilepsy. In 1795, Boissier de Sauvages determined that epilepsy was a chronic disease and separated it from "acute clonic convulsion with insensibility during the paroxysm" which he termed eclampsia [7]. The main distinction between the two was (and remains) the chronicity of epileptic seizures versus the transient nature of eclampsia, which occurred only during pregnancy. By 1800, medical science recognized that there were epileptic seizures both "grand mal" and "petit mal," seizures due to eclampsia, and hysterical seizures which we would today call pseudoseizures or psychogenic seizures. All of the understanding of the time is based on clinical grounds. As early as 1843, it was recognized that proteinuria was seen with eclampsia, and in 1896, Schmorl showed that there were fetal cells in the maternal circulation [8]. In 1857, the first effective treatment for epilepsy was discovered with the use of potassium bromide. The drug could cause impotence in males and it was felt that this might be useful in treating menstrual epilepsy, often known as hysterical epilepsy at the time [9]. This was a fairly effective treatment for epilepsy although quite sedating in many patients. Phenobarbital was developed in 1912 and this was somewhat more effective and less sedating. The use of phenobarbital for epilepsy was an accidental discovery as the drug was intended to be used as a tranquilizer [10]. Magnesium was used for the first time to prevent eclampsia in 1906 and was given intrathecally [11]. It was not until 1933 that magnesium was used in large number of patients with both eclampsia and pre-eclampsia at Los Angeles General Hospital [11,12].

While there were many developments in the field of epilepsy during the nineteenth and early twentieth centuries, social awareness regarding epilepsy lagged far behind. There was a clear connection between epilepsy, mental retardation, and insanity in the mind of the general public that tended to stigmatize epileptics. Oddly enough, at the time when scientific understanding was growing and effective treatment was becoming available, public policy began to move in a different direction. The first law prohibiting marriage of epileptics (and therefore reproduction) in the United States was passed in Connecticut in 1895 [13]. By 1956, 17 states had laws against marriage for epileptics although, to its credit, Connecticut had repealed their version in 1953. The last state to repeal this type of law did so in 1980. These laws were largely ineffective for several reasons. Persons could cross state lines and marry in states that did not have such laws. Medical evaluation was not required to prove a person was epileptic in most of the states that did have these laws. There was no effective way to identify carriers of epilepsy. These facts made the laws ineffective in preventing the birth of epileptics, which was the intent. There was a growing appreciation at the time that there was a limited genetic component to most epilepsy and this eventually led to a repeal of these laws. Contributing equally to stigmatizing epileptics and relating to their reproductive rights were eugenic sterilization laws. The first such law was passed in Indiana in 1907 [14]. Several other states followed suit but all such laws were held unconstitutional until 1927 with the case of *Buck v. Bell.* In a decision authored by Justice J. Holmes it was determined that a woman could be sterilized for the greater good of society. "The principle that sustains compulsory vaccination is broad enough to cover cutting the Fallopian tubes" (*Jacobson v. Massachusetts*, 197 U.S. 11). As stated by Justice Holmes, "Three generations of imbeciles are enough" [15]. Only 4 of 17 states that had such laws in 1956 applied them to epileptics who were not institutionalized. These laws no longer apply to epileptics in any state. The last such law was repealed in 1980.

Today there are successful people in nearly all walks of life who live with epilepsy. There are athletes, members of congress, physicians and lawyers, and persons from nearly every occupation who live normal lives with epilepsy. The disorder has even touched a member of the Supreme Court of the United States [16]. Pregnant women are included in people who have epilepsy but live completely normal lives. Public awareness of epilepsy has improved to the point that the question is now longer *if* a woman with epilepsy can or should have a child, but rather *how* best to do it.

Fertility and Epilepsy

A number of studies have shown that women with epilepsy have fewer children than women in the general population. One study involving women with idiopathic epilepsy showed this number to be reduced to one-third the expected number [17]. Other studies show women with temporal lobe epilepsy having 70–85% of the expected number of children [18]. More recent studies show an improvement in these statistics, which is undoubtedly due to a number of factors, both social and medical. With social factors that reduce the chance of a woman with epilepsy having children set aside, it is clear that both seizures and antiepileptic medications have a role in reproductive dysfunction in women with epilepsy.

Generalized seizures increase the level of prolactin by 3 times within less than 30min of the seizure. Luteinizing hormone (LH) and follicle stimulating hormone (FSH) also increase [19,20]. This well-known endocrine response to a seizure is useful in the diagnosis of psychogenic seizures (pseudoseizures). These increases may also be the key to understanding why women with epilepsy have reproductive endocrine dysfunction more often than the general population. This effect is probably independent of treatment and is due to the seizures themselves [21]. According to the hypothesis of Herzog [22], changes in levels of both FSH and LH can be caused by seizure discharges from the limbic lobe, particularly the amygdala. The amygdala has direct connections with the ventromedial hypothalamus via the stria terminalis. Stimulation of the hypothalamus by both seizures and interictal discharges causes changes in the levels of secreted gonadotrophic releasing factors [23]. In turn, this alters the levels of both LH and FSH, which can cause both polycystic ovarian syndrome and hypothalamic amenorrhea. Both of these conditions are found in increased numbers in women with epilepsy, even if untreated. It has been estimated that one-third of the menstrual cycles in women with epilepsy are anovulatory [24]. Women with polycystic ovarian syndrome and hypothalamic amenorrhea have a reduction in progesterone as well as an increase in androgens. These alterations can alter the ratio of estrogen to progesterone (less progesterone) which may increase seizure discharges in the temporal lobe [25] (Figure 6.1) [26]. It is likely that a positive feedback loop is created where seizures worsen the reproductive dysfunction and this in turn worsens the seizures [27].

Antiepileptic drugs can interfere with normal endocrine function but it is unlikely that they are a direct cause. Some animal studies have failed to show structural changes in the ovaries in animals exposed to valproate that did not have epilepsy [28].

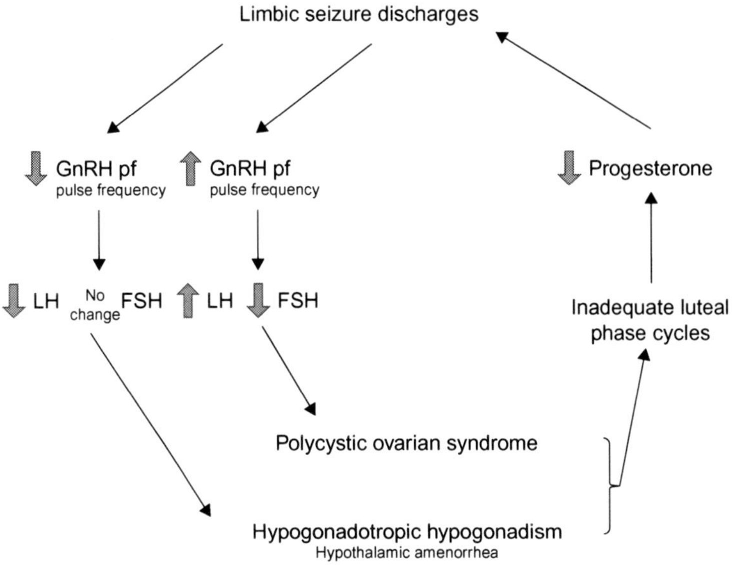

Figure 6.1 Possible mechanisms by which limbic seizure discharges promote reproductive endocrine disorders and how hormonal reproductive hormone levels can influence epilepsy. *Source:* Adapted from Herzog AG et al. Reproductive Endocrine Disorders in Men With Partial Seizures of Temporal Lobe Origin. Arch Neurol 1986;43: 347–350, with permission from American Medical Association.

In contrast, the studies of Isojarvi showed a high incidence of polycystic ovarian syndrome in women who used valproate. The incidence was higher than in women with epilepsy who took other antiepileptic drugs and also higher among women who had started valproate before 20 years of age [29]. Evidence suggests that there is an interaction between valproate and epilepsy in women that produces reproductive dysfunction in women. Studies of women taking valproate for bipolar disorder find a lower rate of polycystic ovarian syndrome than in women taking valproate for epilepsy [30]. As an enzyme inhibitor, valproate can inhibit the conversion of testosterone to estradiol, leading to increased androgen levels that are part of the reproductive dysfunction in women with polycystic ovarian syndrome [31]. It is noted that evaluation of women with bipolar disorder has shown that this population also has a higher incidence of reproductive endocrine dysfunction that makes interpretation of data including the treatment with valproate difficult. Herzog has suggested that enzyme-inducing antiepileptic drugs may promote the metabolism of testosterone and thus minimize the effects of epileptic seizures on reproductive function [23,32,33]. This of course is in addition to the effect of reducing seizures which also would reduce the incidence of polycystic ovarian syndrome. An effective way to block the effects of valproate in promoting polycystic ovarian syndrome in women with epilepsy has not yet been found. In addition, the question of whether valproic acid produces the same degree of reproductive endocrine dysfunction in women whose seizures are very well controlled has not clearly been answered.

Libido is reduced in women with epilepsy. Studies suggest that one-third of women with epilepsy experience sexual dysfunction [34]. There have been few studies that directly address this problem. While most of the evidence for this has been collected by self-report, studies over many years show fairly consistent results in women which contrasts with reporting of sexual dysfunction in men. The incidence of sexual dysfunction in men is estimated at 20%, which is a significantly lower number than previously reported. Some of the discrepancy may ultimately have to do with methods of data collection [35]. In women with temporal lobe epilepsy, sexual dysfunction more often is associated with right-sided lesions as opposed to left-sided lesions [36]. This finding suggests that the problem involves more than the common finding of depression in patients with epilepsy which can produce sexual dysfunction on its own. It appears that lesions of the amygdala and hippocampus can lead to problems with sexuality. Connections from the amygdala to the hypothalamus may play a significant role. It appears that seizures themselves play the major role, as several studies have shown that women with epilepsy had no sexual dysfunction before the onset of the seizures [37,38].

Contraception and Epilepsy

Seizures do not appear to have any significant effect on the effectiveness of birth control, but antiepileptic medications clearly reduce the effectiveness of oral contraceptive pills. According to a recent survey, many physicians are not knowledgeable about this problem, even if they had patients that had experienced oral contraceptive failure [39]. The failure rate for standard oral contraceptive pills is estimated at 0.7 per 100 years in the general population and 3.1 per 100 years in women taking antiepileptic drugs [40]. With the more recent, low-estrogen birth control pills, popular because they reduce side effects, the rate of failure is almost certainly higher. In 1998, the American Academy of Neurology recommended an estradiol dose of 50 μg for 21 days for patients using enzyme-inducing antiepileptic drugs [41]. The original formulation of oral contraceptive pills was 80 μg of estrogen with 1 mg of progestin [40]. It appears that 50 μg of estradiol is inadequate and there are more failures than was initially thought.

The main hepatic system that processes the steroid sex hormones is the P-450 system. Many antiepileptic drugs induce this system (Table 6.1). There is also likely an increase in sex steroid hormone conjugation in the intestinal tract. The result of reducing levels of these hormones is failure to prevent ovulation. Crawford finds that 10% of women have unregulated cycles on low-dose estrogen oral contraceptives [41]. It should be noted that lack of breakthrough bleeding does not guarantee that the birth control is effective [42]. In view of this, it is recommended that a higher dose of estradiol be considered (>50 μg for 21 days) and barrier methods also should be employed. Other methods such as subdermal levonorgestrel (Norplant) and intramuscular medroxyprogesterone are other options, but there is an increase in failure to prevent pregnancy with these methods as well in women taking antiepileptic

Table 6.1 Antiepileptic Drug Effects on Hormonal Contraceptive Agents

Lowers Hormone Levels	No Significant Effect
– Phenobarbital	– Ethosuximide
– Pheytoin	– Valproate
– Carbamazepine	– Gabapentin
– Primidone	– Lamotrigine
– Topiramate	– Tiagabine
– Oxcarbazepine	– Levetiracetam
– Rufinamide	– Zonisamide
• A single study found that Rufinamide decreased estradiol by 22%. The study did not measure markers for ovulation. A more recent review concluded that Rufinamide can compromise oral contraceptive [41].	– Lacosamide

Source: Adapted from [42], with permission from Elsevier, Inc.

drugs [43]. Whether these methods are more successful and safer for women with epilepsy wishing to avoid pregnancy has not yet been determined.

While there are more side effects with higher-dose oral contraceptives that make the newer, lower-dose formulations popular, there also is an effect on antiepileptic drugs. In particular, lamotrigine has been shown to have its levels reduced by oral contraceptive pills. One study showed a 50% reduction in lamotrigine levels after the introduction of birth control [44,45]. Another study showed a 100% increase in lamotrigine levels during the pill-free period [46]. The mechanism appears to be that oral contraceptive pills increase glucuronidation in the liver, which is the main metabolic pathway for elimination of lamotrigine and several other antiepileptic drugs [47]. Lowering serum anticonvulsant levels by increasing the dose of oral contraceptive pills can increase the risk of breakthrough seizures, but the risk may be overstated [48]. Fortunately, if the problem is anticipated, careful monitoring of serum anticonvulsant levels can allow for adjustment in dosage.

The Effect of Pregnancy on Epilepsy

There are a number of factors that can affect seizure frequency in women with epilepsy who are pregnant. The major factors are hormonal changes that accompany the pregnant state, changes in behavior, and changes in metabolism that alter the concentrations of antiepileptic drugs. These will be discussed separately.

Perhaps one-third of women with epilepsy will have an increase in seizures during pregnancy. Ten to twenty percent will have a decrease in seizure frequency. A small number of women will have one or two seizures during pregnancy and never have them at any other time in their life [49]. The majority of women with epilepsy will not have their seizure frequency altered [50]. Studies show that changes in seizure frequency do not depend on the seizure type, age of the mother, duration of epilepsy, or the number of seizures that occurred in a previous pregnancy [51]. In general, it is believed that most seizures will occur toward the end of the pregnancy; however, one-third of seizures can occur in the first trimester [52]. A small percentage of women will have a permanent increase in their seizure frequency following pregnancy [49]. A recent evaluation of previous studies found no clear evidence to state if seizures were increased or decreased in general in pregnant women with epilepsy. For now, women must be treated on a case-by-case basis. The only clear recommendation is that if a woman's seizures are well controlled for a year before pregnancy, there is a 90% chance this will remain during the pregnancy [53].

Maintenance of the placenta requires major changes in the levels of hormones. Estrogens and progesterone increase by 10 times their normal levels during pregnancy. The relationship between these hormones and epilepsy has been fairly well delineated. Estrogens are pro-convulsant in both animal models and human studies while progesterone appears to increase seizure threshold, making seizures less likely [54]. There are several mechanisms for estrogen to decrease seizure threshold. It can increase activity at both *N*-methyl-D-aspartate (NMDA) and non-NMDA glutamate receptors [55]. In the hippocampus, the density of dendritic spines increases in neurons exposed to estrogen. Specifically these are NMDA synapses and the net effect appears to be an increase of excitability [56,57]. Finally, estrogens affect the expression of neurotransmitters in neurons that contain estrogen receptors (highly concentrated in the amygdala) [58]. Progesterone seems to have the exact opposite effect as estrogen on neurons [56]. The effects of estrogen and progesterone begin with menarche. Some previous epidemiologic studies have not been able to show a clear increase in seizures at the time of puberty for women although this has long been suspected. The data on seizure onset and seizure exacerbation related to menarche has been difficult to interpret for a number of reasons. The process of sexual maturation occurs over many years making it difficult to pinpoint a particular vulnerable time. Some epilepsies that have a genetic origin (absence epilepsy) remit during puberty, masking both the incidence of new-onset seizures in the general population or recurrence of previously controlled seizures. Several studies however show that there is an increase in seizure frequency with menarche [59,60]. This appears to be more likely with focal epilepsies. The changes in puberty correlate to rises in hormone levels. Initially there is an increase in the levels of dihydroepiandrosterone sulfate (DHEAS) followed by an increase in estrogens roughly 2 years later. The increase in progesterone levels does not occur until ovulation begins, usually 2–4 years after the increase in estrogen levels [61]. While women during puberty are exposed to high levels of estrogen for a prolonged period, there is no clear data that this fact alone produces epilepsy. Instead, the high estrogen levels may act as a second injury that leads to the development of seizures. Because most focal epilepsy is the result of some type of cerebral insult, it may explain why focal epilepsy is more likely than primary generalized epilepsy to be exacerbated by menarche. This is the "two-hit hypothesis" described by Dichter in 1997 [62]. This possible effect is elegantly demonstrated in animal studies. Female rats castrated before puberty have a lower incidence of seizures than the general population and there is no effect if castration is performed after puberty [54,63,64]. More evidence for the effects of sex hormones on seizure frequency is provided by studies on catamenial epilepsy. Herzog [65] suggests that if the baseline seizure frequency doubles during a woman's menstrual cycle (the phase may differ), this qualifies as catamenial epilepsy. Perhaps one-third of women will fit this definition. What appears to be significant is not the absolute levels of estrogen and progesterone, both of which rise at different times during the menstrual cycle, but their ratio. In spite of all this information, little is known about the direct effect of increased hormone levels during pregnancy on seizures. Ramsey [66] did not find any association between seizure frequency and levels of estrogen, progesterone, or their ratios [67]. In most cases, the effects of increased hormone levels do not translate into more seizures. At this point, there are no practical recommendations regarding management of hormone levels for the purpose of treating seizures.

There are nonhormonal factors that increase the likelihood of seizures during pregnancy. Sleep deprivation is known to be a potential trigger for epileptic seizures and is clearly occurs more frequently during pregnancy. There are physical discomforts that produce this including frequent urination, often at night, fetal movements, and general discomfort that occurs with pregnancy, particularly in the late stages. Stress and anxiety over the health of the infant, marital relationships which are altered during pregnancy, and changes in body image all contribute to anxiety and therefore, insomnia. Related to this is an increase in noncompliance with medication. Many pregnant women are concerned about the effects of antiepileptic medication on the fetus. Particularly if control of seizures is good, there is an increased likelihood that women will discontinue their antiepileptic medication.

A final consideration is the effects of pregnancy on metabolism of antiepileptic drugs. The metabolism of nearly every antiepileptic drug is increased resulting in lower blood levels if adjustments are not made (Table 6.2). The effects of the various changes in maternal metabolism tend to occur after the first trimester but the

Table 6.2 Physiologic Changes During Pregnancy: Effects on Drug Disposition

Parameter	Consequence
Increased total body water and extracellular fluid	Alltered drug distribution
Increased fat stores	Decreased elimination of lipid soluble drugs
Increased cardiac output	Increased hepatic blood flow leading to increased hepatic elimination
Increased renal blood flow and glomerular filtration rate	Increased renal clearance of unchanged drug
Altered cytochrome P-450 activity	Altered systemic absorption and hepatic elimination
Decreased maternal albumin	Altered free drug fraction Increased availability of drug for hepatic extraction

Source: Adapted from [67], with permission from Wolters Kluwer Health Medical Research, Lippincott Williams & Wilkins.

effect on antiepileptic drug levels is unpredictable and depends on the drug being used. For example, highly protein-bound drugs are likely to have their levels altered whereas minimally protein-bound drugs will be little affected by changes in albumin levels. Many neurologists recommend monthly antiepileptic drug levels during pregnancy as changes in blood levels can occur rapidly [68]. Appropriate adjustment for the desired levels can then be achieved. Highly protein-bound antiepileptic drugs should have free drug levels obtained, whereas minimally protein-bound drugs can have total levels obtained. Because the various changes in maternal metabolism do not have predictable results on drug levels except that the levels are nearly always reduced, no formula can be given for adjusting antiepileptic drug levels during pregnancy. Normal metabolism returns 2–3 months after delivery so antiepileptic drug doses have to be adjusted again to avoid overdosing. An exception to this is lamotrigine. Its metabolism returns back to normal within a few weeks requiring a more rapid adjustment (downward) of the dosage [69–71].

The Effects of Epilepsy on Pregnancy

There are a number of complications of pregnancy that are more common in women who have epilepsy. Issues regarding the fetus will be discussed further on. The chance for vaginal bleeding, hyperemesis, eclampsia, and placental abruption are all increased by double over the general population. There is an increased chance of preterm labor and cesarean section as well [72]. Some of these effects are the direct result of seizures while others may be a combination of the effects of antiepileptic drugs and seizures. Maintaining seizure control is still the best way to prevent these complications.

Seizures can be a problem during labor and delivery. Generalized tonic–clonic seizures are particularly troublesome. They can produce acidosis and hypoxia in the mother with subsequent risk to the baby. The fetal heart rate can be lowered by a convulsive seizure, which probably contributes to statistics showing low Apgar scores and other evidence of hypoxia [73]. Nonconvulsive seizures do not carry the same risks but may interfere with a woman's ability to cooperate with a vaginal delivery [74]. Fortunately, convulsive seizures are relatively rare during labor, occurring in only 1% of women who are in labor [74]. These seizures carry with them the risk of stillbirth [75] or developmental delay in the infant [76]. Several factors can contribute to the timing of seizures at the time of delivery. Prolonged labor may be accompanied by sleep deprivation. Drug levels may be low during prolonged labor due to a combination of emesis and impaired absorption. Several studies have shown that most women who do have seizures during pregnancy have subtherapeutic levels of antiepileptic drugs [77,78]. If patients are taking antiepileptic drugs with an intravenous formulation can be switched at an equivalent dose. Levels should be followed during prolonged labor. Seizures can be treated rapidly with benzodiazepines but with a potential risk of respiratory depression in the neonate. There are recent concerns about the use of older anticonvulsants that will cross into the fetal circulation, causing apoptotic cell death [79], but this is generally in the population of asphyxiated babies. There is no clear data on whether these drugs can cause this when given to a mother during labor. Newer antiepileptic drugs such as levetiracetam appear not to have this complication but there is little data on their use for seizures during labor. Women with generalized seizures during labor should be placed on the left side to reduce the chance of aspiration and increase uterine blood flow [80]. They also should be treated with oxygen. The goal of treatment is to avoid convulsive status epilepticus. If the seizures cannot be managed, a cesarean section should be performed rapidly.

A number of antiepileptic drugs can cause vitamin K deficiency in the neonate by inhibiting its transport across the placenta [81]. These drugs include phenobarbital, phenytoin, carbamazepine, ethosuximide, primidone, and diazepam [82]. The newer antiepileptic drugs have not been studied. The potential hemorrhagic complications in the newborn can be serious with a 30% mortality reported [43]. Women taking anticonvulsants that cause this problem should be treated with 10 mg/day of oral vitamin K beginning at 36 weeks of gestation. The newborn should receive 1 mg of intravenous or intramuscular vitamin K at the time of delivery [83]. The mother should receive parenteral vitamin K if she has not been treated in the month preceding labor. If two of the vitamin K dependent coagulation factors in the neonate (II, VII, IX, or X) are below 5% of normal, then fresh frozen plasma should be given [84].

Eclampsia

Eclampsia and pre-eclampsia are disorders that occur only in pregnant women. Pre-eclampsia usually occurs during a woman's first pregnancy. It is a disorder of multiple systems that includes hypertension, proteinuria, generalized edema, hypoalbuminemia, hemoconcentration, abnormalities of hepatic function which can include coagulopathy, and increased levels of urate [85]. Eclampsia is one of several potential complications of this state and involves the development of seizures or unexplained coma in a patient with pre-eclampsia. Most cases occur after 28 weeks of gestation but this is not always the case. Eclampsia has been reported as early as 20 weeks of gestation with 1% of cases occurring even before then. It occurs most frequently antepartum but frequently occurs during labor [86]. It can occur within 48 h after delivery and a few cases have been reported within 4 weeks after delivery. The estimated incidence of eclampsia in Europe and the United States is 1 in 2000 deliveries [87]. Eclampsia is a serious condition with a mortality rate of 1.8–5% [88]. The criteria for pre-eclampsia are listed in Table 6.3.

The pathophysiology of pre-eclampsia is complex, but it appears to be related to the placenta as the symptoms resolve promptly after delivery. In a normal placenta, trophoblast cells invade the spiral arteries of the uterus and destroy the media of the arteries. This transforms relatively small, muscular arteries into large sinusoidal vessels that allow increased perfusion of the placenta [90]. With pre-eclampsia,

Table 6.3 Criteria for Diagnosis of Preeclampsia

- Blood pressure of 140 mm Hg systolic or higher or 90 mm Hg diastolic or higher that occurs after 20 weeks of gestation in a woman with previously normal blood pressure
- Proteinuria, defined as urinary excretion of 0.3 g protein or higher in a 24-hour urine specimen
- *Preeclampsia is a pregnancy-specific syndrome that usually occurs after 20 weeks of gestation.

Diagnosis of Severe Preeclampsia

- Preeclampsia is considered severe if one or more of the following criteria is present:
- Blood pressure of 160 mm Hg systolic or higher or 110 mm Hg diastolic or higher on two occasions at least 6 hours apart while the patient is on bed rest
- Proteinuria of 5 g or higher in a 24-hour urine specimen or 3+ or greater on tweo random urine samples collected at least 4 hours apart
- Oliguria of less than 500 mL in 24 hours
- Cerebral or visual disturbances
- Pulmonary edema or cyanosis
- Impaired liver function
- Thrombocytopenia
- Fetal growth retardation

Source: *Date from Report of the National High Blood Pressure Education Program Working Group Report on High Blood Pressure in Pregnancy. Am J Obstet Gynecol 2000;183:S1–S22
Source: Adapted from American College of Obstetrics and Gynecology with permission

this process of trophoblast invasion of the spiral arteries is incomplete leaving the vessels with a relatively reduced diameter and thicker, more muscular walls than normal. This produces hypertension, a reduction of plasma volume, and hypoperfusion of all vital organs [91]. Inadequate perfusion of the placenta due to the abnormal arteries causes abnormalities in the maternal vascular endothelium with the release of numerous mediators that have widespread effects on circulation in other tissues. This includes thromboxane, endothelin, and superoxide with reductions in nitric oxide and prostacyclin, which function as vasodilators. In addition to widespread vasospasm and activation of both platelets and the coagulation system, there is widespread endothelial dysfunction in the systemic circulation that results in renal dysfunction with increased vascular resistance and hypertension [92]. Immune mechanisms may contribute as well [93]. Finally, there is a certain degree of apoptosis involved in maintenance of normal placental function and it appears that this increases as the pregnancy progresses. If there is inadequate apoptosis it can cause a maternal immune response against the fetus. If there is excessive apoptosis this will damage the normal function of the placenta resulting in placental ischemia [94].

The exact pathogenesis of seizures in eclampsia remains uncertain. The most likely theory centers on abnormal cerebral circulation. It is noted that many of the symptoms of eclampsia and much of the imaging and pathologic data show a marked similarity to hypertensive encephalopathy. In hypertensive encephalopathy there is disruption of the blood–brain barrier in response to rapid, severe elevations in systemic blood pressure. The normal autoregulation of cerebral pressure is overcome and the increased pressure in the cerebral vessels causes breakdown of the blood–brain barrier. During pregnancy there may be changes that predispose cerebral arterioles to dilate at lower than normal pressures, making the brain more susceptible to hyperperfusion with rapid increases in cerebral blood pressure [95]. It has been noted that brain imaging studies usually show abnormalities in the posterior white matter consistent with vasogenic cerebral edema. Pathologic studies of the brain in patients who died with eclampsia show petechial hemorrhages which tend to occur in the parieto-occipital and occipital lobes [96]. The predilection for white matter changes appears related to the structure of this tissue. There is a matrix of glial cells traversed by myelinated fiber tracts and arteries, which is less dense than gray matter. This allows for accumulation of fluid in the extracellular space [97]. White matter in the posterior parietal and occipital regions is supplied by the vertebrobasilar arterial system and this is less well supplied with adrenergic sympathetic input than the carotid system. This may explain why the posterior white matter is more affected in pre-eclampsia than the frontal and central white matter.

The treatment of seizures due to eclampsia has historically been with magnesium. This clearly reduces morbidity and mortality of both the infant and the mother [98]. This has always puzzled neurologists as magnesium was not an anticonvulsant. EEG abnormalities during eclamptic seizures do not resolve with successful treatment with magnesium and often take a week to resolve [99,100]. Magnesium is a potent vasodilator. It is felt that patients with leukoencephalopathy develop intense vasospasm with sudden, severe elevations in systemic blood pressure and this vasospasm can produce cerebral ischemia. Relief of this vasospasm may be the mechanism of action of magnesium in treating eclamptic seizures and the improvement in perfusion of the placenta may improve the outcome of the infant.

Eclampsia should be suspected in any pregnant woman with new-onset seizures. There is a considerable differential diagnosis for new-onset seizures during pregnancy listed in Table 6.4. Many of the conditions listed can be caused by pre-eclampsia. An example would be a cerebral infarct caused by a venous thrombosis secondary to a hypercoagulable state, not uncommon in pregnancy and often seen in severe pre-eclampsia. Because the seizures with eclampsia are potentially life threatening, it is best to recognize pre-eclampsia early and try to prevent its complications. It should be noted that some women who experience seizures postpartum do not have signs of pre-eclampsia that precede eclampsia, so eclampsia must be considered for several weeks postpartum with new-onset seizures. There is evidence that there are markers that may predict pre-eclampsia. Fms-like tyrosine kinase-1 can bind both placental and vascular endothelial growth factor and may have a role in the pathogenesis. Increased levels can be a marker for pre-eclampsia. Urinary placental growth factor can be decreased and this finding also strongly predicts pre-eclapmsia [101].

Table 6.4 Differential Diagnosis of Seizures During Pregnancy

- Epilepsy
  - New onset
  - Pre-existing epilepsy
- Eclampsia
- Cerebrovascular disease
  - Cerebral infarction
  - Central venous thrombosis
  - Subarachnoid or intracerebral hemorrhage
  - Hypertensive encephalopathy
- CNS infection
  - Bacterial meningitis
  - Viral meningoencephalitis
  - Fungal meningitis
- Metabolic abnormality
  - Hyponatremia
  - Hypocalcemia
  - Hypoglycemia or hyperglycemia
  - Hepatic encephalopathy
  - Hypothyroidism
- Collagen vascular disease
  - Systemic lupus erythematosis
- Neoplasm

Source: Collected from various sources, not directly borrowed from any publication.

Careful monitoring of blood pressure and urine protein are routine in the management of pregnant women.

The EEG shows several patterns that may evolve in a patient who progresses from pre-eclampsia to eclampsia. With pre-eclampsia, the EEG is often normal but may show diffuse slowing [102]. Localized abnormalities are not usually seen with pre-eclampsia. Ictal recordings during eclamptic seizures show typical spike wave discharges that are usually generalized as are the seizures. A variety of abnormalities are seen interictally during eclampsia. Most show diffuse, slow-wave activity that is similar to that seen in some women with pre-eclampsia. In many cases this must be due in part to a postictal state. Focal slowing and interictal spikes are seen less frequently [103]. As noted earlier, the interictal EEG abnormalities do not immediately resolve with treatment of the seizures with magnesium and may persist for up to 1 week.

Neuroimaging is probably the most useful study in evaluating eclampsia. Computed tomography (CT) scans are often normal but can show bilateral hypodensities in the white matter (Figure 6.2). These are more often than not symmetric and usually localized to the parieto-occipital white matter. The MRI is the best imaging study for evaluating eclampsia. The characteristic finding is high signal seen in the white matter with a propensity for the parieto-occipital white matter on T2-weighted

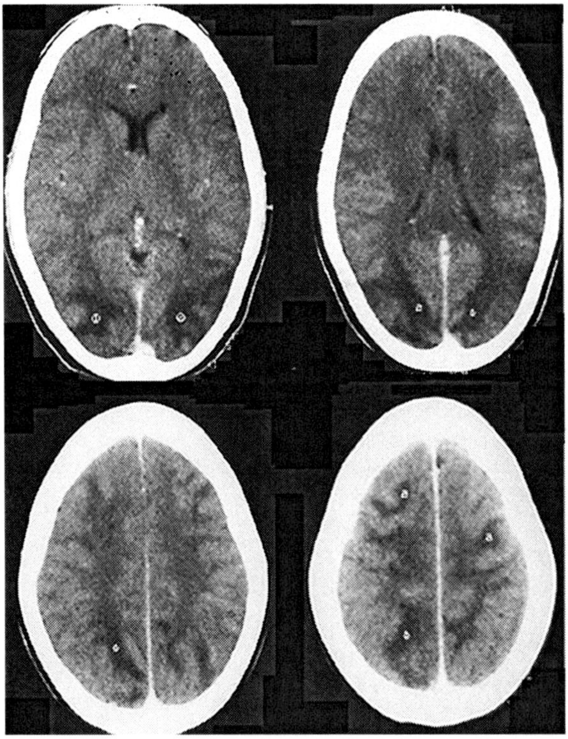

Figure 6.2 Computed tomography (CT) scan of the brain without contrast showing diffuse white matter hypodensity. There is a tendency for the hypodensity to be more prominent in the posterior white matter as seen in the upper two images. With permission from Medlink Neurology Inc.

images and fluid attenuated inversion recovery (FLAIR) sequences [104]. Diffusion-weighted images can help to distinguish vasogenic edema from cytotoxic edema by showing restricted diffusion in the latter. This is helpful in distinguishing the diffuse white matter edema of eclampsia from localized infarction [105]. See Figure 6.3 for MRI of eclampsia noting the lack of restricted diffusion. It was noted in the study of Zeeman et al. that cortical infarcts that were discovered were not accompanied by clinical findings. This could be expected with relatively small lesions in the parieto-occipital region. Cerebral angiography has been performed in some cases of eclampsia and usually shows some degree of spasm in large- and medium-sized arteries [96]. MRI abnormalities seen with eclampsia tend to resolve within 6–8 weeks excluding infarction [106].

After many years of controversy, it appears that magnesium is more effective in the treatment of eclamptic seizures than either phenytoin or diazepam. Women treated with phenytoin were 3 times more likely to have recurrent seizures than women treated with magnesium. In addition, women who develop severe

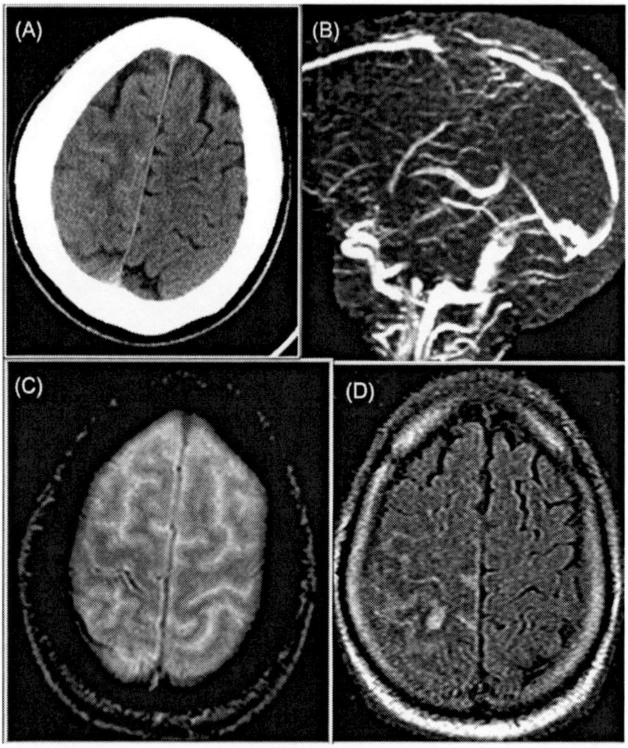

Figure 6.3 Superior sagittal sinus thrombosis in a 30-year-old postpartum female. (A) CT. Transverse slice, showing hyperdensity in the central sulcus and adjacent hypodensity corresponding to edema. (B) Filling defect in the superior sagittal sinus. (C) Magnetic resonance. Gradient echo. Hypointensity in the central sulcus corresponding to blood. (D) Magnetic resonance. Axial FLAIR sequence. Hyperintensity in sulci: hemorrhagic component in this patient with thrombosis of the superior longitudinal sinus (SLS).
Source: From Dr. Toledo.

pre-eclampsia can benefit from prophylaxis with magnesium to prevent the progression to eclampsia [107]. In addition, women who develop severe pre-eclampsia can benefit from prophylaxis with magnesium to prevent the progression to eclampsia [108]. The mechanism of action of magnesium sulfate may involve more than control of vasospasm and treatment of maternal hypertension. Several animal studies have shown that magnesium sulfate reduces the activity of NMDA receptors and blocks calcium entry into the cell mediated by the NMDA receptor. In comparison, phenytoin has not shown any significant effect on calcium channels but acts instead on sodium channels. Animal models have shown that magnesium is more effective in treating seizures that are the result of increased levels of excitatory neurotransmitters [109,110] and in fact exerts a central anticonvulsant effect. Magnesium is ineffective in controlling seizures in amygdala kindled rats, while phenytoin is effective. This model is similar to the condition in adults with focal-onset seizures [111]. These studies suggest that there is a different mechanism for seizures due to eclampsia than women with epilepsy, which would explain the response to a different treatment, and the fact the seizures are usually a transient event and rarely lead to chronic epilepsy. It appears that eclamptic seizures are the result of a generalized excess of excitatory neurotransmitters, which may be the result of a combination of factors previously discussed. It should be noted that the use of antiepileptic drugs in conjunction with magnesium sulfate for the treatment of eclamptic seizures has not been studied.

For severe pre-eclampsia, magnesium sulfate should be used to prevent progression to eclampsia. Altman [112] found that use of magnesium in pre-eclampsia reduces the incidence of eclampsia by about 50% and more than likely reduces maternal mortality as well. It appears superior in this regard than anticonvulsants (although large studies with the newer antiepileptic drugs have not yet been performed) and appears to be superior to nimodipine, a calcium channel blocker that can produce central vasodilatation [113]. The standard dosage for magnesium sulfate is to give a bolus of 5g by intravenous followed by continuous infusion at a rate of 2–3g/h. Alternatively, it can be given as an intermuscular injection of 10g followed by 5g every 4h [87]. The patient must be followed by evaluation of deep tendon reflexes (which are expected to become increased), respiration, and urine output. Magnesium is usually continued for up to 24h after delivery. When the patient develops diuresis in the postpartum period this can serve as an indicator that magnesium can be discontinued [114,115]. Infants delivered with mothers on magnesium can be expected to have low muscle tone which usually clears within 1–2 days as the magnesium clears their system.

Effects of Maternal Seizures on the Developing Fetus

Maternal seizures, particularly generalized tonic–clonic seizure, pose a significant risk to the fetus. A single generalized tonic–clonic seizure can cause both maternal and fetal hypoxia and acidosis. A single generalized tonic–clonic seizure can produce both a miscarriage and intracranial hemorrhage. The fetal heart rate can be reduced for over 20min by a convulsive seizure.

Status epilepticus is particularly dangerous for the fetus and mother. Infant and maternal mortality can approach 50% and 30%, respectively [116]. Injuries due to seizures can provoke a placental abruption. This can occur with relatively minor injuries. The effect of nonconvulsive seizures on the fetus is not clear but more likely than that it is not harmful. As mentioned earlier, this can interfere with labor by rendering the mother unable to cooperate with the delivery process.

The exact risk to the fetus with maternal seizures other than status epilepticus is not known. While the risks to the fetus with the older anticonvulsants are fairly well understood, the exact risk of a generalized tonic–clonic seizure is not. We know the possibilities but not the actual incidence. At this point most researchers believe that the risk of seizures is greater for the fetus that the risk of malformations due to antiepileptic drugs. There is recent evidence to support this conclusion [117–119].

Effects of Epilepsy Treatment on the Developing Fetus

Children of mothers with epilepsy can have a wide variety of problems that are the result of anticonvulsant drugs. These include intrauterine growth retardation (IUGR), minor and major congenital malformations, cognitive dysfunction, and infant mortality. Collectively, these are all grouped under the heading "fetal anticonvulsant syndrome."

The first clear reports of malformations felt to be due to anticonvulsants occurred in the 1960s. An increase in stillbirths was noted in women who were taking antiseizure medication but also cleft palate, congenital heart defects, and microcephaly with developmental delay. It was noted that several of the medications associated with these defects were folic acid antagonists. In a fascinating observation, Meadow [120] noted that children who were exposed to anticonvulsants had many of the same signs as children in whom abortion with folic acid antagonists was attempted but failed. Initially there was an attempt to classify all signs and symptoms into specific syndromes for each drug (fetal hydantoin syndrome). This has proved untenable as all the syndromes overlap. So now the term "fetal anticonvulsant syndrome" is used.

The fetal anticonvulsant syndrome includes some combination of the following signs and symptoms: mental retardation or cognitive dysfunction, microcephaly, minor congenital anomalies, and major congenital anomalies. These will be discussed separately. Some medications are more associated with specific anomalies but only in a general sense.

Minor anomalies are defined as structural abnormalities that do not create a significant risk to the health of the patient. This is somewhat subjective. The chance of a minor anomaly with an infant exposed to antiepileptic medication is roughly 2½ times the risk in the general population. Examples include broad nasal bridge, hypertelorism, epicanthal folds, and a low hairline. Distal digital hypoplasia can occur. The craniofacial abnormalities are often, but not always, outgrown after early childhood.

Major malformations are structural anomalies that either interfere with function or require intervention. In the general population, major malformations occur in 2–3% of births. The rate in children of women with epilepsy taking antiepileptic drugs is 4–7%. It should be noted that although the incidence is increased, it is still a relatively small number. This needs to be understood by both physicians and their patients [40]. The list of malformations includes neural tube defects (ranging from spina bifida to anencephaly); congenital heart defects (atrial septal defect, ventricular septal defect, patent ductus arteriosis, pulmonary stenosis, coarctation of the aorta, and others); cleft lip and or cleft palate; and urogenital defects [121].

Phenytoin (fetal hydantoin syndrome): This syndrome most commonly has hypoplasia of the distal phalanges and growth deficiency. Other signs include cleft lip and palate, hypertelorism, and mental retardation or other cognitive impairment. The digital abnormalities are considered most consistent although not specific to this syndrome. It has been suggested that 11% of infants exposed in utero will develop the full syndrome [122].

Carbamazepine (fetal carbamazepine syndrome): The main feature of this exposure is microcephaly. It often resolves and patients later have a head circumference in the normal range. The incidence of spina bifida appears to be increased by about 10 times the risk of the general population. Cognitive developmental delay has been a common finding but more recently this has been brought into question [123].

Phenobarbital: It was recommended that this need not be called a new syndrome because the features were not specific to phenobarbital exposure in utero. Growth retardation, developmental delay, dysmorphic facies, and minor anomalies were seen. There is a syndrome of vitamin K deficiency in neonates exposed to phenobarbital that was discussed earlier. A withdrawal syndrome has been noted in newborns. Initially there is sedation. This is followed by disturbed sleep, poor feeding, irritability, and an excessive startle reflex. It may take several months to resolve [124]. A similar syndrome can be seen in toddlers withdrawing from the drug who have been on it since birth.

Valproate (fetal valproate syndrome): Following the release of the drug in 1978 there were soon reports of neural tube defects. The fetal valproate syndrome consists of neural tube defects and facial dysmorphic features. Facial features include epicanthal folds; a broad, low nasal bridge; and anteverted nostrils. More significant is a 10- to 20-fold increase in the incidence of neural tube defects as compared to the general population [125,126]. Most concerning are cognitive defects. Seventy percent of patients exposed to valproate monotherapy will have this even without other features of the syndrome. The recent study of Meador et al. is compelling. The IQ of children measured at 3 years of age was compared for children of mothers who had received monotherapy during pregnancy with valproate, lamotrigine, carbamazepine, or phenytoin. The average IQ of children who were exposed to valproate was six to nine points lower than those exposed to other drugs [127]. This effect was dose dependent. This study supported recommendations that valproate need not be used as first-line treatment for women with epilepsy during pregnancy.

The pathogenesis of fetal anticonvulsant syndrome is poorly understood at this time. Few studies have been able to evaluate the problem carefully. There is undoubtedly a variable genetic susceptibility to the effects of the antiepileptic drugs that cannot yet be measured. It is clear that the fetal anticonvulsant syndrome is due to the medications themselves and not the epilepsy or other factors [128]. Evidence points to several possibilities.

Some research has focused on epoxides as promoting teratogenesis. A number of antiseizure drugs are metabolized into epoxides (carbamazepine is metabolized in part to an epoxide metabolite which is responsible for some of the toxicity of the drug). The detoxification of these compounds in the liver requires an epoxide hydrolase and these are relatively deficient in the fetal liver [129]. Studies in rats show that phenytoin toxicity is increased by inhibition of epoxide hydrolase [130] but proving that this is true for humans, and whether it accounts for the fetal anticonvulsant syndrome has been difficult. In 1990, Buehler showed that the levels of epoxide hydrolase was variable in the fetus and genetically determined and measurable with amniocentesis. Low levels predicted a higher risk of fetal anticonvulsant syndrome in patients taking phenytoin [131]. Because drugs that do not have epoxide metabolites (notably trimethadione) still cause the fetal anticonvulsant syndrome, there are likely to be other mechanisms.

It was noted in the late 1960s that the symptoms of fetal anticonvulsant syndrome were similar to the defects seen in infants in whom abortion had been attempted and failed using folic acid antagonists [120]. Many antiseizure medications were studied due to having folic acid antagonism as a mechanism of action. Oddly enough, lamotrigine was initially identified as a possible compound to prevent seizures because of this and it is one of the best anticonvulsants in terms of not causing birth defects. While folic acid is clearly beneficial to pregnant women to reduce the incidence of neural tube defects, it has not been shown to reduce the risk of malformations in women with epilepsy taking antiepileptic medication. It is still recommended that women take folic acid during pregnancy and before pregnancy if it is planned.

There is a growing body of evidence that many of the older anticonvulsant medications used to treat neonatal seizures may promote preprogrammed cell death (apoptosis) [132]. These studies have focused mainly on neonates who have seizures where pathologic studies are able to distinguish apoptotic cell death from cyotoxic cell death. It is felt that the vulnerable period for this effect of antiepileptic drugs is in the final months before birth and the first 1–3 months after delivery. Animal data suggest that carbamazepine and levetiracetam do not cause this problem. Topiramate may not promote apoptosis, however, when combined with phenytoin apoptosis was increased [133]. While it is too early to know if the fetus exposed to the maternal antiepileptic drug levels would experience neuronal apoptosis or not, there is reason for concern. More studies are needed in this area.

Evaluation of a First Seizure in a Pregnant Patient

A woman can experience her first seizure during pregnancy and proceed to develop epilepsy. The incidence of this is not known. Eclampsia certainly accounts for some of these women. Much more common is a breakthrough seizure associated with preexisting epilepsy. The evaluation of a woman with seizures occurring during pregnancy is not significantly different from any patient with new-onset seizures. The differential diagnosis is listed in Table 6.4.

The first step of course is a careful history to determine if the seizure is focal or generalized. Signs and symptoms of intracranial disease must be sought. Physical examination seeks to find localizing signs. Risk factors for epilepsy must be evaluated although pregnancy itself is a considerable risk. Evaluation should include a complete blood count, electrolytes and liver function testing, renal function, and toxicology screen. This is standard for any patient with new-onset seizures and electrolytes should include calcium and magnesium levels. The most common substances of abuse that cause seizures are alcohol and cocaine, so these should be specifically sought [134]. EEG and an MRI scan of the brain are indicated for new-onset seizures unless there is clear evidence that the seizures are due to eclampsia. Any focal signs on examination or the presence of focal seizures makes a diagnosis of eclampsia much less likely. The MRI scan is superior to CT and involves no radiation. There has not been any injury to mother or infant caused by MRI scans with a magnet strength of 1.5T [135]. The MRI scan does involve a longer acquisition time, which may be a consideration if the patient is unstable. After this basic evaluation, further studies and treatment are guided by the differential diagnosis. Pre-eclampsia and eclampsia have been discussed earlier.

Cerebral infarction should be considered in all cases although the incidence is small. It is estimated to be roughly 1 in 25,000 pregnancies in the United States [136]. Both arterial and venous infarctions can occur. There are usually risk factors associated with arterial strokes that can be identified. If there is a patent foramen ovale, then distal venous thrombosis must be considered. There is a wide range of disorders that predispose to arteriopathy and a number of disorders that can produce abnormal blood clotting. The use of diffusion-weighted MRI is invaluable in locating early cerebral ischemia when CT scans and standard MRI sequences show no abnormalities. See Figure 6.4 (A and B) in which the diffusion-weighted image shows evidence of an infarct. The standard MRI sequences did not show any abnormalities at that time. Venous thrombosis can be seen in the absence of any risk factors other than pregnancy. Pregnancy itself can induce a hypercoagulable state and cerebral venous thrombosis must be considered. The syndrome involves some combination of headache, seizures (usually focal) encephalopathy, and lateralized abnormalities on neurological exam [138]. Central venous thrombosis when seizures are involved usually involves the sagittal sinus. Localized infarcts are seen in a watershed distribution on MRI. Magnetic resonance venography (MRV) is the safest way to demonstrate the lesion. See Figure 6.4 (C and D) showing the MRV in the same patient as in Figure 6.4 (A and B).

Cerebral hemorrhage also is rare in pregnant women but pregnancy itself increases the risk. One to five women per 10,000 pregnancies may experience this. Mortality is high [139]. Intracerebral hemorrhage usually is the consequence of hypertension and eclampsia can be included as a cause. Subarachnoid hemorrhage in this population is usually due to an aneurysm or arteriovenous malformation. CT or MRI can be used to show the presence of subarachnoid blood. Standard CT scanners can fail to demonstrate 1–2% of small hemorrhages so lumbar puncture may be indicated if suspicion is high. Blood can also be identified readily on the gradient refocused echo (GRE) sequence and on FLAIR sequences as shown in Figure 6.5. If a blood vessel abnormality is found, standard cerebral arteriography remains the best way to evaluate vascular abnormalities that lead to hemorrhage.

Seizures are a common occurrence with central nervous system (CNS) infections. Pregnant women have a different susceptibility to infection due to alterations in their immune system that block reaction to fetal antigens [140]. The infectious agents most likely to be seen are *Mycobacterium tuberculosis*, *Listeria monocytogenes*, *Coccidioides immitus*, *Toxoplasma*, influenza, and varicella-zoster viruses [141]. There is no difference in the treatment of these infections in pregnant women and seizures are treated in standard fashion as with any CNS infection. In areas where it is endemic, neurocystercosis is a cause of focal-onset seizures. It should

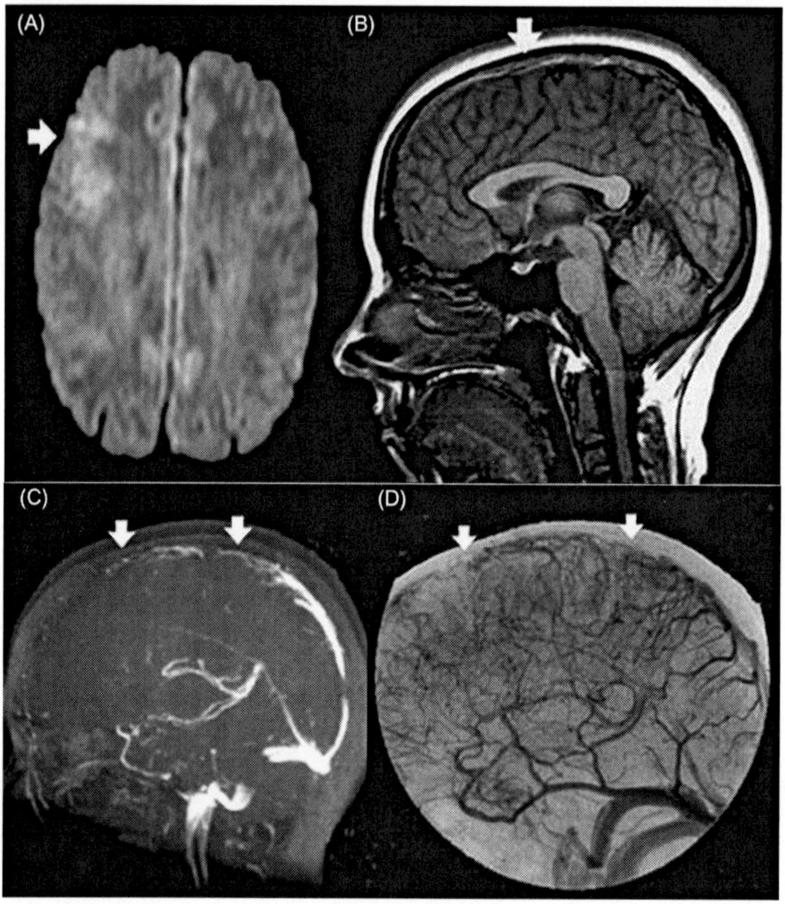

Figure 6.4 A 32-year-old woman who presented with a severe headache and seizure. Diffusion-weighted images (A) confirm an acute right frontal lobe infarct not in the typical arterial distribution (arrow). T1- and T2-weighted images were normal within the first 24 hours of presentation. T1-weighted sagittal (B) images showed an increased signal (Arrow) representing a thrombus within the superior sagittal sinus. *Source:* Adapted from Wolff's Headache 2008 with permission from Oxford University Press.
Magnetic resonance venogram (C) and venous phase angiogram (D) support the diagnosis of superior sagittal thrombosis (arrows indicate occlusion). Risk factors for venous thrombosis include: dehydration, pregnancy, oral contraceptives, trauma, disseminated intravascular coagulation, neoplasms, hypercoagulable states, infections, and idiopathic. *Source:* Adapted from Wolff's Headache 2008 with permission from Oxford University Press.

be discovered with neuroimaging, which is indicated in all cases of focal-onset seizures. Pregnant women do not appear to be more susceptible than the general population.

Neoplasms are not increased in frequency in pregnant women and are of the same type as in all women of this age group. Pregnancy may increase the rate of growth in some tumors. Because most women experience vomiting and "morning sickness"

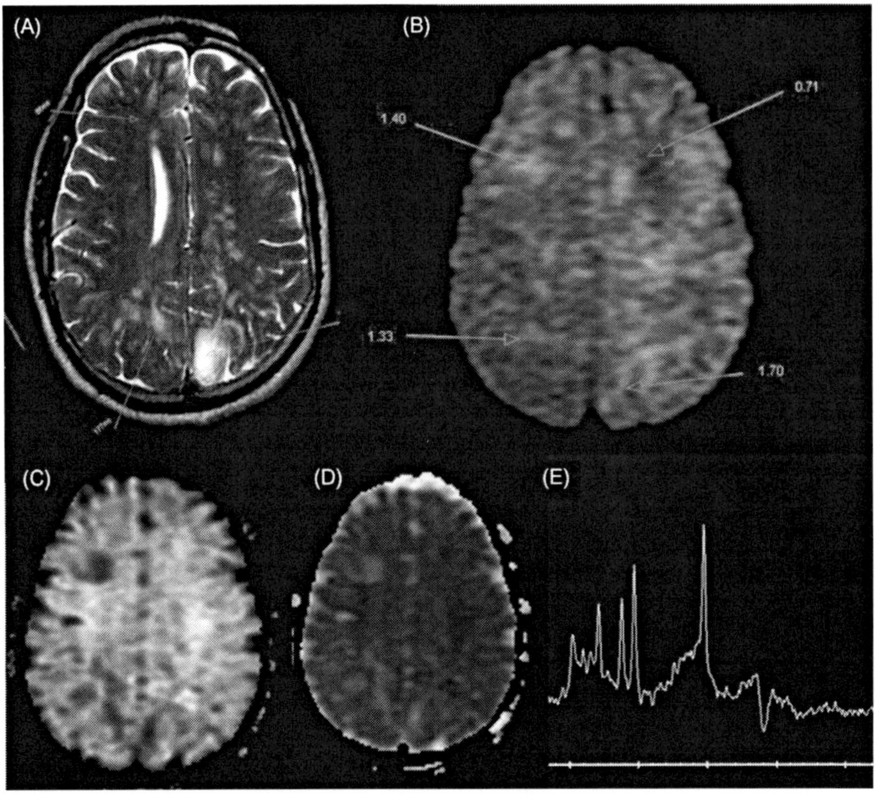

Figure 6.5 Posterior reversible leukoencephalopathy consistent with changes seen in eclampsia. MRI. (A) T2WI. Transverse plane. Multiple hyperintensities in the white matter with prolongued T2 values: 294 ms on the left parieto-occipital, 177 ms in right parieto-occipital, with a value of 86 ms in normal appearing white matter. (B) Diffusion-weighted sequence showing increased diffusion: 1.40 on the right fronto-parietal, 1.33 right parieto-occipital, and 1.70 in left parieto-occipital for a normal value of 0.71, all expressed as $N \times 10^{23}\,mm^2/s$. (C) This can be seen as hyperintensities on ADC map (D) and hyopointensities on exponential diffusion map. The absence of restricted diffusion indicates that this process is reversible, unlike the diffusion-weighted image of an infarction in Figure 6.4 (A and B). (E) Magnetic resonance spectroscopy: presence of lactate indicating anaerobiosis. *Source*: From Dr. Toledo.

during pregnancy, signs of increased intracranial pressure can be missed. MRI will detect neoplasms reliably and is indicated with most new-onset seizures.

Patients with collagen vascular disease often will have an exacerbation of their symptoms during pregnancy. Systemic lupus erythematosus is the most common entity encountered. Lupus can involve the CNS (lupus cerebritis) and usually results in seizures. Antiphospholipid antibodies (lupus anticoagulant) may also occur. These can occur independent of lupus in the primary antiphospholipid antibody syndrome [142]. The presence of these antibodies can lead to arterial or venous thrombosis, stroke, and miscarriage.

A number of metabolic derangements can occur during pregnancy and are listed in Table 6.4. Standard laboratory testing performed during pregnancy should uncover these conditions if present.

Finally, there is a group of patients who develop new-onset epilepsy during pregnancy. This can be considered if a search for other etiologies is negative. The need for long-term antiepileptic therapy must be considered in each case as some women will have seizures during pregnancy and never again.

Summary

Seizures are the most common neurologic problem encountered during pregnancy. Women who have epilepsy can safely have children but there is an increased risk to the mother and especially the child due to the effects of seizures and their treatment. The treatment of epilepsy requires careful consideration of a number of factors in a woman of childbearing age. Epilepsy itself can interfere with a woman's ability to reproduce and antiepileptic drugs may contribute to this. Antiepileptic drugs can interfere with hormonal contraception as well, which affects both the choice of the antiepileptic drug and the method of birth control. Only a fraction of women with pre-existing epilepsy have an increase in seizures during pregnancy. Ideally, decisions regarding antiepileptic drug therapy are made in advance of a woman attempting to conceive. While all antiepileptic drugs carry a risk of birth defects and cognitive delays, it appears that valproate poses the greatest risk and should not be used as a first-line treatment if at all possible [143]. More data is being collected regarding the safest medication to use for seizures but as yet there are no antiepileptic drugs that have category B status. Folic acid is still recommended as a measure to prevent birth defects even though there is data to suggest it does not reduce the risk in women taking antiepileptic drugs. Folic acid should be started at least 1 month before a woman conceives. Medications for seizures need to be monitored closely due to major changes in the clearance of most drugs (particularly lamotrigine). Polypharmacy should be avoided as it appears to increase the risk of fetal anticonvulsant syndrome to the fetus. A pregnant woman has different risk factors for new-onset seizures than women in the general population that are related to the pregnant condition. Evaluation of new-onset seizures requires careful consideration of these risks. MRI has become invaluable in evaluating most causes of new-onset seizures and generally supplants the use of CT. A significant number of women have seizures due to pregnancy alone (eclampsia) and do not go on to have epilepsy after delivery. The management of these seizures differs significantly from epilepsy, as discussed earlier.

References

[1] Pennell P. AES annual course: evidence used to treat women with epilepsy. Epilepsia 2005;47(Suppl. 1):46–53.

[2] Veiby G, Daltveit AK, Engelsen BA, Gilhus NE. Pregnancy, delivery, and outcome for the child in maternal epilepsy. Epilepsia 2009;50(9):2130–9.

[3] Shorvon SD, Tomson T, Cock HR. The management of epilepsy during pregnancy—progress is painfully slow. Epilepsia 2009;50(5):973–4.
[4] Hippocrates. The sacred disease. In: Jones WH, editor. Transl. Cambridge, MA: Harvard University Press; 1984. p. 127–83.
[5] Temkin O. The falling sickness. Baltimore, MD: Johns Hopkins Press; 1945. p. 40.
[6] Temkin O. The falling sickness. Baltimore, MD: Johns Hopkins Press; 1945. p. 183.
[7] Temkin O. The falling sickness. Baltimore, MD: Johns Hopkins Press; 1945. p. 240.
[8] Lapaire O, Holzgreve W, Oosterwijk JC, et al. Georg Schmorl on trophoblasts in the maternal circulation. Placenta 2007;28(1):1–5.
[9] Daras MD, Bladin PF, Eadie MJ, Millett D. Epilepsy: historical perspectives. In: Engel J, Pedley TA, editors. Epilepsy: a comprehensive textbook. 2nd ed. Philadelphia, PA: Lippincott Williams & Wilkins; 2008. p. 23.
[10] Hauptmann A. Luminal bei Epilepsie. Münchner Med Wochenschr 1912;59:1907–9.
[11] Chesley LC. History and epidemiology of preeclampsia–eclampsia. Clin Obstet Gynecol 1984;27:801–20.
[12] Purkerson ML, Vekerdy LA. History of eclampsia, toxemia, and the kidney in pregnancy. Am J Nephrol 1999;19:313–9.
[13] Barrow RL, Fabing HD. Epilepsy and the law. New York, NY: Hoeber-Harper Books; 1956. p. 11.
[14] Barrow RL, Fabing HD. Epilepsy and the law. New York, NY: Hoeber-Harper Books; 1956. p. 28.
[15] *Buck v. Bell.* 274 U.S. 200 1927; 207.
[16] Park A. Does justice roberts have epilepsy? Time.Com 2007 Jul. 31.
[17] Schupf N, Ottman R. Likelihood of pregnancy in individuals with idiopathic/cryptogenic epilepsy: social and biologic influences. Epilepsia 1994;35:750–6.
[18] Webber MP, Hauser WA, Ottman R, Annegers JF. Fertility in persons with epilepsy: 1935–1974. Epilepsia 1986;27:746–52.
[19] Dana-Haeri J, Trimble M, Oxley J. Prolactin and gonadotrophin changes following generalised and partial seizures. J Neurol Neurosurg Psychiatry 1983;46(4):331–5.
[20] Luef G. Hormonal alterations following seizures. Epilepsy Behav 2010;19:131–3.
[21] Bilo L, Meo R, Nappi C, Annunziato L, Striano S, Colao AM, et al. Reproductive endocrine disorders in women with primary generalized epilepsy. Epilepsia 1988;29:612–19.
[22] Herzog AG. A hypothesis to integrate partial seizures of temporal lobe origin and reproductive disorders. Epilepsy Res 1989;3:151–9.
[23] Herzog AG, Coleman AE, Jacobs, Klein P, Friedman MN, Drislane FM, et al. Interictal EEG discharges, reproductive hormones and menstrual disorders in epilepsy. Ann Neurol 2003;54:625–37.
[24] Cummings LN, Giudice L, Morrell MJ. Ovulatory function in epilepsy. Epilepsia 1995;43:341–6.
[25] Backstrom T. Epileptic seizures in women related to plasma estrogen and progesterone during the menstrual cycle. Acta Neurol Scand 1976;54:321–47.
[26] Herzog AG. Disorders of reproduction and fertility. In: Engle J, Pedley TA, editors. Epilepsy A comprehensive Textbook. 2nd ed. Philadephia PA: Lippincott Williams & Wilkins; 2008. p. 2054.
[27] Klein P. Impact of neuroendocrine factors on seizure genesis and treatment. In: Rho JM, Sankar R, Cavazos JE, editors. Epilepsy scientific foundations of clinical practice. New York, NY: Marcel Dekker Inc.; 2004. p. 367.
[28] Ferrin M, Morell M, Xiao E, Kochan L, Qian F, Wright T, et al. Endocrine and metabolic responses to long-term monotherapy with the antiepileptic drug valproate in the normally cycling rhesus monkey. J Clin Endocrinol Metab 2003;88:2908–15.

[29] Isojarvi JIT, Laatkainen TJ, Pakarinen AJ, Juntunen KT, Myllylä VV. Polycystic ovaries and hyperandrogenism in women taking valproate for epilepsy. N Engl J Med 1993;329:1383–8.
[30] Bilo L, Meo R. Polycystic ovary syndrome in women using valproate: a review. Gynecol Endocrinol 2008;24(10):562–70.
[31] Taubll E, Gregoraszczuk EL, Kolodziej A, Kajta M, Ropstad E. Valproate inhibits the conversion of testosterone to estradiol and acts as an apoptotic agent in growing porcine ovarian follicular cells. Epilepsia 2003;44:1014–21.
[32] Herzog AG. Pollycystic ovarian syndrome in women with epilepsy: epileptogenic or iatrogenic? Ann Neurol 1996;39:559–60.
[33] Herzog AG, Schachter SC. On the association between valproate and polycystic ovary syndrome. Epilepsia 2001;42:311–5.
[34] Morrell MJ, Guldner G. Self-reported sexual function in women with epilepsy. Epilepsia 1994;35(S8):108.
[35] Herzog AG. Reproductive endocrine regulation in men with epilepsy: effects on reproductive function and neuronal excitabillity. Ann Neurol 2002;51:539–42.
[36] Herzog AG, Coleman AE, Jacobs AR, Klein P, Friedman MN, Drislane FM, et al. Relationship of sexual dysfunction to epilepsy laterality and reproductive hormone levels in women. Epilepsy Behav 2003;4(4):407–13.
[37] Blumer D, Walker AD. Sexual behavior in temporal lobe epilepsy. Arch Neurol 1967;16:37–43.
[38] Pritchard PB, Hyposexuality A. Complication of complex partial epilepsy. Trans Am Neurol Assoc 1980;105:193–5.
[39] Krauss GL, Brandt J, Campbell M, Plate C, Summerfield M. Antiepileptic medication and oral contraceptive interactions: a national survey of neurologists and obstetricians. Neurology 1996;46(6):1534–9.
[40] Coulam CB, Annegers JF. Do anticonvulsants reduce the efficacy of oral contraceptives? Epilepsia 1979;20:519–26.
[41] Svendsen KD, Choi L, Single-Center Open-Label CBL. Multiple dose pharmacokinetic trial investigating the effect of rufinamide administration on ortho-novum 1/35 in healthy women. Epilepsia 1998;39(Suppl. 6):59.
[42] Pennell PB. Pregnancy in women who have epilepsy. Neurol Clin 2004;22:799–820.
[43] Shane-McWhorter L, Cerveny J, MacFarlane L, Osborne C. Enhanced metabolism of levonorgestrel during phenobarbital treatment and resultant pregnancy. Pharmacotherapy 1998;18:1360–4.
[44] Sabers A, Ohman I, Christensen J, Tomson T. Oral contraceptives reduce lamotrigine plasma levels. Neurology 2003;61:570–1.
[45] Wegner I, Edelbroek PM, Bulk S, Lindhout D. Lamotrigine kinetics within the menstrual cycle, after menopause, and with oral contraceptives. Neurology 2009 Oct. 27;73(17):1388–93.
[46] Sidhu J, Job S, Singh S, Philipson R. The pharmacokinetic and pharmacodynamic consequences of the co-administration of lamotrigine and a combined oral contraceptive in healthy female subjects. Br J Clin Pharmacol. 2006;6:191–9.
[47] Herzog AG, Farina EL, Blum AS. Fluctuation in serum valproate levels with oral contraceptive use. Epilepsia 2005;46:970–1.
[48] Reddy DS. Clinical pharmacokinetic interactions between antiepileptic drugs and hormonal contraceptives. Expert Rev Clin Pharmacol 2010;3(2):183–92.
[49] Knight AH, Rhing EG. Epilepsy and pregnancy: a study of 153 pregnancies in 59 patients. Epilepsia 1975;16:99–110.

[50] Schmidt D, Canger R, Avanzini G. Change in seizure frequency in pregnant epileptic women. J Neurol Neurosurg Psychiatry 1985;46:751–5.
[51] Yerby M. Pregnancy and the mother with epilepsy. In: Engel Jr. J, Pedley T, editors. Epilepsy: a comprehensive textbook. 2nd ed. Philadelphia, PA: Lippincott Williams & Wilkins; 2008. p. 2067.
[52] Cahill WT, Kovilam OP, Pastor D, Khoury JC, Sazaflarski JP, Ficker DM, et al. Neurologic and fetal outcomes of pregnancies of mothers with epilepsy. Epilepsia 2002;43(Suppl. 7):289.
[53] Harden CL, Hopp J, Ting TY, Pennell PB, French JA, Allen Hauser W, et al. American Academy of Neurology; Management issues for women with epilepsy-Focus on pregnancy (an evidence-based review): I. Obstetrical complications and change in seizure frequency: Report of the Quality Standards Subcommittee and Therapeutics and Technology Assessment Subcommittee of the American Academy of Neurology and the American Epilepsy Society. Epilepsia 2009 May;50(5):1229–36.
[54] Wooley DE, Timiras PS. The gonad–brain relationship: effects of female sex hormones on electro-shock convulsions in the rat. Endocrinology 1962;70:196–209.
[55] Smith SS. Estrogen administration increases neuronal responses to excitatory amino acids as a long term effect. Brain Res 1989;503:354–7.
[56] Woolley CS, McEwen BS. Role of estradiol and progesterone in regulation of hippocampal dendritic spine density during the estrous cycle in the rat. J Comp Neurol 1993;336:293–306.
[57] Wooley Cs WH, Schwartzkroin PA. Estradiol increases the frequency of multiple synapse boutons in the hippocampal CA1 region of the adult female rat. J Comp Neurol 1996;373:108–17.
[58] Wallis GJ, Luttge W. Influence of estrogen and progesterone on glutamic acid decarboxylase activity in discrete regions of regions of rat brain. J Neurochem 1980; 34:609–13.
[59] Klein P. Onset of epilepsy at the time of menarche. Neurology 2003;60:495–7.
[60] Morrell MJ, Hamdy SF, Seale CG, Springer A. Self-reported reproductive history in women with epilepsy: puberty onset and effects of menarche and menstrual cycle on seizures. Neurology 1998;50(Suppl. 4):A448.
[61] Klein P. Impact of neuroendocrine factors on seizure genesis and treatment. In: Rho JM, Sankar R, Cavazos JE, editors. Epilepsy scientific foundations of clinical practice. New York, NY: Marcel Dekker Inc., 2004. p. 364.
[62] Dichter M. Basic mechanisms in epilepsy: targets for therapeutic intervention. Epilepsia 1997;38(Suppl. 9):S2–6.
[63] Teresawa E, Timiras P. Electrical activity during the estrous cycle of the rat: cyclic changes in limbic structure. Endocrinology 1968;83:207.
[64] Hom AC, Leppik IE, Rask CA. Effects of estradiol and progesterone on seizure sensitivity in oophorectomized DBA/2J mice and C57/EL hybrid mice. Neurology 1993; 43:198–204.
[65] Herzog AG, Klein P, Ransil BJ. Three patterns of catamenial epilepsy. Epilepsia 1997;38:1082–8.
[66] Ramsey E. Effect of hormones on seizure activity during pregnancy. J Clin Neurophysiol 1987;4:23–5.
[67] Pennell PB. Antiepileptic drug pharmacokinetics during pregnancy and lactation. Neurology 2003;61(6 Suppl. 2):S35–42.
[68] Ohman I, Vitols S, Tomson T. Lamotrigine in pregnancy: pharmacokinetics during delivery, in the neonata and during lactation. Epilepsia 2000;41:709–13.

[69] Pennell PB, Newport D, Stowe ZN, Helmers SL, Montgomery JQ, Henry TR. The impact of pregnancy and childbirth on the metabolism of lamotrigine. Neurology 2004;62:292–5.
[70] Tran TA, Leppik IE, Blesi K, Sathanandan ST, Remmel R. Lamotrigine clearance during pregnancy. Neurology 2002;59:252–5.
[71] Fonager K, Larsen H, Pedersen L, Sorensen HT. Birth outcomes in women exposed to anticonvulsant drugs. Acta Neurol Scand 2000;101:289–94.
[72] Teramo K, Hiilesmaa VK, Bardy A, Saarikoski S. Fetal heart rate during a maternal grand mal epileptic seizure. J Perinat Med 1979;7:3–5.
[73] Delgado-Escueta A, Janz D. Consensus guidelines: preconception counseling, management, and care of the pregnant woman with epilepsy. Neurology 1992;42:149–60.
[74] Higgins TA, Comerford JB. Epilepsy in pregnancy. J Ir Med Assoc 1974;67:317–29.
[75] Leonard G, Andermann E, Pitno A, Schopflocher C. Cognitive effects of antiepileptic drug therapy during pregnancy on school age offspring. Epilepsia 1997;38(S3):170.
[76] Schmidt D, Canger R, Avanzini G, Battino D, Cusi C, Beck-Mannagetta G, et al. Change of seizure frequency in pregnant epileptic women. J Neurol Neurosurg Psychiatry 1983;46:751–5.
[77] Janz D. Antiepileptic drugs and pregnancy: altered utilization patterns and teratogenesis. Epilepsia 1982;23(Suppl. 1):853–63.
[78] Bittigau P, Sifringer M, Ikonomidou C. Antiepileptic drugs and apoptosis in the developing brain. Ann N Y Acad Sci 2003;993:103–14.
[79] Committee on Educational Bulletins of the American College of Obstetricians and Gynecologists Seizure disorders in pregnancy. Int J Gynecol Obstet 1997;56:279–86.
[80] Srinivasan G, Seeler RA, Tiruvury A, Pildes RS. Maternal anticonvulsant therapy and hemorrhagic disease of the newborn. Obstet Gynecol 1982;59:250–2.
[81] Yerby MS. Quality of life, epilepsy advances, and the evolving role of anticonvulsants in women with epilepsy. Neurology 2000;55:21–31.
[82] Report of the Quality Standards Subcommittee of the American Academy of Neurology Practice parameter: management issues for women with epilepsy (summary statement). Neurology 1998;51:944–8.
[83] Yerby MS, Kaplan P, Tran T. Risks and management of pregnancy in women with epilepsy. Cleve Clin J Med 2004;71(Suppl. 2):S25–37.
[84] Lenfant C, Gifford RW, Zuspan FP. Report of the national high blood pressure education program working froup on high blood pressure in pregnancy. Am J Obstet Gynecol 1990;163:1691–712.
[85] Sibai BM. Diagnosis, prevention, and management of eclampsia. Obstet Gynecol 2005;105(2):402–10.
[86] Cunningham FG, MacDonald PC, Gant NF, Leveno KJ, Gilstrap III LC. Hypertensive disorders in pregnancy Williams obstetrics. 19th ed. Norwalk, CT: Appleton & Lange; 1993. p. 763–817.
[87] Douglas KA, Redman CW. Eclampsia in the United Kingdom. Br Med J 1994; 309(6966):1395–400.
[88] Anteby EY, Greenfield C, Natanson-Yaron S, Goldman-Wohl D, Hamani Y, Khudyak V, et al. Vascular endothelial growth factor, epidermal growth factor and fibroblast growth factor-4 and -10 stimulate trophoblast plasminogen activator system and metalloproteinase-9. Mol Hum Reprod 2004;10(4):229–35.
[89] ACOG Committee on Practice Bulletins—Obstetrics. ACOG practice bulletin. Diagnosis and management of preeclampsia and eclampsia. Obstet Gynecol 2002;99(1): 159–67.

[90] Khong TY, DeWolf F, Robertson WB, Brosens I. Inadequate maternal vascular response to placentation in pregnancies complicated by pre-eclampsia and by small-for-gestation age infants. Br J Obstet Gynecol 1986;93:1049–59.
[91] Lyall F. Priming and remodeling of human placental bed spiral arteries during pregnancy— a review. Placenta 2005;26(Suppl. A):S31–36.
[92] Moffett A, Hilby SE. How does the maternal immune system contribute to the development of pre-eclampsia? Placenta 2007;28(Suppl. A):S51–56.
[93] Huppertz B, Hemmings D, Renaud SJ, Bulmer JN, Dash P, Chamley LW. Extravillous trophoblast apoptosis—a workshop report. Placenta 2005;26(Suppl. A):S46–48.
[94] Cipolla MJ, Vitullo L, Delance N, Hammer E. The cerebral endothelium during pregnancy: a potential role in the development of eclampsia. Endothelium 2005;12(1–2):5–9.
[95] Donaldson JO. Eclampsia. In: Devinsky O, Feldman E, Hainline B, editors. Neurological complications of pregnancy. New York, NY: Raven Press; 1994. p. 25–33.
[96] Garg RK. Posterior leukoencephalopathy syndrome. Postgrad Med J 2001;77(903):24–8.
[97] Roberts JM. Magnesium for pre-eclampsia and eclampsia. N Engl J Med 1995;333:250–1.
[98] Thomas SV, Somanathan N, Radhakumari R, Interictal EEG. Changes in eclampsia. Electroencephalogr Clin Neurophysiol 1995;94:271–5.
[99] Sibai BM, Spinnato JA, Watson DL, Lewis JA, Anderson GD. Effect of magnesium sulfate on electroencephalographic findings in pre-eclampsia-eclampsia. Obstet Gynecol 1984;64:261–6.
[100] Levine RJ, Thadhani R, Quian C, Lam C, Lim KH, Yu KF, et al. Urinary placental growth factor and the risk of pre-eclampsia. JAMA 2005;293:77–85.
[101] Sibai BM, Spinnato JA, Watson DL, Lewis JA, Anderson GD. Eclampsia IV. neurological findings and future outcome. Am J Obstet Gynecol 1985;152:184–92.
[102] Morris JA. Effect of magnesium sulfate on electroencephalographic findings in preeclampsia–eclampsia. Obstet Gynecol 1985;65:859–60.
[103] Zeeman GG, Fleckenstein JL, Twickler DM, Cunningham FG. Cerebral infarction in eclampsia. Am J Obstet Gynecol 2004;190(3):714–20.
[104] Fugate JE, Claassen DO, Cloft HJ, Kallmes DF, Kozak OS, Rabinstein AA. Posterior reversible encephalopathy syndrome: associated clinical and radiologic findings. Mayo Clin Proc 2010;85:427–32.
[105] Loureiro R, Leite CC, Kahhale S, Freire S, Sousa B, Cardoso EF, et al. Diffusion imaging may predict reversible brain lesions in eclampsia and severe eclampsia: initial experience. Am J Obstet Gynecol 2003;189:1350–5.
[106] Anonymous Which anticonvulsant for women with eclampsia? Evidence from the collaborative eclampsia trial. Lancet 1995;345(8963):1455–63.
[107] Lucas MJ, Leveno KJ, Cunningham FG. A comparison of magnesium sulfate with phenytoin for the prevention of eclampsia. N Engl J Med 1995;333:201–5.
[108] Lipton SA, Rosenberg PA. Excitatory amino acids as a final common pathway for neurologic disorders. N Engl J Med 1994;330:613–22.
[109] Euser AG, Cipolla MJ. Magnesium sulfate for the treatment of eclampsia: a brief review. Stroke 2009;40(4):1169–75.
[110] Mason BA, Standley CA, Irtenkauf SM, Bardicef M, Cotton DB. Magnesium is more efficacious then phenytoin in reducing *N*-methyl-D-aspartate (NMDA) seizures in rats. Am J Obstet Gynecol 1994;171:999–1002.
[111] Altman D, Carroli G, Duley L, Farrell B, Moodley J, Neilson J, et al. Do women with preeclampsia, and their babies, benefit from magnesium sulphate? The Magpie trial: a randomised placebo-controlled trial. Lancet 2002;359(9321):1877–90.

[112] Belfort MA, Anthony J, Saade GR, Allen Jr. JC, Nimodipine Study Group A comparison of magnesium sulfate and nimodipine for the prevention of eclampsia. N Engl J Med 2003;348(4):304–11.
[113] Isler CM, Barrilleau PS, Rinehart BK, Magann EF, Martin JN Jr. Postpartum seizure prophylaxis: using maternal clinical parameters to guide therapy. Obstet Gynecol 2003;101(1):66–9.
[114] Fontenot MT, Lewis DF, Frederick JB, Wang Y, DeFranco EA, Groome LJ, et al. A prospective randomized trial of magnesium sulfate in severe preeclampsia: use of diuresis as a clinical parameter to determine the duration of postpartum therapy. Am J Obstet Gynecol 2005;192(6):1788–93.
[115] Teramo K, Hiilesmaa V. Pregnancy and fetal complications in epileptic pregnancies: review of the literature. In: Janz D, dam M, editors. Epilepsy pregnancy, and the child. New York, NY: Raven Press; 1982. p. 53–9.
[116] Yi-Hua C, Hung-Yi C, Herng-Ching L, Hsiu-Li L. Affect of seizures during gestation on pregnancy outcomes in women with epilepsy. Archiv Neurol 2009;66(8):979–84.
[117] Harden C. Commentary on affect of seizures during gestation on pregnancy outcomes in women with epilepsy. Epilepsy Curr 2010;10(2):40–1.
[118] Hsiu-Li L, Yi-Hua C, Hsiu-Chen L, Herng-Ching L. No increase in adverse pregnancy outcomes for women receiving antiepileptic drugs. J Neurol 2009;256:1742–9.
[119] Meadow SR. Anticonvulsant drugs and congenital abnormalities. Lancet 1968;2:1296.
[120] Yerby M, Devinsky O. Advances in neurological complications of pregnancy. In: Devinsky O, Feldmanne , Hainline B, editors. Epilepsy and pregnancy. New York, NY: Raven Press; 1994. p. 45–63.
[121] Hansen JW, Myrianthopoulos NC, Harvery MA, Smith DW. Risks to the offspring of women treated with hydantoin anticonvulsants, with emphasis on the fetal hydantoin syndrome. J Pediat 1976;89:662–8.
[122] Yerby MS, Collins SD. Teratogenicity of antiepileptic drugs. In: Wylie E, editor. The treatment of epilepsy: principles and practice. Baltimore, MD: Williams and Wilkins; 1997. p. 785–98.
[123] Desmond MM, Schwanecke RP, Wilson GS, Yasunaga S, Burgdorff I. Maternal barbiturate utilization and neonatal withdrawal symptomatology. J Pediat 1972;80:190–7.
[124] Omtzigt JG, Los FJ, Grobee DE, Pijpers L, Jahoda MG, Brandenburg H, et al. The risk of spina bifida aperta after first-trimester exposure to valproate in a prenatal cohort. Neurology 1992;42:119–25.
[125] Bromfield EB, Dworetsky BA, Wyszinski DF, Smith CR, Baldwin EJ, Holmes LB. Valproate teratogenicity and epilepsy syndrome. Epilepsia 2008;49(12):2122–4.
[126] Meador KJ, Baker GA, Browning N, Clayton-Smith J, Combs-Cantrell DT, Cohen M, et al. Cognitive function at 3 years of age after fetal exposure to antiepileptic drugs. N Engl J Med 2009;360(16):1597–605.
[127] Yerby MS. Teratogenicity of anticonvulsant medication. In: Pellock JM, Dodson WE, Bourgeois BF, editors. Pediatric epilepsy: diagnosis and therapy. 2nd ed. New York, NY: Demos Medical Publishing Co; 2001. p. 357–72.
[128] Pacifici GM, Colizzi C, Giuliani L, Rane A. Cytosolic epoxide hydrolase in fetal and adult human liver. Archiv Toxicol 1983;54:331–41.
[129] Spielberg SP, Gordon GB, Blade DA, Mellits ED, Bross DS. Anticonvulsant toxicity in vitro: possible role of arene oxides. J Pharmacol Exp Ther 1981;217:386–9.
[130] Buehler BA, Delimont D, van Waes M, Finnell RH. Prenatal prediction of risk of the fetal hydantoin syndrome. N Engl J Med 1990;322:1567–72.

[131] Bittigau P, Sifringer M, Ikonomidou C. Antiepileptic drugs and apoptosis in the developing brain. Ann N Y Acad Sci 2003;993:103–14.

[132] Kim J, Kondratyev A, Gale K. Antiepileptic drug induced neuronal cell death in the immature brain: effects of carbamazepine, topiramate, and levetiracetam as monotherapy versus polytherapy. J Pharmacol Exp Ther 2007;323:165–73.

[133] Moroney JT, Allen MH. Cocaine and alcohol use in pregnancy. Adv Neurol 1994;64:231–42.

[134] Schwartz RB. Neurodiagnostic imaging of the pregnant patient. In: Devinsky O, Feldmann E, Hainline B, editors. Neurological complications of pregnancy. New York, NY: Raven Press; 1994. p. 243–8.

[135] Wilterdink JL, Easton HD. Cerebral ischemia. In: Devinsky O, Feldmann E, Hainline B, editors. Neurological complications of pregnancy. New York, NY: Raven Press; 1994. p. 1–11.

[136] Evevoldson T, Ross RR. Cerebral venous thrombosis: new causes for an old syndrome. Q J Med 1990;77:1255–75.

[137] Evans RW, Rozen TD, Mechtler LL. Neuroimaging and and other diagnostic testing in headache. In: Silberstein SD, Lipton RB, Dodick DW, editors. Wolff's headache and other head pain. 8th ed. New York: Oxford University Press; 2008. p. 86.

[138] Wilterdink JL, Feldmann E. Cerebral hemorrhage. In: Devinsky O, Feldmann E, Hainline B, editors. Neurological complications of pregnancy. New York, NY: Raven Press; 1994. p. 13–23.

[139] Gall SA. Maternal adjustments in the immune system in normal pregnancy. Clin Obstet Gynecol 1983;26:521–36.

[140] Johnson RT. Infections during pregnancy. In: Devinsky O, Feldmann E, Hainline B, editors. Neurological complications of pregnancy. New York, NY: Raven Press; 1994. p. 153–62.

[141] Lockwood CJ, Romero R, Feinberg RF, Clyne LP, Coster B, Hobbins JC. The prevalence and biologic significance of lupus anticoagulant and anticardiolipin antibodies in a general obstetric population. Am J Obstet Gynecol 1989;161:369–73.

[142] Vining E. Another nail in the coffin. Epilepsy Curr 2010;10(3):53–4.

[143] Morrell M. Guidelines for the care of women with epilepsy. Neurology 1998;51 (Suppl. 5):S21–27.

7 Movement Disorders and Pregnancy

Natalya Shneyder, Aimee Borazanci, Aronkumar Reddy, Emil Gaitour, Alireza Minagar, Stephen L. Jaffe

Department of Neurology, Louisiana State University Health Sciences Center, Shreveport, LA, USA

Introduction

Co-occurrence of pregnancy and movement disorders is uncommon and poses a significant therapeutic challenge for the treating physician. The existing data regarding the effects of pregnancy on various movement disorders remains limited. Additionally, many medications that are used for the treatment of movement disorders should be stopped before pregnancy to avoid teratogenicity. Pregnancy may uncover a pre-existing movement disorder tendency such as for the development of chorea, or pregnant patients may develop chorea gravidarum (CG). Moreover, pregnancy can have variable effects on the clinical manifestations of such movement disorders as Parkinson's disease (PD). A detailed review of the latest knowledge concerning pregnancy and movement disorders follows.

Parkinson's Disease

PD was initially described by James Parkinson [1] in his famous essay on the "shaking palsy." PD is a progressive neurodegenerative disease that clinically presents with rigidity, resting tremor, bradykinesia, flexed posture, and loss of corrective postural reflexes. Certain clinical manifestations assist clinicians in differentiating PD from other parkinsonian syndromes. Prominent resting tremor, significant therapeutic response to levodopa/carbidopa, initial asymmetry of the basal ganglia manifestations, and minimal imbalance at the early stages of the disease favor a diagnosis of PD. Among the salient clinical features of PD, resting tremor is the most common and affects up to 70% of patients. Other prominent motor symptoms consist of bradykinesia and cogwheel rigidity. Postural instability associated with loss of corrective postural reflexes occurs at later stages of the disease and is a significant cause of falls. Gait disorder is another significant PD feature and is often associated with falls; and gait dysfunction constitutes one of the most disabling features of PD. Postural instability in PD patients is the end product of a number of basal ganglia manifestations including rigidity, akinesia, loss of corrective reflexes, and impairment of postural adjustment.

Neurological Disorders and Pregnancy. DOI: 10.1016/B978-0-12-384911-3.00007-5

Patients with PD suffer from neurobehavioral abnormalities such as depression, sleep disturbances, dementia, and drug-induced hallucinations. Other abnormalities such as restless legs syndrome (RLS), sensory complaints, and akathesia also occur. Autonomic dysfunction including orthostatic hypotension, erectile dysfunction, constipation, urinary incontinence, and thermal dysregulation frequently affect these patients [2,3]. Other PD nonmotor impairments include fatigue, seborrheic dermatitis, and weight loss. PD patients also develop expressionless facies ("masked facies"), hypophonia, and drooling.

Males with PD outnumber females by a ratio of 2:1, and the disease typically develops in the sixth or seventh decade. A small group of patients develop PD before the age of 50. Women usually develop PD at an older age than men, and usually the milder tremor form predominates. The etiologic pathophysiology and curative treatment remains elusive. Neuropathologic examination of the brains of PD patients has revealed selective and severe loss of melanin-containing neurons with intraneuronal Lewy body formation primarily occurring in the ventrolateral section of the pars compacta of the substantia nigra. Lewy bodies contain alpha-synuclein, ubiquitin, and Torsin A [4–6].

Treatment of PD involves symptomatic management of motor and nonmotor manifestations. The available medications include levodopa/carbidopa, dopamine agonists, amantadine, catechol-*O*-methyl transferase (COMT) inhibitors, a combination of levodopa/carbidopa with COMT, and anticholinergics. The dopamine agonists (bromocriptine, pergolide, pramipexole, and ropinirole) are used as either monotherapy in early PD especially in younger patients or as adjunctive therapy with levodopa formulations. COMT inhibitors are used together with carbidopa/levodopa to extend levodopa's half-life and to decrease serum level fluctuations. Anticholinergics are primarily used to reduce tremor.

Cases of pregnancy in the context of PD are rare, and there is not much data concerning the course of the disease through either the pregnancy or the postpartum period. The mechanisms of interaction between pregnancy and PD pathophysiology remain unknown. However, the alteration of medication pharmacokinetics secondary to volume and metabolic changes during pregnancy, as well as the physiologic changes in female hormone levels (i.e., estrogen and progesterone), have been proposed to explain the impact of pregnancy on PD [7,8]. A number of studies have reported worsening of PD during pregnancy [8,9], while others report stabilization of the disease [9–12], or even improvement of the clinical picture [13–15]. Based on the available literature, it appears that in most cases, PD progresses during pregnancy, and this is reflected by the increased severity of the clinical manifestations including deterioration of the Unified Parkinson's Disease Rating Scale (UPDRS) score and the need to increase the dosage of symptomatic medication [7,8,13,16–23]. Additionally, after pregnancy, the patient may not return to her prepregnancy PD symptomatic baseline [8].

Because cases of pregnancy in patients with PD are uncommon, there is not much data in the literature concerning the safety of antiparkinsonian drugs during pregnancy, and much of this data is controversial. Most of the medications that are used for the treatment of PD are denoted "pregnancy class C" because the animal or human data for their teratogenicity potential is not available. Among the medications used for the treatment of PD, amantadine definitely should not be administered during pregnancy. Deep brain stimulation (DBS) is used for the treatment of dystonia as well as PD (see treatment section under dystonia).

In conclusion, patients with PD who plan to become pregnant should be advised of the risk of progression, the possibility of the need to increase PD medication dosage, the possibility of not returning to the prepregnancy PD disease baseline, and the lack of scientific data regarding the impact of PD medications on fetal growth and development.

Chorea Gravidarum

Chorea (derived from the Latin word choreus meaning "dance") is a form of movement disorder that consists of irregular, involuntary, brief, and unpredictable movements resulting from continuous flow of random muscle contractions from one body part to another. Pregnancy may uncommonly present with chorea or chorea may develop during pregnancy, a condition known as chorea gravidarum (CG). CG, originally described in 1661 by Horstius [24], is more common among pregnant women who have a prepregnancy history of Sydenham's chorea. CG has been linked to other causes including the immune-mediated conditions of systemic lupus erythematosus and antiphospholipid antibody syndrome [25,26], as well as infectious diseases such as syphilis and encephalitis [27]. Based on the available literature, in those pregnancies affected by CG, clinical manifestations occur after the first trimester in half of pregnant women [28], spontaneously remits in one-third before delivery, and in most cases resolves after delivery [27,28]. The severity of chorea usually improves as the pregnancy advances [27]. In most cases, CG is not a life-threatening condition; however, severe and unrelenting cases may cause hyperthermia, rhabdomyolysis, myoglobulinuria, and even death [28,29]. Only the severe cases of CG that pose a serious threat to either the mother or the fetus require treatment.

In general, the symptomatic treatment of choreiform disorders in the absence of pregnancy consists of the use of dopamine receptor blockers (phenothiazines and butyrophenones), and dopamine-depleting agents such as reserpine. The use of these medications for the treatment of chorea stems from the hypothesis that increased dopaminergic activity in the striatum is etiologic. Dopamine receptor blockers are categorized as pregnancy class C and should not be administered during the first trimester. Despite such warnings, haloperidol and chlorpromazine are useful for the treatment of CG and are safe if used at low doses [30]. The American Academy of Pediatrics recommends haloperidol over the other neuroleptics due to its less severe maternal anticholinergic, hypotensive, and antihistaminergic side effects [30]. Reserpine is a teratogen and contraindicated in pregnancy. Tetrabenazine, which was approved recently in the United States for treatment of chorea in Huntington's disease (HD), is designated pregnancy class C. Therefore, in summary, treatment of CG is indicated only in severe cases, and haloperidol is the neuroleptic of choice during pregnancy.

Huntington's Disease

HD is an autosomal dominant progressive neurodegenerative disorder with complete penetrance. It is clinically characterized by the triad of movement disorder (mainly chorea), cognitive decline, and psychiatric disorder including depression, apathy, irritability, and personality changes. HD is linked to an unstable polymorphic trinucleotide repeat unit (CAG that codes for the amino acid, glutamine) in the Huntington gene, and was identified in 1983 [31]. The Huntington gene is located on chromosome 4, and huntingtin is the gene protein product although its function is unknown. The number of CAG repeats is an important determinant of the age of onset, and patients with the Westphal variant (juvenile onset disease with rigidity) carry a high number of CAG repeats. Except for this group of patients, the clinical symptoms appear in the fourth and fifth decades. Therefore, most patients with HD manifest symptoms well beyond their childbearing years, and currently, most neurologists are more concerned about genetic counseling and antenatal exclusion testing for presymptomatic, at-risk individuals who can potentially become pregnant. A major reason for genetic counseling is the fact that the ability of HD patients to provide ongoing care for their children can be a significant problem. Therefore, this needs to be discussed with at-risk individuals when the issue of pregnancy is raised. There are no significant concerns about the impact of HD on the actual pregnancy or delivery.

Currently, HD is incurable and its treatment is individualized and only symptomatic. Chorea is treated with antidopaminergic agents or dopamine depletors, and depression is managed with antidepressants. In general, neuroleptics are contraindicated during pregnancy; however if the clinical manifestations are severe, high-potency agents are recommended [32]. For treatment of HD-associated depression, tricyclic antidepressants, for example, nortriptyline and desipramine, are the preferred agents [30].

Dystonia

Dystonia is a hyperkinetic movement disorder characterized by involuntary repetitive motor contractions frequently causing twisting movements or abnormal postures. Dystonia is the product of co-contraction of agonist and antagonist muscles [33]. Because dystonia is a heterogeneous condition, it can be classified based on the age of onset, anatomic distribution, and etiology (primary versus secondary). Dystonia demonstrates a bimodal age of onset with early onset cases (age 9) mainly in genetically inherited dystonias and late onset (age 45) in sporadic cases [34]. Clinically, dystonia has a range of presentations from generalized and disabling contractions which are more frequent in those patients with childhood onset, to more localized and focal contractions which are usually observed with adult-onset forms mainly affecting cervical muscles (torticollis), the arm (writer's cramp), or cranial muscles (blepharospam). Primary or idiopathic dystonia is a form of dystonia with no other additional neurological abnormalities of an underlying neurodegenerative or acquired disease. Secondary dystonia (also known as symptomatic dystonia) is associated with other illnesses and includes inherited forms such as dystonia plus syndromes, toxic and acquired causes (stroke, drugs), and dystonia associated with degenerative parkinsonian disorders.

Acute drug-induced dystonic reactions commonly occur during pregnancy as a number of medications (such as metocloperamide, promethazine, and prochlorperazine) used for treatment of nausea and vomiting associated with the first trimester of pregnancy (such as metocloperamide, promethazine, and prochlorperazine) are associated with such adverse reactions. In general, all dopamine antagonists may acutely generate extrapyramidal manifestations including dystonic-dyskinetic movement disorders. While most of these acute dystonic reactions last a short time and resolve spontaneously, cases of death after dystonic reactions have been reported [35]. Dystonia gravidarum describes dystonia that arises during pregnancy without any obvious cause and usually resolves before or shortly after delivery [36].

A number of case reports have addressed the impact of pregnancy on existing dystonia [37,38]. Gwinn-Hardy et al. [37] assessed the effect(s) of female hormonal variations on the severity of dystonia. The investigators surveyed 279 women with dystonia at Mayo Clinic Scottsdale over a 6-year period, of whom 204 responded. The participants were asked questions about their reproductive and menstrual histories and dystonia severity with emphasis on deteriorating or relieving factors. Most of the women did not report any consistent effect on dystonia severity. However, of the 62 premenopausal women with dystonia, 27 reported at least one pregnancy since the dystonia onset. Only four women described alterations in their clinical manifestations during pregnancy.

Dopaminergic agents, principally levodopa, are used for treatment of cases of dopamine-responsive dystonia. While levodopa has not been formally assigned to pregnancy class, levodopa/carbidopa has been assigned to pregnancy class C by the Federal Drug Administration (FDA).

Botulinum toxin A (Botox) and B (Myobloc) injections are used for treatment of focal dystonias. Currently, there is not sufficient clinical data from controlled human clinical trials regarding the treatment of pregnant patients with these forms of botulinum toxins. So far, Myobloc has not been connected to fetal harm in humans but is assigned as pregnancy class C. Botox has been given to pregnant mice and rats [39] during organogenesis and at high doses was associated with low birth weights and delayed ossification.

DBS is used for the treatment of dystonia and PD. Paluzzi et al. [40] reported three patients with dystonia who became pregnant after insertion of bilateral globus pallidus internus stimulators and completed the pregnancies successfully with vaginal delivery of healthy children. DBS does not pose any risks to pregnant women during investigation by routine ultrasound or fetal monitoring.

Essential Tremor

Essential tremor (ET) is one of the most common movement disorders encountered in neurology clinics, and is characterized by involuntary rhythmic movements of fingers, hands, and forearms as a result of alternating contractions of flexor and extensor muscles at approximately 6 Hz. ET has an estimated prevalence ranging from 0.4% to 4.8% [41], and its incidence dramatically increases with age [42]. Patients with ET usually have a positive family history with the inheritance pattern appearing to be autosomal dominant with incomplete penetrance. Several candidate genes have been identified which include FET1 and ETM2 [43,44], and LINGO 1 [45]. Head, legs, and voice may be involved. Tremor is characterized as either postural (occurring with maintenance of posture) or kinetic (occurring or increased during target-oriented movements). Tremor ranges from mild to severe, and can interfere with most daily living activities including food intake [46]. Patients usually seek medical treatment when the tremor is moderate to severe.

Currently, there is no cure for ET, but there are several very effective symptomatic treatments. Both pharmacologic and nonpharmacologic modalities are available. Mild tremor is usually not treated. Propranolol and primidone are the most widely used medications. Both are usually well tolerated, and medically as well as cost effective. Second-line drugs include gabapentin, topiramate, nimodipine, clozapine, and clonidine [47]. Botulinum toxin injections can be very effective in skilled hands [48]. Thalamotomy and thalamic DBS are surgical procedures that have been shown to be effective in severe limb tremor not responsive to pharmacologic treatment, or when medication side effects are intolerable. But the risk of complications such as hemorrhage, infection, and dysarthria should be carefully considered.

There is not much data concerning management, prevalence, or development of ET during pregnancy in the literature. The drug primidone is listed as pregnancy category D; propranolol, topiramate, and gabapentin are designated pregnancy category C. There are several animal studies that have shown the potential teratogenicity of topiramate. Therefore, the general recommendation would be to avoid pharmacologic treatment of ET during pregnancy if possible. Women of childbearing age diagnosed with ET should be advised about the possible teratogenic effects of available drugs [49].

Wilson's Disease

Wilson's disease (WD), also known as hepatolenticular degeneration, is a rare autosomal recessive neurodegenerative disorder associated with abnormal copper metabolism and excessive deposition of copper in the liver, brain, and cornea. Clinically, WD manifests with neuropsychiatric and hepatic abnormalities. Mutations in the WD gene located in the 13q chromosomal region produces an abnormal ATP7B protein/enzyme that is a P-type copper-transporting ATPase [50–52]. The age of onset of WD clinical manifestations ranges from the first to fifth decade, and many patients are thus in the childbearing age-range. Pregnancy does not have any significant effect on the clinical course or clinical manifestations of WD; however, the disease itself may increase the chance of miscarriage.

Sinha et al. [53] performed a retrospective analysis of data from a large cohort of patients with both treated and untreated WD in order to evaluate the various aspects of fertility in 16 women with WD. This series of 16 patients had conceived on 59 occasions and had 30 successful pregnancies, 24 spontaneous abortions, 2 medical terminations, and 3 stillbirths. Recurrent abortions were more frequent among pregnant patients with untreated WD. According to these authors, pregnancy did not affect WD adversely, and teratogenicity was not observed in this patient series treated with low-dose penicillamine and zinc sulfate. The authors also hypothesized that uterine copper deposition impairs embryonic implantation, and injury to other organs secondary to abnormal copper metabolism may play a role in this process. Treatment of WD includes chelation therapy using D-penicillamine, trientine, and tetrathiomolybdate. While Sinha et al. [53] did not report teratogenicity when using low-dose D-penicillamine in their pregnant patients, others have reported D-penicillamine and trientine teratogenicity [54,55]. Therefore, pregnant women with WD should probably be treated solely with zinc, as teratogenicity has not been reported with this pharmacologic.

Restless Legs Syndrome

RLS, also known as Ekbom syndrome, is the most frequent movement disorder associated with pregnancy and affects up to 23% of pregnancies, usually in the third trimester [56]. Clinically, RLS is characterized by the presence of paresthesias or dysesthesias occurring mainly in the lower extremities associated with an irresistible urge to move the legs. As a result, RLS often produces sleep-onset insomnia [57]. The symptoms of RLS are typically relieved by activity and increased by rest. Genetic variants in four chromosomal regions have been recognized to increase the risk of developing RLS. Increase in the frequency of RLS during pregnancy may be due to the physiologic, hormonal, and anatomic changes associated with pregnancy [58]. Manconi et al. [59] performed a large and comprehensive epidemiologic study of RLS during pregnancy and the puerperium. The authors reported that RLS first appeared or increased in severity during the third trimester of pregnancy, followed by remission of clinical manifestations during the ninth month or after delivery. The authors concluded that pregnancy is associated with transient RLS.

Tourette's Syndrome

Tourette's syndrome (TS) is a chronic and relatively common movement disorder clinically characterized by motor and vocal tics as well as behavioral disorders. TS begins before age 18 and is commonly associated with obsessive–compulsive disorder and attention-deficit hyperactivity disorder. Because many tics are initiated and fixed in childhood or adolescence and improve with age, some women with TS are in the childbearing age-range. However, because TS is more common in men, current knowledge concerning this movement disorder and pregnancy is limited. Existing clinical observations suggest that tics are not aggravated by pregnancy. Schwabe and Konkol [60] conducted a survey of 47 women of all ages with TS. Twenty-six percent of surveyed women reported premenstrual aggravation of tics, indicating a hormonal effect. However, pregnancy was not associated with a change in tic frequency. In another retrospective study of 8 women with TS including 11 pregnancies, Stern et al. [61] found no adverse impact on the pregnancies, and improvement of TS clinical manifestations were reported during five of the pregnancies. In three pregnancies, symptoms deteriorated; and in three pregnancies, there were no changes.

Tics in patients with TS are treated with neuroleptics such as haloperidol, pimozide, and resperidol. In general, neuroleptics should not be used during pregnancy. However, haloperidol is recommended by the American Academy of Pediatrics despite its association with extrapyramidal presentations in the neonate [30].

Conclusions

Our knowledge about the relationship between movement disorders and pregnancy is mainly anecdotal. However based on the existing literature, it appears that with the exception of RLS and CG, movement disorders are uncommon during pregnancy. Pharmacologic treatment of pregnant patients with movement disorders is a major challenge for the treating neurologist. Familiarity with side effects of the utilized medications as well as their potential for teratogenicity is imperative. Presently due to the paucity of systematic studies on this subject, many questions remain about the management of these patients. Therefore, any therapeutic decisions for pregnant patients with movement disorders become an individualized process, resting on the treating neurologist's clinical judgment and familiarity with the effects of utilized pharmacological agents as determined from both human and animal studies.

References

[1] Parkinson J. An essay on the shaking palsy. Med Classics 1817;10(2):964–97.
[2] Mathers SE, Kempster PA, Law PJ, Frankel JP, Bartram CI, Lees AJ, et al. Anal sphincter dysfunction in Parkinson's disease. Arch Neurol 1989;46(10):1061–4.
[3] Martignoni E, Micieli G, Cavallini A, Pacchetti C, Magri M, Nappi G. Autonomic disorders in idiopathic parkinsonism. J Neural Transm Suppl 1986;22:149–61.
[4] Andersen JK. What causes the build-up of ubiquitin-containing inclusions in Parkinson's disease? Mech Ageing Dev 2000;118(1–2):15–22.
[5] Lücking CB, Brice A. Alpha-synuclein and Parkinson's disease. Cell Mol Life Sci 2000;57:1894–908.
[6] Shashidharan P, Good PF, Hsu A, Perl DP, Brin MF, Olanow CW. Torsin A accumulation in Lewy bodies in sporadic Parkinson's disease. Brain Res 2000;877:379–81.
[7] Robottom BJ, Mullins RJ, Shulman LM. Pregnancy in Parkinson's disease: case report and discussion. Expert Rev Neurother 2008;8:1799–805.
[8] Shulman LM, Minagar A, Weiner WJ. The effect of pregnancy in Parkinson's disease. Mov Disord 2000;15:132–5.
[9] Hagell P, Odin P, Vinge E. Pregnancy in Parkinson's disease: a review of the literature and a case report. Mov Disord 1998;13:34–8.

[10] Ball MC, Sagar HJ. Levodopa in pregnancy. Mov Disord 1995;10:115.
[11] Benito-Leon J, Bermejo F, Porta-Etessam J. Pregnancy in Parkinson's disease: a review of the literature and a case report. Mov Disord 1999;14:194.
[12] Cook DG, Klawans HL. Levodopa during pregnancy. Clin Neuropharmacol 1985; 8:93–5.
[13] Golbe LI. Parkinson's disease and pregnancy. Neurology 1987;37:1245–9.
[14] De Mari M, Zenzola A, Lamberti P. Antiparkinsonian treatment in pregnancy. Mov Disord 2002;17:428–9.
[15] Kupsch A, Oertel WH. Selegiline, pregnancy, and Parkinson's disease. Mov Disord 1998;13:175–6.
[16] Allain H, Bentue-Ferrer D, Milon D, Moran P, Jacquemard F, Defawe G. Pregnancy and parkinsonism. A case report without problem. Clin Neuropharmacol 1989;12:217–9.
[17] Gershanik OS, Leist A. Juvenile onset Parkinson's disease. Adv Neurol 1987;45: 213–6.
[18] Jacquemard F, Palaric JC, Allain H, Giraud JR. Parkinson disease and pregnancy. Apropos of a case. J Gynecol Obstet Biol Reprod (Paris) 1990;19:461–3.
[19] Kanzato N, Nishihira T, Murao H, Takara H. Case of juvenile parkinsonism in pregnancy. Rinsho Shinkeigaku 2006;46:400–3.
[20] Routiot T, Lurel S, Denis E, Barbarino-Monnier P. Parkinson's disease and pregnancy: case report and literature review. J Gynecol Obstet Biol Reprod (Paris) 2000;29:454–7.
[21] Scott M, Chowdhury M. Pregnancy in Parkinson's disease: unique case report and review of the literature. Mov Disord 2005;20:1078–9.
[22] Tobiassen C, Brasso K, Kohler OM. Pregnancy and Parkinson disease. Ugeskr Laeger 1991;153:1210–1.
[23] Bauherz G. Pregnancy and Parkinson's disease: a case report. New Trends Clin Neuropharmacol 1994;8:142.
[24] Wilson P, Preece AA. Chorea gravidarum. Arch Inten Med 1932;49:471–533.
[25] Wolf RE, McBeath JG. Chorea gravidarum in systemic lupus erythematosus. J Rheumatol 1985;12:992–3.
[26] Mujic F, Cuadrado MJ, Lloyd M, Khamashta MA, Page G, Hughes GR. Primary antiphospholipid syndrome evolving into systemic lupus erythematosus. J Rheumatol 1995;22:1589–92.
[27] Cardoso F. Chorea gravidarum. Arch Neurol 2002;59:868–70.
[28] Donaldson JO. Neurologic emergencies in pregnancy. Obstet Gynecol Clin North Am 1991;18:199–212.
[29] Ichikawa K, Kim RC, Givelber H, Collins GH. Chorea gravidarum. Report of a fatal case with neuropathological observations. Arch Neurol 1980;37:429–32.
[30] American Academy of Pediatrics Committee on Drugs Use of psychoactive medication during pregnancy and possible side effects on the fetus and the newborn. Pediatrics 2000;105:880–7.
[31] Gusella JF, Wexler NS, Conneally PM, Naylor SL, Anderson MA, Tanzi RE, et al. A polymorphic DNA marker genetically linked to Huntington's disease. Nature 1983;306:234–8.
[32] Altshuler LL, Szuba MP. Course of psychiatric disorders in pregnancy. Dilemmas in pharmacologic management. Neurol Clin 1994;12:613–35.
[33] Fahn S. Concept and classification of dystonia. Adv Neurol 1998;50:1–8.
[34] Bressman SB, de Leon D, Brin MF, Risch N, Burke RE, Greene PE, et al. Idiopathic dystonia among Ashkenazi Jews: evidence for autosomal dominant inheritance. Ann Neurol 1989;26:612–20.

[35] Bateman DN, Rawlins MD, Simpson JM. Extrapyramidal reactions with metoclopramide. Br Med J (Clin Res Ed) 1985;291:930–2.
[36] Lim EC, Seet RC, Wilder-Smith EP, Ong BK. Dystonia gravidarum: a new entity? Mov Disord 2006;21:69–70.
[37] Gwinn-Hardy KA, Adler CH, Weaver AL, Fish NM, Newman SJ. Effect of hormone variations and other factors on symptom severity in women with dystonia. Mayo Clin Proc 2000;75:235–40.
[38] Rogers JD, Fahn S. Movement disorders and pregnancy. In: Devinsky O, editor. Advances in neurology, vol. 64: Neurological complications of pregnancy. New York: Raven Press; 1994. p. 163–78.
[39] Botox® [package insert]. Irvine, CA: Allergan Inc.; 2010.
[40] Paluzzi A, Bain PG, Liu X, Yianni J, Kumarendran K, Aziz TZ. Pregnancy in dystonic women with in situ deep brain stimulators. Mov Disord 2006;21:695–8.
[41] Lorenz D, Deuschl G. Update on pathogenesis and treatment of essential tremor. Curr Opin Neurol 2007;20:447–52.
[42] Elble RJ. Diagnostic criteria for essential tremor and differential diagnosis. Neurology 2000;54(11 Suppl. 4):S2–6.
[43] Glucher JR, Jónsson P, Kong A, Kristjánsson K, Frigge ML, Karason A, et al. Mapping of a familial essential tremor gene, FET1, to chromosome 3q13. Nat Genet 1997;17:84–7.
[44] Higgins JJ, Pho LT, Nee LE. A gene (ETM) for essential tremor maps to chromosome 2p22-p25. Mov Disord 1997;12:859–64.
[45] Stefansson H, Steinberg S, Petursson H, Gustafsson O, Gudjonsdottir IH, Jonsdottir GA, et al. Variant in the sequence of the LINGO1 gene confers risk of essential tremor. Nat Genet 2009;41(3):277–9. Epub 2009 Feb 1. Erratum in: Nat Genet. 2009;41:504.
[46] Bain PG, Findley LJ, Thompson PD, Gresty MA, Rothwell JC, Harding AE, et al. A study of hereditary essential tremor. Brain 1994;117(Pt 4):805–24.
[47] Connor GS. A double blind placebo-controlled trial of topiramate treatment for essential tremor. Neurology 2002;59:132–4.
[48] Zesiewicz TA, Elble R, Louis ED, Hauser RA, Sullivan KL, Dewey RB Jr. et al. Practice parameter: therapies for essential tremor: report of the quality standards subcommittee of the American academy of neurology. Neurology 2005;64:2008–20.
[49] Bordelon Y, Smith M. Movement disorders in pregnancy. Semin Neurol 2007;27:467–75.
[50] Bull PC, Thomas GR, Rommens JM, Forbes JR, Cox DW. The Wilson disease gene is a putative copper transporting P-type ATPase similar to the Menkes gene. Nat Genet 1993;5:327–37.
[51] Bonné-Tamir B, Frydman M, Agger MS, Bekeer R, Bowcock AM, Hebert JM, et al. Wilson's disease in Israel: a genetic and epidemiological study. Ann Hum Genet 1990;54(Part 2):155–68.
[52] Yamaguchi Y, Heiny ME, Gitlin JD. Isolation and characterization of a human liver cDNA as a candidate gene for Wilson disease. Biochem Biophys Res Commun 1993;197:271–7.
[53] Sinha S, Taly AB, Prashanth LK, Arunodaya GR, Swamy HS. Successful pregnancies and abortions in symptomatic and asymptomatic Wilson's disease. J Neurol Sci 2004;217(1):37–40.
[54] Pinter R, Hogge WA, McPherson E. Infant with severe penicillamine embryopathy born to a woman with Wilson disease. Am J Med Genet A 2004;128A:294–8.

[55] Yalaz M, Aydogdu S, Ozgenc F, Akisu M, Kultursay N, Yagci RV. Transient fetal myelosuppressive effect of D-penicillamine when used in pregnancy. Minerva Pediatr 2003;55:625–8.

[56] Lee KA, Zaffke ME, Baratte-Beebe K. Restless legs syndrome and sleep disturbance during pregnancy: the role of folate and iron. J Womens Health Gend Based Med 2001;10:335–41.

[57] Trenkwalder C, Paulus W. Restless legs syndrome: pathophysiology, clinical presentation and management. Nat Rev Neurol 2010;6:337–46.

[58] Sahota PK, Jain SS, Dhand R. Sleep disorders in pregnancy. Curr Opin Pulm Med 2003;9:477–83.

[59] Manconi M, Govoni V, De Vito A, Economou NT, Cesnik E, Casetta I, et al. Restless legs syndrome and pregnancy. Neurology 2004;63:1065–9.

[60] Schwabe MJ, Konkol RJ. Menstrual cycle-related fluctuations of tics in Tourette syndrome. Pediatr Neurol 1992;8:43–6.

[61] Stern JS, Orth M, Robertson MM. Gilles de la Tourette syndrome in pregnancy: a retrospective series. Obstet Med 2009;2:128–9.

8 Psychiatric Disorders and Pregnancy

Nadejda Alekseeva[1,2], *Rita Horton*[3], *Felix Geller*[3], *Jeanie McGee*[1], *Alireza Minagar*[1]

[1]Department of Neurology, Louisiana State University Health Sciences Center, Shreveport, LA, USA
[2]Overton Brooks VA Medical Center, Shreveport, LA, USA
[3]Department of Psychiatry, Louisiana State University Health Sciences Center, Shreveport, LA, USA

Introduction

During the past two decades the complex interactions among psychiatric disorders and reproductive processes such as menarche, pregnancy, delivery, lactation, and menopause have been elucidated, making more accurate information available for treating physicians and other health care providers who are involved in management of pregnant and breast-feeding psychiatric patients. In general, women are at great risk of developing psychiatric disorders during their reproductive years of life (between ages 18 and 45 years). Therefore, a large number of women may develop a new psychiatric illness or experience worsening of their existing psychiatric disorder during pregnancy or lactation. The two most common psychiatric disorders among women are depression and anxiety disorders. Other less prevalent psychiatric illnesses include schizophrenia, eating disorders, and bipolar disorders (BPD). In general, management of these psychiatric disorders during pregnancy poses a significant challenge to treating psychiatrists and successful treatment outcomes require familiarity with the course of these disorders during pregnancy and thorough knowledge of the potential effects of psychiatric medications on the fetus.

Schizophrenia and Pregnancy

Schizophrenia is a severe and complex mental disorder which includes chronic or relapsing psychotic episodes and long-term compromise of the individual's functional capacity. Schizophrenia affects 1% of individuals worldwide and primarily is characterized by abnormalities in perception or expression of reality. Many female patients with schizophrenia are in their childbearing years. This chronic psychiatric disorder, with typical onset in young adulthood, manifests clinically with severe social withdrawal, auditory hallucinations, disorganized thought process, paranoid and bizarre delusions, and misinterpretation of reality. Diagnostic criteria for schizophrenia are presented in Table 8.1. Psychiatric symptoms of schizophrenia are classified as positive

Neurological Disorders and Pregnancy. DOI: 10.1016/B978-0-12-384911-3.00008-7

Table 8.1 Diagnostic Criteria for Schizophrenia

A. *Characteristic symptoms*: Two (or more) of the following, each present for a significant portion of time during a 1-month period (or less if successfully treated):

1. delusions
2. hallucinations
3. disorganized speech (e.g., frequent derailment or incoherence)
4. grossly disorganized or catatonic behavior
5. negative symptoms, i.e., affective flattening, alogia, or avolition

Note: Only one Criterion A symptom is required if delusions are bizarre or hallucinations consist of a voice keeping up a running commentary on the person's behavior or thoughts, or two or more voices conversing with each other.

B. *Social/occupational dysfunction*: For a significant portion of the time since the onset of the disturbance, one or more major areas of functioning such as work, interpersonal relations, or self-care are markedly below the level achieved before the onset (or when the onset is in childhood or adolescence, failure to achieve expected level of interpersonal, academic, or occupational achievement).

C. *Duration*: Continuous signs of the disturbance persist for at least 6 months. This 6-month period must include at least 1 month of symptoms (or less if successfully treated) that meet Criterion A (i.e., active-phase symptoms) and may include periods of prodromal or residual symptoms. During these prodromal or residual periods, the signs of the disturbance may be manifested by only negative symptoms or two or more symptoms listed in Criterion A present in an attenuated form (e.g., odd beliefs, unusual perceptual experiences).

D. *Schizoaffective and mood disorder exclusion*: Schizoaffective disorder and mood disorder with psychotic features have been ruled out because either (1) no major depressive, manic, or mixed episodes have occurred concurrently with the active-phase symptoms; or (2) if mood episodes have occurred during active-phase symptoms, their total duration has been brief relative to the duration of the active and residual periods.

E. *Substance/general medical condition exclusion*: The disturbance is not due to the direct physiologic effects of a substance (e.g., a drug of abuse, a medication) or a general medical condition.

F. *Relationship to a pervasive developmental disorder*: If there is a history of autistic disorder or another pervasive developmental disorder, the additional diagnosis of schizophrenia is made only if prominent delusions or hallucinations are also present for at least a month (or less if successfully treated).

Classification of longitudinal course (can be applied only after at least one year has elapsed since the initial onset of active-phase symptoms):

Episodic with interepisode residual symptoms (episodes are defined by the re-emergence of prominent psychotic symptoms); also specify if: With prominent negative symptoms

Episodic with no interepisode residual symptoms

Continuous (prominent psychotic symptoms are present throughout the period of observation); also specify if: With prominent negative symptoms

Single episode in partial remission; also specify if: **With prominent negative symptoms**

Single episode in full remission

Other or unspecified pattern

Source: Reprinted with permission from the Diagnostic and Statistical Manual of Mental Disorders, Fourth Edition, Text Revision, © 2000. American Psychiatric Association.

(such as perceiving things which other individuals cannot see or hear) and negative (such as loss of motivation and apathy). Schizophrenic patients also suffer from cognitive decline with impairment of abstract thinking, lack of focus and attention, memory loss, and difficulty with carrying on a meaningful conversation. Other symptoms consist of mood instability, impaired executive function, and impaired language processing. Magnetic resonance imaging of patients with schizophrenia reveals reduction of the volumes of the hippocampus–amygdala complex and parahippocampal gyrus.

Schizophrenia differs in women versus men in various aspects. The risk of schizophrenia may be lower in women [1] and its peak age of onset is later in women with a second smaller peak between 45 and 49 years of age. In addition, women are more likely than men to finish school, start an occupation, and be married with children by the time of clinical diagnosis of schizophrenia. Family histories of schizophrenia and affective disorders are more common among schizophrenic females compared to males [2]. The doses of antipsychotics needed to treat schizophrenic women may be smaller because of the higher females' body fat which accumulates lipophilic antipsychotics and higher blood levels of antipsychotics in women [2].

A significant number of pregnancies in females with schizophrenia are unplanned and unwanted [3]; therefore, these fetuses may already be exposed to mother's poor nutritional status, nicotine, drug abuse, and high concentrations of antipsychotics during the first trimester of pregnancy. In addition, many of these pregnant schizophrenic women are not married and have restricted social support [4]. Studies of the outcome of pregnancy in schizophrenic patients reveal significantly elevated risks of stillbirth, infant death, premature labor, low birth weight, newborns who are small for gestational age, and lower APGAR scores [4–6]. A significant issue about the pregnancy outcome in schizophrenia is that psychosis is harmful to the fetus. Nilsson et al. [5] assessed the pregnancy and birth outcomes in 1438 mothers with schizophrenia and reported higher adverse pregnancy outcomes (which included stillbirth, prematurity, small size for gestation, and death) in women who developed a psychotic attack during pregnancy. Apart from psychosis and its adverse impact on pregnancy and its outcomes, the mother's stress and agitation, particularly during the third trimester, is associated with long-term effect on the baby's hypothalamic–pituitary–adrenal axis [7] and may increase the possibility of congenital malformations [8] and low birth weight [9]. Therefore, when one considers treating pregnant schizophrenic patients, the risks to the fetus in untreated psychosis should be compared to the risks and benefits of using antipsychotics and exposing the fetus to these medications.

Course of Schizophrenia During Pregnancy and Postpartum

The course of schizophrenia during pregnancy varies, and it remains unknown whether physiologic changes associated with pregnancy and lactation alter the course and symptomatology of this chronic psychiatric illness. Therefore, these pregnancies should be regarded as high risk [4]. Women with schizophrenia usually have less contact with psychiatric hospitals and their admission rates during pregnancy are lower compared to periods pre- and postdelivery [10]. Although some patients may experience improvement of their symptoms, others may experience more delusions and psychotically deny the pregnancy and attempt to harm the unborn child [11]. In addition, pregnant women with schizophrenia do not demonstrate a need for smaller doses of maintenance medications [12]. Many schizophrenic women who wish to have children may discontinue their medication(s) abruptly in order to avoid any potential harmful effect of these medications on the fetus. Such a poorly planned disruption in treatment may result in further deterioration of the disease.

While the prevalence of postpartum psychosis in the general population is 1–2 per 1000 childbirths, this rate is 100 times higher in women who suffer from BPD or have a past history of postpartum psychosis [13]. Patients with schizophrenia demonstrate a higher prevalence of postpartum psychosis [14,15]. Within a 6-month period following delivery, 16% of schizophrenic patients are admitted to the hospital due to postpartum psychosis. The etiology of such elevated rates of postpartum psychosis in schizophrenic patients remains unknown; however, an abrupt drop in serum levels of female hormones and increased dopaminergic activity following postpartum estrogen drop may play a pathogenic role [16]. Postpartum psychosis in schizophrenic patients is a psychiatric emergency and hospital admission is necessary to secure the safety of both mother and child. In cases of medication-resistant psychosis or psychosis in a breast-feeding patient electroconvulsive therapy should be considered.

Antipsychotic Medications and Pregnancy

Pregnant women with psychiatric disorders are frequently treated with antipsychotics [17]. Psychotropic medications diffuse across the placenta during pregnancy; therefore, use of antipsychotics during pregnancy is associated with potential teratogenic complications as well as obstetric complications and neurobehavioral and neonatal toxicity [17–19]. Currently, the data on the efficacy and safety of use of antipsychotics during pregnancy is limited. After the launching of the atypical antipsychotics, pregnancy rates in schizophrenic women have increased [17] and despite the paucity of safety data, these medications are being used commonly for treatment of pregnant women with psychosis [17–19]. Practically, the fundamental task for both the treating psychiatrist and psychotic pregnant patient is to weigh the risks versus benefits of treating these patients and protecting the unborn fetus against complications including developmental problems that may arise during infancy. A summary of mechanisms of actions of the atypical and typical antipsychotics are presented in Tables 8.2 and 8.3.

Most of the existing data on the impact of typical antipsychotics on pregnant women stems from their application for treatment of hyperemesis gravidarum. Of course, the required doses for treating this condition are smaller than doses used for treatment of schizophrenia. Altshuler et al. [20] reviewed the literature regarding the effects of prenatal exposure to psychotropic agents on fetal outcome and performed

Table 8.2 Mechanisms of Atypical and Second-Generation Antipsychotic Medications

Medication	Mechanism of Action	Indications	FDA Class	Side Effects
Clozapine	D2 antagonist D4 antagonist 5HT2A antagonist 5HT2C antagonist Alpha 1 antagonist M1 antagonist M3 antagonist H1 antagonist	Schizophrenia Resistant mania TD	B: No teratogenic effect in animals given upto 4 times the human dose	Weight gain Sedation Orthostasis Hypersalivation Agranulocytosis Myocarditis Pulmonary embolism Eosinophilia
Risperidone	D2 antagonist Alpha 1 antagonist	Schizophrenia BPD Irritability in autism	C: Extra-pyramidal symptoms (EPS) and withdrawal symptoms in neonates. Increase in rat stillborns	Orthostasis EPS TD
Olanzapine	D2 antagonist 5HT2A antagonist 5HT2C antagonist Alpha 1 antagonist M1 antagonist M3 antagonist H1 antagonist	Schizophrenia Bipolar mania Acute agitation	C: Decreased fetal viability in animal studies	Sedation Weight gain Orthostasis
Quetiapine	D2 antagonist 5HT2A antagonist NET antagonist 5HT2C antagonist 5HT1A partial agonist H1 antagonist M1 antagonist M3 antagonist	Schizophrenia, bipolar depression, bipolar type II, bipolar mania	C: Increase in fetal pup death with excessive dosage	Sedation Weight gain Cataracts Hyperlipidemia Orthostasis
Ziprasidone	D2 antagonist 5HT2A antagonist 5HT2C antagonist 5HT1D antagonist Serotonin and norepinephrine reuptake inhibition	Schizophrenia BPD	C: Animal studies exhibit toxicity when given small doses compared to humans	Akathesia Dystonia Sedation Orthostasis
Aripiprazole	D2 partial agonist 5HT2A antagonist 5HT1A partial agonist	Schizophrenia BPD Adjunct depression	C: Diaphragmatic hernia, delayed skeletal ossification	Akathesia Orthostasis

(*Continued*)

Table 8.2 Mechanisms of Atypical and Second-Generation Antipsychotic Medications

Medication	Mechanism of Action	Indications	FDA Class	Side Effects
Iloperidone	D2 antagonist 5HT2A antagonist 5HT1A partial agonist Alpha 1 receptor	Schizophrenia	C	Orthostasis Dry mouth Somnolence Dyspepsia QTc prolongation
Asenapine	D2 antagonist D4 antagonist 5HT2A antagonist 5HT1A partial agonist	Schizophrenia BPD	C: Decreased fetal pup survival	Metallic taste Somnolence Weight gain
Lurasidone	D2 antagonist 5HT2A antagonist 5HT7 antagonist Alpha1 antagonist Alpha 2c antagonist Alpha 2a antagonist 5HT1A partial agonist No affinity for H1 or M1 receptors	Schizophrenia	B: No teratogenicity in rabbits or rats when given doses ranging from 3 to 12 times the average human dose	Neonatal withdrawal. Secreted in rat breast milk, unknown whether secreted in human milk. Nausea Akathisia Somnolence Agitation Parkinsonism

Abbreviations: **BPD**: bipolar disorder; **TD**: tardive dyskinesia; **NMS**: neuroleptic malignant syndrome; **N/V**: nausea and vomiting; **QTc**: corrected QT interval. Please see text for appropriate references.

Table 8.3 Mechanism(s) of Action of the First Generation of Antipsychotics

	Mechanism of Action	Indications	FDA Class	Side Effects
Chlorpromazine	D2 antagonist, M1 cholinergic antagonist, H1 histamine antagonist, alpha 1 antagonist	Nausea and Vomiting (N/V), psychosis, preoperational sedation, intractable hiccups, adjunct treatment for tetanus, acute intermittent porphyria	C: Cleft palate, skeletal, cerebellar, and eye abnormalities in animal studies. Increased risk of EPS, withdrawal, GI complications, and poor respiration in human neonates	Sedation, lowering of seizure threshold, QT Interval (QTc) prolongation, postural hypotension, NMS, and EPS TD

(*Continued*)

Table 8.3 Mechanism(s) of Action of the First Generation of Antipsychotics

	Mechanism of Action	Indications	FDA Class	Side Effects
Thioridazine	D2 antagonist, M1 cholinergic antagonist, H1 histamine antagonist, alpha 1 antagonist	Schizophrenia	C: Cleft palate in animal studies when treated with excessive doses of the medication	Sedation, lowering of seizure threshold, QTc prolongation, postural hypotension, NMS, and EPS TD
Fluphenazine	High potency D2 antagonist	Schizophrenia, bipolar mania	C: Cleft palate, impairment of in ossification of skull bones, increased incidence of dilated cerebral ventricles, rhinorrhea in humans	EPS Decreased seizure threshold NMS TD
Perphenazine	D2 antagonist, H1 antagonist, M1 antagonist	Schizophrenia, bipolar mania, N/V	C: Increase in cleft palates in animal studies	EPS Sedation Orthostasis NMS TD
Trifluoperazine	D2 antagonist, H1 antagonist, M1 antagonist	Schizophrenia Bipolar mania Nonpsychotic anxiety	C: Sporadic congenital skeletal and internal organ anomalies occur	EPS Orthostasis Sedation QTc prolongation NMS TD
Prochlorperazine	D2 antagonist, H1 antagonist, M1 antagonist	Schizophrenia Nonpsychotic anxiety N/V	C: Increased risk of cleft palates in animal studies. Slight association with cardiac septal defects	EPS Orthostasis Sedation QTc prolongation NMS TD
Promethazine	D2 antagonist, H1 antagonist, M1 antagonist	N/V Psychosis Motion sickness	C	EPS Sedation Orthostasis NMS TD

(*Continued*)

Table 8.3 Mechanism(s) of Action of the First Generation of Antipsychotics

	Mechanism of Action	Indications	FDA Class	Side Effects
Thiothixene	D2 antagonist, H1 antagonist, M1 antagonist	Schizophrenia Bipolar mania Anxiety	C: Case reports of small left colon syndrome. Decrease in conception, and increase in resorption rate	EPS Sedation Orthostasis NMS TD
Haloperidol	D2 antagonist Alpha 1 antagonist	Schizophrenia Bipolar mania Tourette disorder	C: Cleft palate in animal studies. Micromelia in animals and one case in humans	EPS Withdrawal NMS Dystonia NMS TD
Pimozide	D2 antagonist	Schizophrenia Tourette	C: Cleft palate and limb anomalies	EPS Withdrawal NMS Dystonia QTc prolongation TD
Loxapine	D2 and possible D4 antagonist	Schizophrenia Bipolar mania	C: Few studies to date	EPS Withdrawal NMS Dystonia Orthostasis TD
Malindone	D2 antagonist	Schizophrenia Bipolar mania	C	EPS TDl NMS Dystonia Orthostasis

Abbreviations: BPD: bipolar disorder; TD: tardive dyskinesia; NMS: neuroleptic malignant syndrome; N/V: nausea and vomiting; QTc: corrected QT interval.

a meta-analysis on published literature between 1966 and 1995. The results of this study revealed that three primary effects were associated with medication use during pregnancy: teratogenicity, perinatal syndromes, and postnatal behavioral sequelae. The authors concluded that there was a small but statistically important increase in the risk of congenital anomalies on babies exposed to the low-potency antipsychotics during the first trimester. Based on their study, there was no specific pattern of anomalies. Information on the behavioral sequelae in children who were exposed to antipsychotics during pregnancy is scarce. Two different studies by Kris [21] and Stika et al. [22] did not establish any significant behavioral or cognitive abnormalities in children who were exposed to chlorpromazine or chlorprothixene in utero.

The typical older antipsychotics possess many side effects, including parkinsonian syndrome and tardive dyskinesia (TD). Other adverse effects consist of weight gain, cardiac conduction disorders, postural hypotension, and cognitive decline. The atypical antipsychotics used in schizophrenia include risperidone, olanzepine, quetiapine, ziprasidone, aripiprazole, and clozapine. The benefits of the atypical antipsychotics over the older-generation medications include better responses of some patients who are resistant to the first-generation antipsychotics, improvement of negative symptoms and cognitive decline, and decreased potential for development of short-term acute or long-term parkinsonism, dystonia, or akathesia. Significant side effects of atypical antipsychotics consist of weight gain, their impact on the insulin and leptin effects, which increases the chance of obesity and diabetes, sedation, and hypertension. The obesity which is associated with treatment with atypical antipsychotics in turn may be associated with higher rates of obstetric complications such as gestational diabetes, preeclampsia, and cesarean delivery [23].

So far, there are no randomized or blinded evaluations to assess and determine the birth outcome measures following treatment of pregnant psychotic patients with atypical antipsychotics. One prospective study by McKenna et al. [17] assessed the rates of major malformations, spontaneous and therapeutic abortions, rates of stillbirth, birth weight, and gestational age in patients treated with olanzepine, risperidone, quetiapine, and clozapine and reported that only one malformation in one baby exposed to olanzepine was detected. While the group exposed to the atypical antipsychotics did not show any statistically significant differences in the rates of miscarriage, stillbirth, prematurity, congenital malformation, and perinatal syndromes compared to the healthy controls, their results indicated an increased rate of low birth weight babies.

BPD and Pregnancy

While pregnancy has historically been referred to as a period of emotional well-being and more stability, a number of studies indicate that mood disorders may manifest or continue during this unique stage of life [24–27]. Mood disorders are common among women of childbearing years and carry a chronic or relapsing course [28]. The impact of pregnancy on the natural course of bipolar mood disorder remains largely unrecognized; however, available references indicate that pregnancy does not have much lessening effect on risk for recurrence of mania and depression in females with bipolar mood disorder [29] and there is a significant risk of relapses following sudden cessation of the mood stabilizers [30,31]. In female patients with BPD, the negative impact of episodes of mania or depression during pregnancy should be assessed against the risk of medication exposure to the fetus in a patient who continues taking a mood stabilizer in order to avoid any relapses. In addition, the issue of "not treating" the depressed pregnant woman and the impact of such a decision on the mother and the baby should be carefully assessed [32,33] because depression during pregnancy is the strongest predictor of postpartum depression. Currently, the long-term impact on the infant of many mood-stabilizing medications used during pregnancy remains unknown, and because sudden withdrawal of the medications increases the risk of recurrence of the mood disorder, pregnant patients with mood disorders should be educated about the risks versus benefits of receiving treatment during pregnancy. In many instances, pregnant patients with acute major depressive disorders are not treated [34] which may in turn have an adverse effect on the mother and infant development [35,36].

Diagnosing depression during pregnancy may be a difficult task because certain symptoms such as sleep disturbances (insomnia or hypersomnia), weight gain, and fatigue also exist during pregnancy. Certain clinical manifestations such as feelings of guilt and worthlessness, anhedonia, hopelessness, thoughts of death and suicidal ideation, and psychomotor difficulties must alert the clinician to a diagnosis of major depressive disorder. Additionally, if these symptoms interfere with a patient's daily living activities the case for treatment is even stronger. While psychotherapy can be a useful treatment for depressive disorders, some patients may be unable to access such services. In other cases, psychotherapy alone may be an insufficient treatment, causing physicians to consider psychopharmacologic interventions.

Treatment of BPD during pregnancy requires in-depth knowledge of the potential side effects and teratogenicity of the mood stabilizers. Prenatal use of lithium carbonate has been associated with higher rates of cardiovascular anomalies (e.g., Epstein anomaly) [37]. However, more recent assessment of the cardiovascular malformations associated with prenatal use of lithium indicates a smaller risk (1/2000 versus 1/1000) [25]. Currently, examination with high-resolution ultrasound and fetal echocardiography are suggested during the first and second trimester to detect cardiac malformations associated with in utero exposure to lithium. Another mood stabilizer, lamotrigine, is particularly being used for prevention of relapses. Use of lamotrigine during the prenatal period, particularly the first trimester, is associated with cleft lips/palate [38]. In utero exposure to other anticonvulsants, carbamazepine and valproic acid, which are administered as mood stabilizers, carries higher risks for teratogenicity with development of certain abnormalities such as neural tube defects (spina bifida), midface hypoplasia, congenital heart disease, and microcephaly [39–41]. Therefore, due to potential risks of teratogenicity, anticonvulsants should be used as mood stabilizers with great caution during pregnancy. Physicians should treat patients with the lowest effective dose, and serum levels should be monitored carefully in order to adjust the dosage of the anticonvulsant. In addition, screening ultrasounds during weeks 18–22 are recommended to detect any organ malformations following in utero exposure to anticonvulsants. The data about safety of more recent anticonvulsants such as gabapentin, oxcarbazepine, and topiramate is limited.

Another issue in the treatment of BPD is that in many cases, patients are not on monotherapy and they are also treated with typical or atypical antipsychotics. As discussed earlier, the data on the safety of these agents during pregnancy is limited. In general, treatment of bipolar mood disorder with typical conventional antipsychotics is recommended because there is more knowledge of their safety profile compared to the atypical antipsychotics. In cases where the patient has only a history of mania with full resolution and no further attacks, one may consider the cessation of the mood-stabilizing agent before conception [25,29]. However, there is always the risk for subsequent relapses. In more complicated patients with a history of frequent relapses of mania or bipolar depression, one choice is to continue the mood stabilizer until pregnancy is confirmed, then taper the medication. This strategy also carries the risk of relapse following discontinuing the treatment. Patients who undergo discontinuation of treatment during pregnancy should be followed closely in order to capture and treat relapse of the mood disorder in a timely fashion. Re-establishment of treatment with mood stabilizers in stable patients who successfully tapered their medication requires clinical judgment and depends on a mutual agreement between the patient and the treating physician as to when to resume the treatment. In severe cases of bipolar mood disorder in a patient who is psychotic with suicidal ideation, continuation of the therapy is the safest approach.

Postpartum Depression

The postpartum period carries a significant risk for development of affective disorders, particularly postpartum depression [12]. The presence of untreated prenatal depression is a strong risk factor for postpartum depression. Other risk factors for postpartum depression include a previous history of postpartum psychosis, a history of BPD (particularly antenatal depression) [42], and the emergence of depressive symptoms during pregnancy [12,43]. Postpartum depressive disorders can be classified as postpartum blues, nonpsychotic major depression, and puerperal psychosis. The postpartum blues are common, not indicative of an underlying psychopathology, and affect 50–85% of women before delivery [44,45]. Postpartum blues do not affect a woman's daily living activities and do not require any treatment. However, if the clinical manifestations continue more than 2 weeks, the patient should be assessed for a depressive disorder.

Postpartum depression presents within 2–3 months after delivery and manifests with depressed mood, irritability, and loss of interest in daily functions. Sleep and appetite disturbances occur. In certain cases, postpartum depression may co-occur with generalized anxiety and obsessive manifestations [46]. Postpartum depression, particularly the untreated cases, may affect the child's health and development [47,48]. Before treatment of postpartum depression, medical causes of depression such as hypothyroidism must be excluded. Conventional antidepressive agents such as fluoxetine, venlafaxine, and sertraline are effective and well-tolerated therapies for postpartum depression [49–53]. Selective serotonin reuptake inhibitors (SSRIs) are excellent therapies as they possess anxiolytic and nonsedating properties. Addition of a benzodiazepine such as lorazepam or clonazepam also improves coexisting anxiety. In severe cases of postpartum depression, particularly if the patient is suicidal, inpatient admission to the hospital is necessary. Electroconvulsive therapy is a relatively safe procedure which should be considered in cases of severe postpartum depression. A summary of the effects of antidepressants on the embryo and fetus is presented in Table 8.4.

Table 8.4 The Effects of Antidepressants on the Fetus and Embryo

Effects on the Fetus		
Measure	**TCA**	**SSRI/SNRI**
Miscarriage	No study available	No study available
Preterm birth		Increased risk with fluoxetine
Birth weight	Increased risk of Large for gestational age (LGA)	Decreased birth weight with fluoxetine. Infants tend to be low birth weight, but not small for gestation
Intrauterine growth	Slightly increased risk of preterm delivery, with increased duration of TCA use	Decreased birth weight and length with fluoxetine Slightly increased risk of preterm delivery, with increased duration of SSRI use
Intrauterine death	No evidence of increase	No evidence of increase
Effects on the Embryo		
Measure	**TCA**	**SSRI/SNRI**
Malformations	Increased risk of VSD/Atrial septal defect (ASD) and cardiovascular defects	Also increased risk of cardiovascular defects (VSD) and Persistent pulmonary hypertension of the newborn (PPHN), especially paroxetine Increased risk of minor congenital anomalies with fluoxetine
Respiratory	Decreased respiratory drive	OR for SSRI (fluoxetine) respiratory adversity less than SNRI. Increased risk of persistent pulmonary hypertension, especially with exposure during late pregnancy
Low APGAR	Lower APGAR than SSRI	SSRI (fluoxetine) lower APGAR than SNRI
Hypoglycemia	Significant increase in OR	SNRI more significant increase in OR than SSRI
Convulsions	OR>7.0 as compared to SSRI	SSRI<SNRI
Excitation	More significant than SSRI	SSRI (fluoxetine) withdrawal is significantly increased. SNRI data not available

Abbreviations: TCA: tricyclic antidepressants; SSRI: selective serotonin reuptake inhibitors; SNRI: seratonin/norepinephrine reuptake inhibitors; VSD: ventricular septal defect; ASD: atrial septal defect; PPHN: persistent pulmonary hypertension of the newborn; OR: odds ratio. Please see text for appropriate references.

Postpartum psychosis presents with mania, restlessness, paranoia, sleep abnormalities, delusions, impulsivity, and dangerous behavior that may endanger the mother or the child. Patients with postpartum psychosis must be admitted to the hospital and may be treated with mood stabilizers, antipsychotics, benzodiazepines, and/or electroconvulsive therapy. Due to the significance of the postpartum mood disorders, psychosis, and anxiety, one should always consider prophylactic treatment which can either be initiated at 36 weeks of gestation or no later than 48 h after delivery [54–56]. Postpartum depression may be prevented by initiating treatment with antidepressants (either tricyclic antidepressants or SSRIs) within the 48 h of parturition.

Anxiety Disorders and Pregnancy

While pregnancy and the perinatal period are happy chapters of life for many women, some patients develop or experience worsening of emotional distress. A number of previous observations indicate improvement and lessening of psychiatric disorders during pregnancy [57,58]; however, more recent literature points toward worsening of anxiety disorders during pregnancy [59]. Five major types of anxiety disorders include generalized anxiety disorder (GAD), obsessive–compulsive disorder (OCD), panic disorder, post-traumatic stress disorder (PTSD), and social phobia (or social anxiety disorder). The prevalence of anxiety disorders in nonpregnant women ranges from 8.7% to 30% [60–62], which in turn reflects the differences in screening and diagnostic tools to execute these studies. Clinical observations suggest that symptoms of anxiety frequently occur during pregnancy and postpartum period [63,64] and the mother's anxiety during pregnancy predicts the child's behavioral and emotional problems independently of postnatal depression [64]. Increased activity of mother's hypothalamic–pituitary–adrenal axis has been implicated in adverse events observed in fetuses born to anxious mothers. For example, elevated levels of cortisol may lead to premature labor and delivery [65,66].

GAD is a chronic condition characterized by at least 6 months of frequent worry and anxiety along with three or more of the following symptoms: restlessness or feeling keyed up or on edge, being easily fatigued, irritability, poor concentration, muscle tension, and sleep disturbance [67]. GAD affects almost 5% of the general population [68] and the clinical manifestations should be present for at least 6 months before establishing a diagnosis [67]. A number of clinical observations have assessed the prevalence of GAD during the perinatal period. One study reported a rate of 8.5% during the third trimester of pregnancy [69] and three other studies that investigated the prevalence of GAD or adjustment disorder with anxiety during the postpartum period reported prevalence rates of 4.4–8.2% [70–72]. Based on the diagnostic and statistical manual of mental disorders, III revised (DSM-III-R) report in 1994 [73] the 1-year prevalence for GAD is almost 1.6% in a community sample and the lifetime prevalence rate is 5.1% of the US population aged 15–45 years [73]. The findings indicate that postpartum generalized anxiety carries a higher prevalence than postpartum depression [71] and GAD and adjustment disorder may be more common in postpartum females than in the general population. There is no epidemiologic data on the risk factors for or predictors of

GAD during the perinatal period. In addition, not much is known about the course of pre-existing GAD during the perinatal period. One Australian study demonstrated that 1.9–3.1% of postpartum females develop symptoms of GAD with postpartum onset [74]. Treatment of perinatal GAD includes cognitive–behavioral therapy (CBT) and if pharmacotherapy is used, antidepressants are preferred over benzodiazepines due to their better safety profile for the growing fetus [75,76].

Panic disorder is characterized by a period of unexpected intense fear or discomfort, during which the individual experiences physical symptoms such as palpitations, shortness of breath, sweating, shaking, or a feeling of choking. Other diagnostic features include fear of upcoming attacks, fear and discomfort about the consequences of the attack, and alteration of behavior as a consequence of the attack. Those with agoraphobia develop anxiety about being in locations or circumstances from which escape may be difficult.

PTSD is an anxiety disorder which is recognized by exposure to a traumatic event or ordeal, which results in psychological trauma. The painful traumatic event may consists of the threat of death or serious injury to oneself or others [77]. The individual's response involves hopelessness, fear, or a sense of horror. The painful event is followed by re-experiencing the original trauma or nightmares and flashbacks reliving the experience. Victims of PTSD persistently avoid stimuli associated with trauma and develop hyperarousal (such as irritability, hypervigilance, and insomnia). Based on the formal diagnostic criteria of DSM-IV-TR, the duration of the disturbance is more than 1 month. PTSD has been reported to occur in association with painful and traumatic medical and surgical procedures [78], invasive procedures [79], and obstetric and gynecologic procedures [80]. Pregnant women who have been victims of sexual abuse may experience the painful recollections in response to delivery procedures, which in turn may lead to avoidance of certain medical procedures such as internal examination [81–83]. Some evidence suggests that pregnancy and childbirth procedures may aggravate the manifestations of PTSD if pregnancy is the result of rape or the delivery resurrects the recollections of previous sexual traumatic experience. There is not much data about new onset PTSD across the prenatal period.

OCD is characterized by the presence of unwanted intrusive thoughts, images, ideas, or impulses (obsessions) that raise anxiety and the attempts to neutralize these obsessions or reduce the stress by executing repetitive or ritualistic behaviors or thought patterns (compulsions). The diagnostic criteria for OCD are presented in Table 8.5 [67]. OCD is believed to possess a robust neurobiologic basis with cortico-striatal-cortical circuits and is closely associated with Tourette syndrome. A number of clinical studies have assessed the prevalence of OCD during pregnancy and postpartum periods [69,70] and the findings of these studies indicate a lower prevalence of OCD during pregnancy (0.2–1.2%) than during the postpartum period (2.7–3.9%). Existing data suggest that obsessions in perinatal women often consist of intrusive fears about the child's well-being with concerns about intentionally or accidentally hurting the fetus or the child [84,85]. A number of clinical observations have shown that in up to 40% of cases of OCD, the onset occurs during pregnancy [86–88] and in up to 30% of the cases, the disorder manifests in the postpartum period [84,85].

The obsessive ideas about hurting the child have been reported in more than 40% of women with postpartum depression [89,90]. In a study of 41 pairs of parents who

Table 8.5 Diagnostic Criteria for Obsessive-Compulsive Disorders

A. Either obsessions or compulsions:

Obsessions as defined by (1), (2), (3), and (4):

1. Recurrent and persistent thoughts, impulses, or images are experienced at some time during the disturbance as intrusive and inappropriate and cause marked anxiety and distress. Those with this disorder recognize the craziness of these unwanted thoughts (such as fears of hurting their children) and would not act on them, but the thoughts are very disturbing and difficult to tell others about
2. The thoughts, impulses, or images are not simply excessive worries about real-life problems
3. The person attempts to suppress or ignore such thoughts, impulses, or images or to neutralize them with some other thought or action
4. The person recognizes that the obsessional thoughts, impulses, or images are a product of his/her own mind (not imposed from without, as in thought insertion).

Compulsions are defined by (1) and (2):

1. The person performs repetitive behaviors (e.g., hand washing, ordering, checking) or mental acts (e.g., praying, counting, repeating words silently) in response to an obsession or according to rules that must be applied rigidly
2. The behaviors or mental acts are aimed at preventing or reducing distress or preventing some dreaded event or situation; however, these behaviors or mental acts either are not connected in a realistic way with what they are meant to neutralize or prevent or they are clearly excessive

B. At some point during the course of the disorder, the person recognizes that the obsessions or compulsions are excessive or unreasonable. This does not apply to children

C. The obsessions or compulsions cause marked distress; are time consuming (take >1 h/d); or significantly interfere with the person's normal routine, occupational or academic functioning, or usual social activities or relationships

D. If another Axis I disorder is present, the content of the obsessions or compulsions is not restricted to it (e.g., preoccupation with food and weight in the presence of an eating disorder, hair pulling in the presence of trichotillomania, concern with appearance in body dysmorphic disorder, preoccupation with drugs in substance use disorder, preoccupation with having a serious illness in hypochondriasis, preoccupation with sexual urges in Paraphilia; or guilty ruminations in the presence of major depressive disorder.

E. The disturbance is not due to the direct physiologic effects of a substance (e.g., a drug of abuse, a medication) or general medical condition.

Specify if:

With Poor Insight: if, for most of the time during the current episode, the person does not recognize that the obsessions and compulsions are excessive or unreasonable

Source: Reprinted with permission from the Diagnostic and Statistical Manual of Mental Disorders, Fourth Edition, Text Revision, © 2000. American Psychiatric Association.

were interviewed two weeks after birth of their infant, 32% of the interviewed parents reported having had thoughts of harming the child [91]. One study found 6.5% of the healthy mothers had experienced passing thoughts of harming their child [89 as referenced in 92]. Clinicians must differentiate obsessive–compulsive-related obsessions of infant harm from the ideas of hurting or even killing the child, which occurs in patients with postpartum psychosis and severe postpartum depression. In fact, there is evidence that there is a connection between postpartum depression and symptoms of OCD, which includes ideas of hurting the newborn child [89,90]. The major difference between these two groups is that patients with OCD typically have insight and are aware of the unwanted urges and make an effort not to execute them. On the contrary, females with postpartum psychosis do not have any fear about their thoughts and lack insight into the nature of the problem and if left untreated, may act based on their delusion or hallucination and harm the newborn or themselves [93]. Indeed, patients who present with ideas of harming their child with concurrent postpartum psychosis or postpartum depression need urgent inpatient admission to prevent any injuries to themselves or others. However, females with OCD with no concurrent depression or psychosis require only reassurance and usually can be managed without hospital admission [94].

Treatment approaches to anxiety disorders during pregnancy mainly consist of nonpharmacologic approaches rather than biologic agents. Nonpharmacologic approaches include CBT and interpersonal therapy (IPT). Both of these methods are ideal approaches to pregnant patients because they are safe. However, there are no controlled studies of these methods in pregnant women with anxiety disorders.

In the absence of any strong evidence to support the role of nonpharmacologic treatments for anxiety disorders during pregnancy and based on the fact that untreated anxiety disorders may have adverse effects on the mother and the fetus, using pharmacologic agents for their treatment during pregnancy is an important option. The major problem with use of pharmacologic agents such as SSRIs or serotonin norepinephrine reuptake inhibitors (SNRIs) during pregnancy is that these medications are secreted into the amniotic fluid and readily cross the placenta to enter the body of the growing fetus [95]. Use of older antidepressants such as tricyclic antidepressants and monoamine oxidase inhibitors (MAOIs) are limited due to their side effects and the fact that in utero MAOI exposure restricts fetal growth [96].

While a number of studies have assessed the effects of SSRIs on pregnancy, a study by Oberlander et al. [97] using population-based linked health data demonstrated that the duration of in utero exposure rather than the stage of pregnancy at which in utero exposure occurred increased the risk of respiratory distress and lower birth weight and gestational age. In a more recent prospective longitudinal study Oberlander et al. [98] assessed whether prenatal use of SSRIs impacts behavior in 3 year olds of pregnant anxious or depressed mothers and if the risk of such impact was moderated by a serotonin transporter promoter (SLC6A4) genotype. The investigators studied mothers and their 3-year-old children (33 subjects exposed to SSRIs during pregnancy and 42 nonexposed). The results of this study indicated that prenatal exposure to both maternal depressed mood and SSRI antidepressants increased internalizing behaviors during childhood, while present maternal mood increased the risk for externalizing behaviors. The authors concluded that exposure to prenatal SSRIs and maternal mood exerted distinct effects on child behavior at 3 years of age, reflected in an increased level of internalizing behaviors. The effect of prenatal maternal anxiety on the child's mood was mediated by the child SLC6A4 genotype and despite SSRI therapy for prenatal maternal mood disturbances, childhood behavior at 3 years of age remained at risk. Apart from this, prenatal exposure to SSRIs may increase the risk of congenital malformations [99]. Of course, more detailed and controlled studies are needed to identify the effects of the SSRIs and

SNRIs on the fetus. While there are a significant number of reports that support the negative impact of SSRI exposure during the prenatal period on pregnancy outcomes, withdrawal of these medications in pregnant women also carries risk of adverse effects on mother and child. In fact, a significant issue about SSRIs and SNRIs is the issue that neonates who have been exposed to these medications in utero may manifest symptoms of withdrawal recognized by irritability, rigidity, tremor, and respiratory distress once the in utero exposure has decreased [100]. Therefore, use of SSRIs and SNRIs during pregnancy for treatment of anxiety disorders and depressive disorders is based on a mutual decision between the treating physician and the patient. In making such a decision, the existing data about these medications along with risk versus benefit analysis should be presented to the patient so an educated decision will be made to protect both mother and fetus against the negative impact of the untreated psychiatric disorders and the negative impact of SSRIs and SNRIs on the pregnancy and on the child in the long run.

Eating Disorders and Pregnancy

Eating disorders are common among women and affect about 5–7% of women of childbearing age [101]. Despite great interest in eating disorders their cause remains unknown and the lifetime prevalence is approximated to be up to 10% [102]. A number of clinical retrospective case–control studies have proposed possible risk factors for eating disorders which include female gender, gestation and delivery complications, anxiety, perfectionism, insufficient contact with parents, family influences such as high parental expectations from the children, parental alcoholism, overanxious parents, parental obesity, being teased about weight and body shape, and childhood obesity [103–113]. The three major groups of eating disorders are anorexia nervosa, bulimia nervosa, and eating disorders not otherwise specified. Anorexia nervosa is recognized by refusal to maintain normal body weight for age and height along with pervasive fear of weight gain or becoming obese even when the individual is underweight. There is often an unrealistic view and perception of body weight and shape despite having a starved appearance. Patients deny the seriousness of the low body weight (which in turn translates to being less than 85% of the proposed weight for age and height), experience amenorrhea for 3 months, or never resume menses. Anorexia nervosa is further categorized based on the compensatory weight loss mechanisms into: restricting and binge–purge subtypes. Patients with restricting subtype of anorexia nervosa have periods of starvation, excessive exercise, and food intake restriction, while patients with binge–purge subtype take purgatives (laxatives/diuretics), and self-induce vomiting to lose weight. Many female patients with anorexia lose excessive amounts of body weight and develop amenorrhea.

Bulimia nervosa is also observed in women who overestimate their body size and shape and is recognized by recurrent episodes of binge eating at least twice weekly for 3 months with inappropriate compensatory behavior such as vomiting or excessively exercising in order to avoid weight gain and obesity and a sense of self-evaluation which is unduly influenced by body shape and weight [67]. This abnormal pattern of eating is followed by feelings of losing control and guilt which pushes the individual toward purging behavior to undo the binge episode. Bulimia nervosa has two subtypes: the purging type during which the patient uses laxatives, diuretics, or enemas or self-induced vomiting to compensate for the binge eating; and the nonpurging type during which the patient is fasting or excessively exercising to burn the calorie intake.

The group of eating disorders not otherwise specified, including binge-eating disorder, are those eating disorders that do not meet the criteria for any other specific-eating disorder. They are believed to be common and more than 50% of patients under treatment in eating disorders clinics are diagnosed with eating disorders not otherwise specified [114,115].

A number of clinical studies have assessed the impact of pregnancy on the symptoms of eating disorders. The effects of pregnancy on the symptomatology of eating disorders cover a full range of outcomes from complete resolution to an acute worsening of the symptoms [116,117]. In many cases, a mother's concern and care for the fetus' health is believed to be responsible for the improvement of the symptoms. The observed improvement of the symptomatology may range from reduction to complete resolution and this alteration may be temporary or permanent and may recur after delivery [117]. In one study, patients who demonstrated improvement or cessation of their symptoms experienced better outcomes and delivered heavier babies with higher 5-min APGAR scores [118]. On the contrary, patients who relapsed or experienced worsening of their symptoms during pregnancy based on the fear of becoming obese delivered smaller children with lower 5-min APGAR scores [118].

It is important to realize that pregnant patients with anorexia nervosa or bulimia nervosa even before pregnancy may suffer from severe malnutrition and this by itself may exert unfavorable effects on the fetus. Therefore, it has been shown that pregnant women with these eating disorders may have higher risks of delivering babies with intrauterine growth retardation and low birth weight, and carry higher rates of perinatal mortality [119] and microcephaly [120]. In order to have better outcomes, management of eating disorders during pregnancy should be based on a multidisciplinary approach to provide medical, psychiatric, and nutritional treatment. In addition, the psychiatric care should be done along with the obstetric care to secure the best possible outcomes. In cases of persistence or deterioration of symptoms during pregnancy, it is necessary to educate the mother about the need for adequate nutrition in order to improve the fetus' growth and development.

Conclusion

Despite the fact that many patients with psychiatric disorders become pregnant while in treatment, most physicians feel uncomfortable treating these patients. This feeling of uneasiness stems from the fact that most psychiatric disorders deteriorate during pregnancy and our knowledge about the safety profile of psychiatric medications is very limited. The authors conclude that in most cases pregnancies in the context of psychiatric disorders should be considered as "high-risk" pregnancies and any decision about discontinuing, initiating, or continuing psychotropic medications in pregnant patients should be undertaken with great caution so both mother and the newborn are protected against the underlying disease or the adverse effects of the offered treatments.

References

[1] Aleman A, Kahn RS, Selten JP. Sex differences in the risk of schizophrenia: evidence from meta-analysis. Arch Gen Psychiatry 2003;60:565–71.

[2] Yaeger D, Smith HG, Altshuler LL. Atypical antipsychotics in the treatment of schizophrenia during pregnancy and the postpartum. Am J Psychiatry 2006;163:2064–70.

[3] Rudolph B, Larson GL, Sweeny S, Hough EE, Arorian K. Hospitalized pregnant psychotic women: characteristics and treatment issues. Hosp Community Psychiatry 1990;41:159–63.

[4] Howard LM. Fertility and pregnancy in women with psychotic disorders. Eur J Obstet Gynecol Reprod Biol 2005;119:3–10.

[5] Nilsson E, Lichtenstein P, Cnattingius S, Murray RM, Hultman CM. Women with schizophrenia: pregnancy outcome and infant death among their offspring. Schizophr Res 2002;58(2–3):221–9.

[6] Jablensky AV, Morgan V, Zubrick SR, Bower C, Yellachich LA. Pregnancy, delivery, and neonatal complications in a population cohort of women with schizophrenia and major affective disorders. Am J Psychiatry 2005;162:79–91.

[7] O'Connor TG, Ben Shlomo Y, Heron J, Golding J, Adams D, Glover V. Prenatal anxiety predicts individual differences in cortisol in pre-adolescent children. Biol Psychiatry 2005;58:211–7.

[8] Hansen D, Lou HC, Olsen J. Serious life events and congenital malformations: a national study with complete follow-up. Lancet 2000;356:875–80.

[9] Field T, Diego M, Hernandez-Reif M, Schanberg S, Kuhn C, Yando R, et al. Pregnancy anxiety and comorbid depression and anger: effects on the fetus and neonate. Depress Anxiety 2003;17:140–51.

[10] Seeman M, Lang M. The role of estrogens in schizophrenia gender differences. Schizophr Bull 1990;16:185–94.

[11] Miller LJ. Psychotic denial of pregnancy: phenomenology and clinical management. Hosp Community Psychiatry 1990;41:1233–7.

[12] Kendell RE, Chalmers JC, Platz C. Epidemiology of puerperal psychoses. Br J Psychiatry. 1987;150:662–73.

[13] Stewart DE, Klompenhouwer JL, Kendell RE, van Hulst AM. Prophylactic lithium in puerperal psychosis. The experience of three centres. Br J Psychiatry 1991;158:393–7.

[14] Sit D, Rothschild AJ, Wisner KL. A review of postpartum psychosis. J Womens Health (Larchmt) 2006;15:352–68.

[15] Spinelli MG. Postpartum psychosis: detection of risk and management. Am J Psychiatry 2009;166:405–8.

[16] Grigoriadis S, Seeman MV. The role of estrogen in schizophrenia: implications for schizophrenia practice guidelines for women. Can J Psychiatry 2002;47:437–42.

[17] McKenna K, Koren G, Tetelbaum M, Wilton L, Shakir S, Diav-Citrin O, et al. Pregnancy outcome of women using atypical antipsychotic drugs: a prospective comparative study. J Clin Psychiatry 2005;66:444–9.

[18] Trixler M, Gáti A, Fekete S, Tényi T. Use of antipsychotics in the management of schizophrenia during pregnancy. Drugs 2005;65:1193–206.

[19] Littrell KH, Johnson CG, Peabody CD, Hilligoss N. Antipsychotics during pregnancy. Am J Psychiatry. 2000;157:1342.

[20] Altshuler LL, Cohen L, Szuba MP, Burt VK, Gitlin M, Mintz J. Pharmacologic management of psychiatric illness during pregnancy: dilemmas and guidelines. Am J Psychiatry 1996;153:592–606.

[21] Kris EB. Children of mothers maintained on pharmacotherapy during pregnancy or postpartum. Curr Ther Res Clin Exp 1965;7:785–9.

[22] Stika L, Elisová K, Honzáková L, Hrochová H, Plechatová H, Strnadová J, et al. Effects of drug administration in pregnancy on children's school behaviour. Pharm Weekbl Sci 1990;12:252–5.

[23] Brost BC, Goldenberg RL, Mercer BM, Iams JD, Meis PJ, Moawad AH, et al. The preterm prediction study: association of cesarean delivery with increases in maternal weight and body mass index. Am J Obstet Gynecol 1997;177:333–7.

[24] Evans J, Heron J, Francomb H, Oke S, Golding J. Cohort study of depressed mood during pregnancy and after childbirth. BMJ 2001;323(7307):257–60.

[25] Cohen LS, Friedman JM, Jefferson JW, Johnson EM, Weiner ML. A reevaluation of risk of in utero exposure to lithium. JAMA 1994;271:146–50.

[26] O'Hara MW. Social support, life events, and depression during pregnancy and the puerperium. Arch Gen Psychiatry 1986;43:569–73.

[27] Frank E, Kupfer DJ, Jacob M, Blumenthal SJ, Jarrett DB. Pregnancy-related affective episodes among women with recurrent depression. Am J Psychiatry 1987;144: 288–93.

[28] Kessler RC, McGonagle KA, Swartz M, Blazer DG, Nelson CB. Sex and depression in the National Comorbidity Survey. I: Lifetime prevalence, chronicity and recurrence. J Affect Disord 1993;29:85–96.

[29] Viguera AC, Cohen LS, Bouffard S, Whitfield TH, Baldessarini RJ. Reproductive decisions by women with bipolar disorder after prepregnancy psychiatric consultation. Am J Psychiatry 2002;159:2102–4.

[30] Viguera AC, Nonacs R, Cohen LS, Tondo L, Murray A, Baldessarini RJ. Risk of recurrence of bipolar disorder in pregnant and nonpregnant women after discontinuing lithium maintenance. Am J Psychiatry 2000;157:179–84.

[31] Newport DJ, Brennan PA, Green P, Ilardi D, Whitfield TH, Morris N, et al. Maternal depression and medication exposure during pregnancy: comparison of maternal retrospective recall to prospective documentation. BJOG 2008;115:681–8.

[32] Wisner KL, Appelbaum PS, Uhl K, Goldkind SF. Pharmacotherapy for depressed pregnant women: overcoming obstacles to gathering essential data. Clin Pharmacol Ther 2009;86:362–5.

[33] Wisner KL, Zarin DA, Holmboe ES, Appelbaum PS, Gelenberg AJ, Leonard HL, et al. Risk–benefit decision making for treatment of depression during pregnancy. Am J Psychiatry 2000;157:1933–40.

[34] Marcus SM. Depression during pregnancy: rates, risks and consequences—Motherisk Update 2008. Can J Clin Pharmacol 2009;16:e15–22.

[35] Wisner KL, Peindl KS, Gigliotti T, Hanusa BH. Obsessions and compulsions in women with postpartum depression. J Clin Psychiatry 1999;60:176–80.

[36] di Scalea TL, Wisner KL. Pharmacotherapy of postpartum depression. Expert Opin Pharmacother 2009;10:2593–607.

[37] Weinstein MR, Goldfield M. Cardiovascular malformations with lithium use during pregnancy. Am J Psychiatry 1975;132:529–31.

[38] Holmes LB, Baldwin EJ, Smith CR, Habecker E, Glassman L, Wong SL, et al. Increased frequency of isolated cleft palate in infants exposed to lamotrigine during pregnancy. Neurology 2008;70(22 Pt 2):2152–8.

[39] Wyszynski DF, Nambisan M, Surve T, Alsdorf RM, Smith CR, Holmes LB. Antiepileptic Drug Pregnancy Registry. Increased rate of major malformations in offspring exposed to valproate during pregnancy. Neurology 2005;64:961–5.

[40] Lammer EJ, Sever LE, Oakley Jr. GP. Teratogen update: valproic acid. Teratology 1987;35:465–73.
[41] Omtzigt JG, Los FJ, Grobbee DE, Pijpers L, Jahoda MG, Brandenburg H, et al. The risk of spina bifida aperta after first-trimester exposure to valproate in a prenatal cohort. Neurology 1992;42(4 Suppl. 5):119–25.
[42] Dean C, Williams RJ, Brockington IF. Is puerperal psychosis the same as bipolar manic-depressive disorder? A family study. Psychol Med 1989;19:637–47.
[43] Cohen LS, Wang B, Nonacs R, Viguera AC, Lemon EL, Freeman MP. Treatment of mood disorders during pregnancy and postpartum. Psychiatr Clin North Am 2010;33:273–93.
[44] O'Hara MW, Zekoski EM, Philipps LH, Wright EJ. Controlled prospective study of postpartum mood disorders: comparison of childbearing and nonchildbearing women. J Abnorm Psychol 1990;99:3–15.
[45] Handley SL, Dunn TL, Waldron G, Baker JM. Tryptophan, cortisol, and puerperal mood. Br J Psychiatry 1980;136:498–508.
[46] Hendrick V, Altshuler L, Strouse T, Grosser S. Postpartum and nonpostpartum depression: differences in presentation and response to pharmacologic treatment. Depress Anxiety 2000;11:66–72.
[47] Murray L, Cooper P. Effects of postnatal depression on infant development. Arch Dis Child 1997;77:99–101.
[48] Hayworth J, Little BC, Carter SB, Raptopoulos P, Priest RG, Sandler M. A predictive study of post-partum depression: some predisposing characteristics. Br J Med Psychol 1980;53:161–7.
[49] Suri R, Altshuler L, Hendrick V, Rasgon N, Lee E, Mintz J. The impact of depression and fluoxetine treatment on obstetrical outcome. Arch Womens Ment Health 2004 Jul;7(3):193–200.
[50] Appleby L, Warner R, Whitton A, Faragher B. A controlled study of fluoxetine and cognitive-behavioural counselling in the treatment of postnatal depression. BMJ 1997;314:932–6.
[51] O'Hara MW, Stuart S, Gorman LL, Wenzel A. Efficacy of interpersonal psychotherapy for postpartum depression. Arch Gen Psychiatry 2000;57:1039–45.
[52] Suri R, Burt VK, Altshuler LL, Zuckerbrow-Miller J, Fairbanks L. Fluvoxamine for postpartum depression. Am J Psychiatry 2001;158:1739–40.
[53] Nonacs RM, Soares CN, Viguera AC, Pearson K, Poitras JR, Cohen LS. Bupropion SR for the treatment of postpartum depression: a pilot study. Int J Neuropsychopharmacol 2005;8:445–9.
[54] Austin MP, Ross M, Murray C, O'Carroll RE, Ebmeier KP, Goodwin GM. Cognitive function in major depression. J Affect Disord 1992;25:21–9.
[55] Stewart DE. Thyroid function and postpartum depression. Am J Psychiatry 1991;148(6):816.
[56] Cohen LS, Sichel DA, Robertson LM, Heckscher E, Rosenbaum JF. Postpartum prophylaxis for women with bipolar disorder. Am J Psychiatry 1995;152:1641–5.
[57] Altshuler LL, Hendrick V, Cohen LS. Course of mood and anxiety disorders during pregnancy and the postpartum period. J Clin Psychiatry 1998;59(Suppl. 2):29–33.
[58] Cowley DS, Dager SR, Dunner DL. Lactate response in patients with primary major depression. Psychiatry Res 1989;27:357–8.
[59] Elliott SA, Rugg AJ, Watson JP, Brough DI. Mood changes during pregnancy and after the birth of a child. Br J Clin Psychol 1983;22(Pt 4):295–308.
[60] Birndorf CA, Madden A, Portera L, Leon AC. Psychiatric symptoms, functional impairment, and receptivity toward mental health treatment among obstetrical patients. Int J Psychiatry Med 2001;31:355–65.

[61] Kelly RH, Russo J, Katon W. Somatic complaints among pregnant women cared for in obstetrics: normal pregnancy or depressive and anxiety symptom amplification revisited? Gen Hosp Psychiatry 2001;23:107–13.

[62] Stuart S, Couser G, Schilder K, O'Hara MW, Gorman L. Postpartum anxiety and depression: onset and comorbidity in a community sample. J Nerv Ment Dis 1998;186:420–4.

[63] Heron J, O'Connor TG, Evans J, Golding J, Glover V. ALSPAC Study Team. The course of anxiety and depression through pregnancy and the postpartum in a community sample. J Affect Disord 2004;80:65–73.

[64] O'Connor TG, Heron J, Glover V, Alspac Study Team. Antenatal anxiety predicts child behavioral/emotional problems independently of postnatal depression. J Am Acad Child Adolesc Psychiatry 2002;41:1470–7.

[65] Sandman CA, Wadhwa PD, Dunkel-Schetter C, Chicz-DeMet A, Belman J, Porto M, et al. Psychobiological influences of stress and HPA regulation on the human fetus and infant birth outcomes. Ann N Y Acad Sci 1994;739:198–210.

[66] Wadhwa PD, Sandman CA, Porto M, Dunkel-Schetter C, Garite TJ. The association between prenatal stress and infant birth weight and gestational age at birth: a prospective investigation. Am J Obstet Gynecol 1993;169:858–65.

[67] American Psychiatric Association Diagnostic and statistical manual of mental disorders: DSM-IV-TR. Washington, DC: American Psychiatric Publishing, Inc.; 2000.

[68] Carter AS, Garrity-Rokous FE, Chazan-Cohen R, Little C, Briggs-Gowan MJ. Maternal depression and comorbidity: predicting early parenting, attachment security, and toddler social-emotional problems and competencies. J Am Acad Child Adolesc Psychiatry 2001;40:18–26.

[69] Sutter-Dallay AL, Giaconne-Marcesche V, Glatigny-Dallay E, Verdoux H. Women with anxiety disorders during pregnancy are at increased risk of intense postnatal depressive symptoms: a prospective survey of the MATQUID cohort. Eur Psychiatry 2004;19:459–63.

[70] Wenzel A, Haugen EN, Jackson LC, Brendle JR. Anxiety symptoms and disorders at eight weeks postpartum. J Anxiety Disord 2005;19:295–311.

[71] Wenzel A, Haugen EN, Jackson LC, Robinson K. Prevalence of generalized anxiety at eight weeks postpartum. Arch Womens Ment Health 2003;6:43–9.

[72] Ballard CG, Stanley AK, Brockington IF. Post-traumatic stress disorder (PTSD) after childbirth. Br J Psych 1995;166:525–8.

[73] Wittchen HU, Zhao S, Kessler RC, Eaton WW. DSM-III-R generalized anxiety disorder in the National Comorbidity Survey. Arch Gen Psychiatry 1994;51(5):355–64.

[74] Matthey S, Barnett B, Howie P, Kavanagh DJ. Diagnosing postpartum depression in mothers and fathers: whatever happened to anxiety? J Affect Disord 2003;74:139–47.

[75] Ross LE, Murray BJ, Steiner M. Sleep and perinatal mood disorders: a critical review. J Psychiatry Neurosci 2005;30:247–56.

[76] Rubinchik SM, Kablinger AS, Gardner JS. Medications for panic disorder and generalized anxiety disorder during pregnancy. Prim Care Companion J Clin Psychiatry 2005;7:100–5.

[77] Breslau N, Davis GC, Peterson EL, Schultz L. Psychiatric sequelae of posttraumatic stress disorder in women. Arch Gen Psychiatry 1997;54:81–7.

[78] Fisch RZ, Tadmor O. Iatrogenic post-traumatic stress disorder. Lancet 1989; 2(8676):1397.

[79] Shalev AY, Schreiber S, Galai T, Melmed RN. Post-traumatic stress disorder following medical events. Br J Clin Psychol 1993;32(Pt 2):247–53.

[80] Menage J. Women's perception of obstetric and gynecological examinations. BMJ 1993;306(6885):1127–8.

[81] van der Kolk BA, Pelcovitz D, Roth S, Mandel FS, McFarlane A, Herman JL. Dissociation, somatization, and affect dysregulation: the complexity of adaptation of trauma. Am J Psychiatry 1996;153(Suppl. 7):83–93.
[82] Crompton J. Post-traumatic stress disorder and childbirth. Br J Midwifery 1996;4:290–3.
[83] Ross LE, McLean LM. Anxiety disorders during pregnancy and the postpartum period: a systematic review. J Clin Psychiatry 2006;67:1285–98.
[84] Sichel DA, Cohen LS, Rosenbaum JF, Driscoll J. Postpartum onset of obsessive–compulsive disorder. Psychosomatics 1993;34:277–9.
[85] Arnold LM. A case series of women with postpartum-onset obsessive–compulsive disorder. Prim Care Companion J Clin Psychiatry 1999;1:103–8.
[86] Neziroglu F, Anemone R, Yaryura-Tobias JA. Onset of obsessive–compulsive disorder in pregnancy. Am J Psychiatry 1992;149:947–50.
[87] Williams KE, Koran LM. Obsessive–compulsive disorder in pregnancy, the puerperium, and the premenstruum. Clin Psychiatry. 1997;58:330–4; quiz 335–6.
[88] Labad J, Menchón JM, Alonso P, Segalàs C, Jiménez S, Vallejo J. Female reproductive cycle and obsessive-compulsive disorder. J Clin Psychiatry 2005;66:428–35.
[89] Jennings KD, Ross S, Popper S, Elmore M. Thoughts of harming infants in depressed and nondepressed mothers. J Affect Disord 1999;54(1–2):21–8.
[90] Wisner KL, Peindl KS, Gigliotti T, Hanusa BH. Obsessions and compulsions in women with postpartum depression. J Clin Psychiatry 1999;60:176–80.
[91] Leckman JF, Mayes LC, Feldman R, Evans DW, King RA, Cohen DJ. Early parental preoccupations and behaviors and their possible relationship to the symptoms of obsessive-compulsive disorder. Acta Psychiatr Scand Suppl 1999;396:1–26.
[92] Abramowitz JS, Schwartz SA, Moore KM, Luenzmann KR. Obsessive–compulsive symptoms in pregnancy and the puerperium: a review of the literature. J Anxiety Disorder 2003;17:461–78.
[93] Spinelli MG. Maternal infanticide associated with mental illness: prevention and the promise of saved lives. Am J Psychiatry 2004;161:1548–57.
[94] Brandes M, Soares CN, Cohen LS. Postpartum onset obsessive–compulsive disorder: diagnosis and management. Arch Womens Ment Health 2004;7:99–110.
[95] Kim J, Riggs KW, Misri S, Kent N, Oberlander TF, Grunau RE, et al. Stereoselective disposition of fluoxetine and norfluoxetine during pregnancy and breast-feeding. Br J Clin Pharmacol 2006;61:155–63.
[96] Misri S, Kendrick K. Treatment of perinatal mood and anxiety disorders: a review. Can J Psychol 2007;52:489–98.
[97] Oberlander TF, Warburton W, Misri S, Aghajanian J, Hertzman C. Neonatal outcomes after prenatal exposure to selective serotonin reuptake inhibitor antidepressants and maternal depression using population-based linked health data. Arch Gen Psychiatry 2006;63:898–906.
[98] Oberlander TF, Papsdorf M, Brain UM, Misri S, Ross C, Grunau RE. Prenatal effects of selective serotonin reuptake inhibitor antidepressants, serotonin transporter promoter genotype (SLC6A4), and maternal mood on child behavior at 3 years of age. Arch Pediatr Adolesc Med 2010;164:444–51.
[99] Wogelius P, Nørgaard M, Gislum M, Pedersen L, Munk E, Mortensen PB, et al. Maternal use of selective serotonin reuptake inhibitors and risk of congenital malformations. Epidemiology 2006;17(6):701–4.
[100] Koren G, Boucher N. Adverse effects in neonates exposed to SSRIs and SNRI in late gestation—Motherisk Update 2008. Can J Clin Pharmacol 2009;16:e66–67.

[101] Micali N, Treasure J, Simonoff E. Eating disorders symptoms in pregnancy: a longitudinal study of women with recent and past eating disorders and obesity. J Psychosom Res 2007;63:297–303.

[102] Jacobi C, Hayward C, de Zwaan M, Kraemer HC, Agras WS. Coming to terms with risk factors for eating disorders: application of risk terminology and suggestions for a general taxonomy. Psychol Bull 2004;130:19–65.

[103] Fairburn CG, Doll HA, Welch SL, Hay PJ, Davies BA, O'Connor ME. Risk factors for binge eating disorder: a community-based, case–control study. Arch Gen Psychiatry 1998;55:425–32.

[104] Fairburn CG, Cooper Z, Doll HA, Welch SL. Risk factors for anorexia nervosa: three integrated case–control comparisons. Arch Gen Psychiatry 1999;56:468–76.

[105] Fairburn CG, Welch SL, Doll HA, Davies BA, O'Connor ME. Risk factors for bulimia nervosa. A community-based case–control study. Arch Gen Psychiatry 1997;54:509–17.

[106] Striegel-Moore RH, Dohm FA, Kraemer HC, Schreiber GB, Taylor CB, Daniels SR. Risk factors for binge-eating disorders: an exploratory study. Int J Eat Disord 2007;40:481–7.

[107] Bulik CM, Sullivan PF, Fear JL, Joyce PR. Eating disorders and antecedent anxiety disorders: a controlled study. Acta Psychiatr Scand 1997;96:101–7.

[108] Foley DL, Thacker 2nd LR, Aggen SH, Neale MC, Kendler KS. Pregnancy and perinatal complications associated with risks for common psychiatric disorders in a population-based sample of female twins. Am J Med Genet 2001;105:426–31.

[109] Shoebridge P, Gowers SG. Parental high concern and adolescent-onset anorexia nervosa. A case–control study to investigate direction of causality. Br J Psychiatry 2000;176:132–7.

[110] Vize CM, Cooper PJ. Sexual abuse in patients with eating disorder, patients with depression, and normal controls. A comparative study. Br J Psychiatry 1995;167:80–5.

[111] Welch SL, Doll HA, Fairburn CG. Life events and the onset of bulimia nervosa: a controlled study. Psychol Med 1997;27:515–22.

[112] Welch SL, Fairburn CG. Sexual abuse and bulimia nervosa: three integrated case–control comparisons. Am J Psychiatry 1994;151:402–7.

[113] Pike KM, Hilbert A, Wilfley DE, Fairburn CG, Dohm FA, Walsh BT, et al. Toward an understanding of risk factors for anorexia nervosa: a case–control study. Psychol Med 2008;38:1443–53.

[114] Fairburn CG, Harrison PJ. Eating disorders. Lancet 2003;361(9355):407–16.

[115] Patton GC, Coffey C, Sawyer SM. The outcome of adolescent eating disorders: findings from the Victorian Adolescent Health Cohort Study. Eur Child Adolesc Psychiatry 2003;12(Suppl. 1):125–129.

[116] Lemberg R, Philips J. The impact of pregnancy on anorexia nervosa and bulimia. Int J Eat Disord 1989;8:285–95.

[117] Blais MA, Becker AE, Burwell RA, Flores AT, Nussbaum KM, Greenwood DN, et al. Pregnancy: outcome and impact on symptomatology in a cohort of eating-disordered women. Int J Eat Disord 2000;27:140–9.

[118] Stewart DE, Raskin J, Garfinkel PE, MacDonald OL, Robinson GE. Anorexia nervosa, bulimia, and pregnancy. Am J Obstet Gynecol. 1987;157:1194–8.

[119] Stewart DE. Reproductive functions in eating disorders. Ann Med 1992;24(4):287–91.

[120] Koubaa S, Hällström T, Lindholm C, Hirschberg AL. Pregnancy and neonatal outcomes in women with eating disorders. Obstet Gynecol 2005;105:255–60.

[121] Reich T, Winokur G. Postpartum psychoses in patients with manic depressive disease. J Nerv Ment Dis 1970;15:60–8.

9 Neuromuscular Diseases in Pregnancy

Kourosh Rezania

Department of Neurology, The University of Chicago Medical Center, Chicago, IL, USA

Neuromuscular diseases often occur in pregnant women. Some of these diseases result from the physiologic changes of pregnancy and postpartum period, whereas others arise as complications of labor and delivery. On the other hand, an underlying neuromuscular disease may adversely affect the outcome of the pregnancy or jeopardize the health of the parturient. This chapter is divided into three sections: pathophysiology; neuromuscular complications that result from pregnancy, labor, delivery, and postpartum period; and pregnancy in a woman with an underlying neuromuscular disease.

Pathophysiology

Physiologic changes associated with pregnancy often result in musculoskeletal pathology (i.e., back pain and mononeuropathy) in a susceptible individual. The course and natural history of an underlying neuromuscular disease also may change as a result of hormonal or immunologic changes of a normal pregnancy. Below are some of the pregnancy-associated changes that are pertinent to certain kinds of neuromuscular diseases.

Fluid retention: Pregnancy results in a 30–50% increase in plasma and extracellular fluid volume. This is due to a primary renal sodium and water retention as well as a generalized vasodilation [1]. Fluid retention may result in soft-tissue edema, thus predisposing to nerve entrapments, including carpal tunnel syndrome (CTS) and possibly Bell's palsy (BP).

Weight gain: Physiologic weight gain during pregnancy is due to fluid retention, uterine enlargement, and the growing fetus. It results in a compensatory lumbar lordosis to adjust the center of the gravity [2]. Weight gain and lordosis result in increased mechanical stress on the spine, thus contributing to the high prevalence of back pain in pregnant women. Weight gain is also a predisposing factor for meralgia paresthetica (MP).

Relaxin: Relaxin is a polypeptide hormone, and its elevation in pregnancy is thought to be involved in the ligamentous laxity of the sacroiliac, sacrococcygeal, and pubic joints [3]. Elevated relaxin has been proposed in the pathogenesis of CTS

Neurological Disorders and Pregnancy. DOI: 10.1016/B978-0-12-384911-3.00009-9

by such mechanisms as fluid retention in the perineural connective tissue and relaxation of the flexor retinaculum [4–6]. It has also been suggested that relaxin makes the intervertebral discs more vulnerable to stress, resulting in back and pelvic pain [6–8]. However, the pathogenetic role of relaxin in the above-mentioned conditions remains controversial, as other studies have failed to demonstrate correlation of relaxin levels and joint laxity [9,10].

Compression of the pelvic floor neural structures: The enlarging uterus and the fetal head may compress the lumbar or sacral plexi, sciatic, obturator, and femoral nerves later in the pregnancy. Occasionally this results in plexopathy or mononeuropathy, especially at labor and delivery, when the compression of neural elements is more severe.

Labor and delivery: Forceps application may increase the risk of ischemic plexopathy and mononeuropathy due to prolonged compression of the pelvic floor neural elements. Prolonged lithotomy position, especially with excessive leg extension and external hip rotation is another risk factor for post-labor mononeuropathy. In a study of 991 patients who underwent a surgical procedure in the lithotomy position, 15 had unilateral or bilateral mononeuropathy [11]. In that study, the obturator, lateral femoral cutaneous, sciatic, and peroneal nerves were involved in different patients. Furthermore, neuroaxial blockade (including epidural anesthesia), which is commonly used for labor or cesarean section, rarely results in lumbar radiculopathy or other neurologic deficits [12].

Altered immune responses: Autoimmune diseases commonly affect women of childbearing age. Activity of an autoimmune disease often changes as a result of pregnancy-related alterations of the immune responses. Improvement of some of the autoimmune diseases during pregnancy may be the result of increased tolerance to the autoantigens. Animal evidence suggests changes in the maternal T-cell immunoreactivity to accommodate the tolerance to the developing fetus [13,14]. Furthermore, a human study found reduction of interleukin 2 (IL2) and increased soluble tumor necrosis factor (TNF) receptors in the third trimester of pregnancy, while the level of TNF-α and IL1 were unchanged [15]. This suggests down-regulation of Th1 pathway responses during pregnancy. On the contrary, other lines of evidence suggest an increased susceptibility to autoimmunity in the pregnant women. Fetal-derived cells have been shown to circulate in the maternal blood during, and even long after the pregnancy (microchimerism) [16]. Microchimerism is hypothesized to result in autoimmune disease in some cases, as the cells of fetal origin may be the target of an immune response, or they may act as immune effector cells against the mother's autoantigens [16].

Altered respiratory function: Physiologic changes in the respiratory function during pregnancy may adversely affect the outcome of the gestation in a patient with an underlying respiratory muscle weakness. Although the total lung capacity is preserved or mildly decreased in a normal pregnancy, the functional residual capacity (FRC) decreases by 10–25%, starting at twelfth week of gestation [17,18]. The reduction in FRC is due to 35–40% decrease in chest wall compliance [17,19]. On the other hand, the efficiency of diaphragmatic function improves in the parturient due to the increased area of opposition of the diaphragm and the chest wall [20].

Pregnancy does not significantly alter forced expiratory volume in second 1 (FEV1), or forced vital capacity (FVC), and abnormal FEV1, FVC, or their ratio should not be attributed to the pregnancy alone [17].

Neuromuscular Diseases that Result from Pregnancy, Labor, and the Postpartum Period

Carpal tunnel syndrome (CTS): CTS is the most common pregnancy-related entrapment neuropathy. CTS results from the median nerve entrapment in the carpal tunnel, that is, the space between the flexor retinaculum and the distal radius and the carpal bones. Nocturnal hand dysesthesia that mainly involves the palmar surface of the first three fingers and improves with shaking of the hands is the most common presenting symptom. More severe stages are characterized by constant pain and numbness, and abnormal two-point discrimination in the median nerve distribution. Thenar atrophy and weakness of the thumb abduction, flexion, and opposition are seen in very severe cases. Other signs of CTS include Tinel's sign: a radicular pain in the first three fingers with tapping on the median nerve at the wrist; and Phalen's maneuver: paresthesia in the distribution of the median nerve with wrist flexion for 30–60 s.

Association of CTS and pregnancy, as well as the first case of transection of the carpal ligament during pregnancy, was first reported by Wallace and Cook in 1957 [21]. In a longitudinal study by Melvin et al. [22], 31% of a cohort of 58 unselected pregnant women complained of symptoms suggestive for CTS, and 7% had diagnostic abnormalities in the nerve conduction study. All of the patients who were diagnosed with CTS in that study had at least one abnormal sensory nerve action potential, while abnormal motor nerve distal latency was present in only half of the patients with CTS. Bilateral CTS was noted in more than half of the affected subjects in that study. In a more recent, prospective study of 2364 pregnant women, only 2% were diagnosed with CTS [23]. Symptoms were bilateral in about 70% and started in the third trimester in 85% of the women with CTS. Factors that are suggested to predispose to CTS in pregnancy include weight gain, primiparity, age of the mother, and presence of generalized edema [23,24].

Pregnancy-related CTS generally has a good prognosis and therefore is treated conservatively in most cases. Conservative treatment of CTS in nonpregnant patients includes wrist splints, nonsteroidal anti-inflammatory agents, low-salt diet, and hydrocortisone injections. Nonsteroidal anti-inflammatory agents should not be used late in pregnancy due to potential risk of premature constriction of the ductus arteriosus [25]. In a longitudinal study by the Italian CTS study group on 37 untreated pregnant women with CTS, the symptoms resolved in 30% soon after delivery, 11% during lactation, and 5% after interruption of lactation [26]. Interestingly, severe baseline symptoms were associated with a higher probability of later improvement, which could be due to greater behavior modification when the symptoms are more severe. In the study by Turgut et al. [23], 60% of the patients had resolution of the symptoms after delivery with the conservative treatment.

Only 4% had symptoms 1 year postpartum and needed surgical decompression. In another study, conservative management of CTS with splinting of the wrist made 82% of pregnant women with CTS symptom free. Only 7% needed decompression surgery during or after the pregnancy [24].

Other upper extremity mononeuropathies: Pregnancy-related ulnar and radial neuropathies are rare compared to CTS. A patient with postpartum bilateral radial neuropathy was reported due to improper use of the birthing bars [27]. Another patient had bilateral ulnar and radial neuropathy due to compression at the axilla, after the use of a birthing stool [28].

Intercostal neuralgia: Intercostal neuralgia usually manifests in the third trimester of pregnancy with radicular pain in the distribution of one or two thoracic nerve roots [29,30]. It has been attributed to mechanical stretching from the enlarging uterus [31]. A pregnant patient was reported to have intercostals neuralgia in right T8/9 distribution, which completely improved after delivery and recurred in a subsequent pregnancy [32]. Herpes zoster infection, diabetic truncal polyradiculopathy, and structural lesions such as herniated thoracic discs are the main differential diagnosis. Amitryptiline and lidocaine patch (class B medication) and epidural anesthesia have been used to alleviate pain [6,30,32].

Bell's palsy (BP): The association of BP and pregnancy was first suggested by Charles Bell in 1830 [33]. BP is characterized by paresis or complete paralysis of the facial nerve. Other associated symptoms may include pain, dry eyes, hyperacusis, impaired taste sensation in the anterior tongue, and reduced salivation. BP is usually unilateral, but bilateral and recurrent cases have been reported in pregnancy [34,35]. Typically, BP presents with an acute onset over 1–2 days; progression may continue up to 1 week and may result in complete paralysis of facial innervated muscles.

A study by Hilsinger et al. [36], estimated the frequency of BP in pregnancy to be 45 per 100,000, which is higher than the general population (17 per 100,000). On the other hand, Vrabec, et al. have speculated that BP is not more common in the parturient than the general population [37]. Pregnancy-associated BP is more likely to occur in the third trimester of pregnancy and the postpartum period [36–40]. In the study by Hilsinger et al. [36], 74% of pregnancy-related BP occurred in the third trimester and another 12% in the first 2 weeks postpartum.

Fluid retention during the pregnancy may result in perineural edema and therefore, compression neuropathy of the facial nerve. In a retrospective study of 41 women with BP during pregnancy, 29.3% had pre-eclampsia or gestational hypertension, which is about 5 times the expected rate for the general population [39]. Other potential pathogenesis includes reactivation of the herpes simplex virus in the geniculate ganglion, hypercoagulability, and hormonal changes [37].

The differential diagnosis of BP includes leptomeningitis (e.g., Lyme disease and neurosarcoidosis), myasthenia gravis, otitis media, cholesteatoma, malignant infiltration, herpes zoster oticus, and arteriovenous malformation [34,36,37]. Diagnosis usually can be made solely on the clinical grounds in the typical cases. Atypical features include bilateral involvement, insidious or progressive course, severe ear pain, tinnitus, otorrhea, hearing loss, vestibular symptoms, or other cranial or peripheral nerve involvement. The presence of these atypical features should prompt a diagnostic workup, including a brain MRI, CSF examination, Lyme and myasthenia gravis serology, and nerve conduction study and electromyography.

One of the most important aspects of the treatment include prophylactic treatment of eye dryness with artificial tears during the daytime and a thicker ointment at night, eyelid taping or patching, or use of a moisture chamber [37]. As treatment with steroids is suggested to improve the prognosis of BP in the general population, a course of oral prednisone (1 mg/kg for 5 days followed by a taper) has been recommended in complete BP beyond the first trimester of pregnancy [37,41]. The fetal risks of steroids in later stages of pregnancy include adrenal suppression and low birth weight. The use of steroids is not recommended in the first trimester due to increased risk of cleft palate in the fetus [42]. Another treatment option is nucleoside analogue antivirals such as valacyclovir and famciclovir. A study on BP in nonpregnant patients showed a better outcome with the combination of these antivirals and steroids compared to the steroids alone [9,10]. The maximal efficacy of these medications is when they are started within 3 days of the onset of symptoms. Furthermore, the above mentioned antivirals are class B medications and unlikely to be teratogenic, making the risk to benefit ratio more favorable in pregnant women with BP. Facial nerve decompression has been performed in patients with severe axonal BP and has been suggested to improve the long-term prognosis [43]. The prognosis of incomplete facial palsy is excellent, but a persistent deficit may be present in up to 50% of the patients with complete BP [37,44].

Backache and lumbar radiculopathy: More than 50% of pregnant women complain of back pain [45,46]. It usually starts between the fifth and eighth months of the pregnancy, and radicular pain is reported in more than 40% of the patients [45,46]. Pregnancy-related backache is often accompanied by a pelvic girdle pain which often radiates to the symphisis pubis or the posterior thigh. Ligamentous laxity of the pelvis and spine, lordotic posture, and weight of the uterus have been implicated as the predisposing factors [6,47–49].

In a study by Mantle et al. [46], the prevalence of severe back pain increased 5% for every 5 years of increase in maternal age; and there was no association with obesity, weight gain, and the weight of the fetus.

Despite the high prevalence of backache in pregnancy, herniated disc has only been reported in 1/10,000 of the parturient [50]. Lumbar radiculopathy usually is unilateral, and affects the L5 or S1 nerve roots. Herniation of the nucleus pulposus commonly occurs posterolaterally, resulting in radicular pain that is often sudden in onset and exacerbated with coughing or straining. Segmental weakness or sensory or reflex changes may be present. A central disc herniation, on the other hand, may cause bilateral lumbar of sacral radiculopathy and sphincter dysfunction (cauda equine syndrome). Spinal and epidural anesthesia rarely result in a lumbar radiculopathy or other neurologic complications such as epidural hematoma when the tip of the needle touches the dural cuff and damages the nerve root or the artery that enters the intervertebral foramen [7].

Although backache and lumbar radiculopathy in pregnancy are often treated conservatively with bed rest and analgesics, surgical intervention should be considered in pregnant women with severe or progressive neurologic dysfunction or incapacitating pain due to lumbar radiculopathy [7,51–53]. Patients with radicular pain and segmental weakness or numbness should undergo a timely workup, including electromyography and MRI study. MRI is the imaging method of choice in the parturient, as it does not expose the fetus to radiation, however, contrast injection should be avoided unless absolutely necessary [6,54].

Another less common cause of back pain in the postpartum period and even during the pregnancy is sacral fracture [55–57]. In a retrospective study of 236 nonpregnant patients with sacral fractures secondary to trauma, Denis et al. showed that about 6% had neurological findings. The same study suggested that fractures that involve the sacral ala can result in L5 nerve root entrapment between the displaced fragment of the ala and the transverse process of L5 [58]. More commonly, a radiculopathy does not occur with sacral fractures, and the symptoms are groin, buttock, and low back pain and tenderness on deep palpation of the sacrum, with a negative straight leg raising test [57]. Sacral fracture in pregnancy may be secondary to an underlying metabolic bone disease such as a transient osteoporosis which is often associated with the pregnancy and lactation [57]. It should be noted that plain X-ray has a low sensitivity for detecting a sacral fracture. Fracture line is seen better in a CT scan, while MRI study best shows the concomitant bone marrow edema [57].

Lumbar and sacral plexopathy: Plexopathy may result during a vaginal delivery from the compression of the plexi by the fetal head (specially the head of a macrosomic infant) or application of obstetric forceps (especially mid-forceps). Plexopathy is probably the most common cause of acute foot drop after the labor. In a study by Katirji et al. [59], six of seven patients with postdelivery foot drop had short stature and the other had a large newborn. Other predisposing factors for a plexopathy include a straight sacrum, a flat posterior pelvis, and prominent ischial spines [7,60].

Lumbar plexopathy presents with weakness of the hip adductors, hip flexors, and quadriceps. It should be differentiated from femoral neuropathy, which manifests with weakness of quadriceps with or without hip flexion; and obturator neuropathy (weakness of the hip adductors only). Psoas and retroperitoneal hematoma should be considered in patients with lumbar plexopathy. Although hematoma occurs more commonly in the setting of anticoagulation, it has also been reported after normal vaginal delivery [61,62].

Sacral plexopathy can be differentiated from sciatic neuropathy by the presence of weakness of the gluteus medius (hip abduction), gluteus maximus (hip extension), and anal sphincter in the former.

Labor-related lumbar and/or sacral plexopathy are usually treated conservatively as the neuropathic lesion is usually demyelinating, and complete recovery over a period of 5–6 months is expected [59,63]. A less-favorable prognosis can be anticipated if severe axonal degeneration (i.e., absent or markedly abnormal compound muscle action potential (CMAP) amplitude) is detected in the nerve conduction study.

Meralgia paresthetica (MP): MP is a mononeuropathy of the lateral femoral cutaneous nerve. Lateral femoral cutaneous nerve is a purely sensory branch derived from the lumbar plexus (L2–3). It is predisposed to compression and stretch injury at the level of anterior superior iliac spine, under or in the inguinal ligament [64,65]. MP is characterized by dysesthesia, pain, and numbness in the anterolateral thigh without weakness or reflex changes. Symptoms often deteriorate with prolonged standing and improve with sitting. Often there is exacerbation of symptoms with tapping on the upper part of the inguinal ligament near the anterior superior iliac spine, and with hip extension, which stretches the nerve [65]. The main differential diagnosis of MP is a lumbar radiculopathy. The presence of such findings as motor weakness, reflex changes, or a positive straight leg raise testing should prompt a diagnostic workup, including an MRI study of the lumbar spine [65]. Otherwise, MP can be diagnosed based on the clinical presentation. MP can be spontaneous or iatrogenic. Spontaneous MP can be caused by stretching of the nerve in the setting of increased intra-abdominal pressure, such as pregnancy. Other predisposing factors for MP include weight gain, diabetes, and hypothyroidism [64,65]. Spontaneous MP can occur at any time during the pregnancy or the postpartum period. It is usually unilateral, and bilateral involvement is seen in 8–12% of patients [64]. Iatrogenic MP is caused by a number of orthopedic and pelvic operations, including cesarean section [66,67]. Treatment of pregnancy-related MP is almost always conservative, such as minimizing periods of standing, and avoiding tight clothing. The patient should be reassured that the symptoms usually improve after delivery. More severe pain can be treated with local injection of methylprednisolone at the lateral border of the inguinal ligament.

Sciatic and peroneal neuropathy: The sciatic nerve is the largest branch of the sacral plexus and is derived from branches of L4–S3. It is deep to the gluteus maximus in its superior part, where it could be injured because of deep intramuscular injections. Other risk factors for a postpartum sciatic neuropathy include prolonged lithotomy position with knee extension and external hip rotation, and prolonged lateral tilt position during anesthesia [7,68,69]. The prognosis of postpartum sciatic neuropathy is generally favorable [68,69].

The sciatic nerve divides to common peroneal and tibial nerve branches proximal to the knee joint. Peroneal neuropathy usually presents with unilateral or rarely bilateral postpartum foot drop and numbness and paresthesia in the lateral aspect of the leg and dorsum of the foot [70]. A peroneal neuropathy can be differentiated from a sciatic neuropathy or L5 radiculopathy by the lack of weakness of the ankle inversion in the former. An electromyography (EMG) and nerve conduction study may help differentiating these potential causes of postpartum foot drop as well as predicting the prognosis. The peroneal nerve can be injured during labor by inappropriate leg positioning, hyperflexion of the knees, prolonged squatting, manual pressure on the knees during the labor, and prolonged second stage of labor [6,70–72]. The postpartum peroneal neuropathy is usually predominantly demyelinating, and the prognosis is favorable.

Femoral neuropathy: The femoral nerve arises from the posterior divisions of L2–4 spinal roots and emerges from the psoas muscle. It then descends under the inguinal ligament to innervate the iliacus, sartorius, pectineous, and quadriceps femoris. It also provides sensation to the medial aspect of the thigh and leg through its terminal branch, the saphenous nerve. A femoral neuropathy should be distinguished from a lumbar radiculopathy or plexopathy (see lumbar and sacral plexopathy). Femoral neuropathy usually manifests by painless weakness of hip flexion, and severe weakness of the quadriceps. Thigh numbness or attenuated knee jerk also could be present. Femoral neuropathy rarely presents in the third trimester of pregnancy [73]; but the majority of pregnancy-related cases occur during the labor and delivery, with an estimated frequency of 1.5/1000 deliveries [74]. Cephalopelvic disproportion, prolonged labor, primiparity, and prolonged lithotomy position are predisposing factors [11,75]. As postpartum femoral neuropathy is usually demyelinating in nature, the treatment is conservative and the prognosis generally is good, and complete recovery is expected in the majority of patients within a 6-month period [7].

Obturator neuropathy: The obturator nerve is a branch of the lumbar plexus which arises from the anterior divisions of L2–4. Its anterior division innervates the pectineus, gracilis, and the adductor longus and brevis, as well as sensation to the medial aspect of mid and lower thigh. The posterior division provides innervation to adductor magnus and obturator externus. The obturator nerve is vulnerable to compression against the lateral wall of the pelvis as it crosses the upper margin of the obturator internus [76]. In a retrospective study, only one of the 22 patients with obturator neuropathy was postpartum nature [77]. Compression by the fetal head especially in the setting of cephalopelvic disproportion, forceps application, and prolonged lithotomy position are the predispoing factors [76,78]. Obturator neuropathy often presents with neuropathic pain in the medial thigh which often radiates to the knee. Other symptoms include gait impairment due to hip adductor weakness [76]. The treatment of obturator neuropathy is conservative and prognosis is generally good [77]. A patient with severe neuropathic pain was successfully treated with obturator nerve block and steroid injection at the obturator foramen [78].

Pudendal neuropathy: The pudendal nerve arises from the sacral plexus (ventral divisions of S2–4) and innervates the perineal muscles, external urethral and anal sphincter, and skin of the perineum and labia major. Pudendal neuropathy may complicate a normal vaginal delivery due to compression by the fetal head, forceps application, or large episiotomies [79–81]. It may result in pelvic floor weakness and urinary or fecal incontinence.

Muscle Cramps

A cramp is referred to a sudden, painful, involuntary muscle contraction which lasts for seconds to a few minutes. A cramp often begins and ends with fasciculations. Stretching of the affected muscles generally results in immediate resolution of a cramp. Pregnant women commonly experience cramps in the legs, which are more troublesome at night. Potential causes include pregnancy-related changes in fluid and electrolyte parameters or the compression of the pelvic neural structures by the enlarged uterus or fetal head. Such causes as hypothyroidism, uremia, and hyponatremia must be excluded. Regular exercise, multivitamin and mineral supplements, and magnesium lactate or citrate could be effective for the muscle cramps in the parturient [82].

Pregnancy and Underlying Neuromuscular Disease

Pregnancy may cause exacerbation or flare-up of a variety of autoimmune neuromuscular diseases because of changes in the immune responses. Furthermore, it is speculated that pregnancy could affect the natural history of some of the genetic neuromuscular diseases.

Furthermore, pregnancy-related physiologic changes of respiratory function (mentioned earlier) may have deleterious effects on the outcome of a pregnancy, and even prove to be life threatening to the parturient [83]. Abnormal respiratory function in the neuromuscular diseases may be the result of respiratory muscle weakness and/or kyphoscoliosis [83]. Managing a pregnant patient with respiratory muscle weakness may prove to be challenging and needs a multidisciplinary approach. Noninvasive positive pressure ventilation (NPPV) is often used and elective cesarean section is often considered to avoid the need for intubation and mechanical ventilation. Successful pregnancies have been reported with forced vital capacity of 50% and even much lower [84–86].

Inflammatory Neuropathies

Guillain–Barré syndrome (GBS): GBS is an autoimmune, acute, monophasic polyradiculoneuropathy. Most of the cases in the United States and Europe are of the sensorimotor demyelinating type (acquired inflammatory demyelinating polyneuropathy; AIDP). Axonal subtypes, acute motor axonal neuropathy (AMAN), and acute motor and sensory axonal neuropathy occur in less than 10% of cases in the North America and Europe [87]. AMAN is particularly common in China and another variant, Miller Fisher syndrome (MFS) is more prevalent in Japan [87–90]. AIDP is characterized by progressive weakness, with maximal weakness present within 4 weeks, but usually within 2 weeks, after the onset [91,92]. The weakness typically affects both proximal and distal limb muscles and frequently the truncal and respiratory muscles. Reflexes are typically absent early in the course. Facial neuropathy is seen in 70% of patients [87]. Oculomotor involvement is less common, except in patients who are positive for GQ1b antibody, including those with MFS. Sensory symptoms are commonly present, including severe pain in some patients.

A history of a respiratory or gastrointestinal tract infection 3 weeks or less before the onset is present in about two-thirds of patients with AIDP [87]. Molecular mimicry is the possible explanation for this association; that is, the immune response directed towards an infectious organism also is directed to the peripheral nerve antigens (e.g., gangliosides). *Campylobacter jejuni* is the most common pathogen in the nonpregnant population [93,94]. AIDP associated with *C. jejuni* infection is also associated with seropositivity to IgG GM1, an axonal form, and less-favorable prognosis [95,96]. Cytomegalovirus is the second most common infection associated with GBS [93,94]. Cytomegalovirus infection and associated seropositivity to GM1 and GM2 antibodies has been associated with GBS in early and late pregnancy [97–99]. Other more commonly encountered pathogens are Epstein–Barr virus, *Mycoplasma pneumoniae*, human immunodeficiency virus, and *Haemophilus influenzae*.

The incidence of GBS in pregnancy is estimated to be 0.75–2 in 100,000, similar to the general population [100,101]. Although AIDP can present any time in a pregnancy, it is more common in the second and third trimesters, and in the first month of the postpartum period [101]. There appears to be an increased frequency of GBS in the first 30 days postpartum compared to the general population [101]. The occurrence of AIDP in the later stages of pregnancy often results in maternal respiratory failure and premature birth [102,103]. However, the fetal survival rate was reported to be 96% in a review of 29 cases [104]. Luijckx et al. [99] reported a rare case of GBS in a newborn of a GBS patient with recent CMV infection.

Multidisciplinary care is needed to prevent potentially fatal complications. About 25% of patients with GBS who are unable to walk will need mechanical ventilation [87]. Therefore, the vital capacity and respiratory rate must be closely monitored. Other important management issues include prophylaxis for deep vein thrombosis and appropriate treatment of fluctuations in the blood pressure, ileus, and urinary retention.

Plasma exchange (PE) and intravenous immunoglobulins (IVIG) are both proven to be effective in the treatment of GBS [89,105]. PE and IVIG can safely be used in pregnancy [102,106,107]. PE is more effective when it is given early in the course, and the usual regimen is a total exchange of 200–250 mL/Kg over a period of 10 days to 2 weeks [89,108]. Hemodynamic changes (especially hypotension) often complicate PE. Other potential side effects of PE include septicemia, pneumonia, abnormal clotting, transfusion reactions including anaphylaxis and urticaria, and rarely transfusion-related infections [108].

IVIG has replaced PE as the preferred method of treatment in many hospitals, after a large randomized clinical trial showed its equal efficacy to PE [109]. The usual dose is 2 g/kg over a 5-day period [108]. A prospective study on 84 IVIG treatment courses in patients with neurologic diseases showed that the most common side effect was headache (30% of treatment courses). The treatment had to be stopped in 4% of the patients due to more severe side effects like thrombosis of the jugular vein, allergic reaction, and retrosternal pressure [110]. Other common side effects of IVIG include nausea or vomiting, meningismus, exacerbation of chronic renal failure, hypercoagulability, and painful erythema at the infusion site [108].

The more severe cases of GBS who are bed-bound or require artificial ventilation have a worse prognosis than those who have less disability at the peak of their weakness [111]. Other predictors of a poor outcome are rapid onset and axonal features (such as absent motor responses) in the nerve conduction study [89].

AIDP is not considered an indication for cesarean section or therapeutic abortion [103,112]. The uterine contractions probably are not affected, however, cesarean section was performed in 61% of 23 patients with third-trimester AIDP [102]. Both epidural and general anesthesia can be used. Caution should be exercised with the use of depolarizing neuromuscular blockers (e.g., succinylcholine) in patients with AIDP and other diseases that affect the lower motor neurons, because of potentially severe hyperkalemia [113]. The proposed reason for this complication is proliferation of the postsynaptic acetylcholine receptors in diseases of the lower motor neurons. Depolarizing neuromuscular blockers may therefore result in increased release of potassium from the muscle in patients with these diseases [113,114].

Chronic inflammatory demyelinating polyneuropathy (CIDP): CIDP is classically characterized by symmetrical weakness of the proximal and distal muscles of the upper and lower extremities. The disease progression should exceed 2 months, an important feature that differentiates CIDP from GBS (which is a monophasic, self-limited illness) [115]. Other features of CIDP include sensory impairment, absent or attenuated deep tendon reflexes, demyelinating features in the nerve conduction study, elevation of CSF protein, and signs of demyelination in the nerve biopsy [115,116]. Relapsing polyneuropathy was reported with pregnancy and oral contraceptive use even before the diagnostic criteria for CIDP were defined [116–118]. In the patient reported by Calderon-Gonzalez et al., severe relapsing polyneuropathy occurred during the second or third trimesters of three subsequent pregnancies, with complete remission after the delivery each time. That patient probably had CIDP, as she had elevation of CSF protein level, very slow conduction velocities (<14 m/s), and segmental demyelination in a sural nerve biopsy [117]. In a more recent study by McCombe et al. [119] on nine women with CIDP who became pregnant, the onset of the neuropathy was during a pregnancy in 45%, and others had more relapses while pregnant. The symptoms generally worsened in the last trimester and the postpartum period in that study. Maintenance IVIG treatment has been shown to be effective for CIDP and should be considered in the parturient with this condition. Prednisone and intravenous methylprednisolone are category C medications, and can be used. Steroid-sparing agents such as mycophenolate mofetil, cyclosporine, and azathoiprine (all category D medications) must be used with extreme caution, if at all [6].

Multifocal motor neuropathy (MMN): MMN is an autoimmune demyelinating neuropathy that is characterized by slowly progressive, asymmetrical weakness, and presence of conduction block in the motor nerves. Sensory nerves are typically not affected. Thirty to eighty-five percent of the patients with MMN are seropositive for IgM GM1 antibodies [120]. An observational study showed deterioration of neuropathy and involvement of the unaffected nerves in three pregnant patients with MMN [121]. The patients were treated with IVIG, and strength improved to the baseline level after delivery. As steroids may result in the exacerbation of weakness in the patients with MMN, it was suggested that increased disease activity could have been the result of endogenous corticosteroid secretion.

Hereditary Neuropathies

Hereditary motor and sensory neuropathies (Charcot–Marie–Tooth disease; CMT) are a genetically heterogenous group of progressive peripheral neuropathies that often affect the women in the childbearing age. CMT is caused by a number of mutations that affect the peripheral nerve myelination (CMT 1,4) or result in a primarily axonal degeneration (CMT2) [122]. CMT is clinically characterized by pes cavus, symmetrical weakness and atrophy of muscles of the feet and legs, and to a lesser extent, weakness and atrophy of the hand muscles. The sensory symptoms are less prominent than the other neuropathies.

Association of CMT and pregnancy was first reported by Bellina and Deming [123], who reported a patient with increasing weakness and atrophy of the distal muscles in five subsequent pregnancies but no progression between the pregnancies.

Pregnancy-related exacerbations were also noted in the patient's sister. Pollock et al. [124], reported a previously asymptomatic patient with CMT who developed severe neuropathic pain in the third trimester of pregnancy, that resulted in an elective cesarean section. The patient improved 3 months after the delivery. The authors proposed increasing pressure of the enlarging uterus and the estrogen-induced endoneural edema as the potential causes of the observed deterioration.

In a retrospective study by Rudnik-Schoneborn et al. [125], childhood and juvenile onset but not the adult onset CMT, were predisposed to exacerbation of neuropathy symptoms. In that study, 38% of the patients reported exacerbation of weakness during at least one pregnancy, and in 65% of the patients who deteriorated, the deficits persisted after delivery. On the other hand, there was no adverse effect on the outcome of the pregnancy. In another study on 108 gestations of patients with CMT, the patients had a higher rate of fetal presentation abnormalities, including breech or abnormal cephalic presentations which resulted in increased rate of interventions like the use of forceps [126]. That finding was hypothesized to be due to abnormal mobility of the fetuses, but involvement of the fetuses was not reported in that study.

Anesthetic management of the parturient with CMT depends on the severity of the disease. Patients with mild CMT may have a normal vaginal delivery with local or epidural anesthesia [127,128]. On the other hand, if kyphoscoliosis and significantly impaired respiratory function are present, NPPV may have to be started in later stages of pregnancy and elective cesarean section should be considered [128]. Depolarizing neuromuscular blockers should be avoided as there is a risk of severe hyperkalemia (see Guillain Barre Syndrome).

Autoimmune Inflammatory Myopathies

Dermatomyositis (DM) and polymyositis (PM) are the most common autoimmune inflammatory myopathies that affect women of childbearing age. Pregnancy is uncommon in DM/PM, as the two peaks of the onset are in the childhood and over the age of 45 [129]. Flare-up of the underlying DM/PM often occurs in pregnancy or the postpartum period, although a fatal outcome for the mother has only rarely been reported [129–132]. Four of the seven pregnant women with DM/PM had the onset, and three others had an exacerbation of their disease during pregnancy in a study by Gutierrez et al. [133]. The outcome of the pregnancy in DM/PM depends on the disease activity, as well as the age of onset of the myositis. In a study on 28 women with DM/PM, 4 became pregnant, 2 of the 4 with an active disease had abortions, whereas the other 2 with an inactive disease had good fetal outcomes [134]. In yet another retrospective study, only 42% of the pregnancies in DM/PM resulted in normal deliveries, with a strong correlation between the outcome of the pregnancy and the activity of the myositis [135]. The risk of getting pregnant should be discussed with the patients of childbearing age, and pregnancies are better planned when the disease is in remission [129,133]. Muscle strength, respiratory muscle function, and serum CPK should be closely followed during the pregnancy, and flare-ups of the myositis should be treated aggressively [6,129]. Prednisone (starting at 1 mg/kg) is a category C medication and usually is the first line of treatment for DM and PM during pregnancy. IVIG should also be considered a second line of treatment [105]. Some authors have suggested that because DM and PM could have a very aggressive course during pregnancy, such steroid-sparing agents as azathioprine and cyclosporive have to be considered in the more severe cases [129]. DM/PM generally do not affect the uterine contractility, but forceps or vacuum extraction has to be considered if there is generalized muscle weakness [6].

Hereditary Myopathies

Muscular Dystrophies

Duchenne muscular dystrophy (DMD) is an X-linked recessive disease which is caused by a deletion or mutation in the dystrophin gene. DMD is the most common form of muscular dystrophy, with an estimate of 1 in 3300 male births. The frequency of heterozygous female carriers is estimated to be 1 in 6000–10,000. Although the female heterozygote carriers of DMD are usually asymptomatic, about 70% of them have significantly elevated serum CPK levels [136,137]. The heterozygous female carriers rarely have a slowly progressive proximal myopathy that starts in the second or third decade [138]. Besides its genetic implications, the carrier statehood of DMD may affect the outcome of the pregnancy. In a retrospective study on 35 gestations of DMD carrier women, 17% of the newborns had a breech presentation, which is about 5 times the rate of the normal population [139]. The authors suggested a uterine wall abnormality (rather than a fetal factor) as the explanation for their finding.

Myotonic dystrophy type 1 (DM1) is the most common muscular dystrophy that is encountered in pregnant women with an estimated prevalence of 1/8000 adults [6]. DM1 is a multisystem disease which is characterized by clinical and electrophysiologic myotonia and distal predominant muscle weakness and atrophy. Other common features include insulin resistance, cardiac arrhythmias, gonadal dysfunction, cataracts, and cognitive dysfunction. DM1 is caused by a CTG repeat expansion within the dystrophia myotonia protein kinase (*DMPK*) gene [140]. The number of CTG repeats is normally 5–38. Minimally affected patients at least have 50 repeats, and the severity of the disease correlates with the number of the repeats [140]. DM1 is often subclinical and it is not uncommon for a woman to be diagnosed with DM1 only after delivering a child with the congenital form [141]. Myotonic dystrophy type 2 (DM2) results from CCTG repeat expansion within the zinc finger 9 gene and patients have the same phenotype as DM1 [142,143]. The congenital form of DM2 has not so far been reported. Although infertility is common in the males with DM1, some of the women with DM1 have normal fertility. Whether DM1 women have a lower fertility rate than the general population is a controversial issue [83]. Pregnancy may exacerbate the weakness in patients with DM1 and DM2. Thirty percent of pregnant patients with DM1 reported increase of weakness which was reversible after delivery; in some it was attributed to weight gain [144]. Pregnancy in DM1 and 2 should be considered high risk because of potentially serious complications.

Early miscarriage was present in 11% of DM1 and 13% of DM2 pregnancies in two large retrospective studies [141,145]; this is comparable to the frequency of miscarriage in the general population. Ectopic pregnancy and postpartum hemorrhage are more frequent in the DM1 gestations, raising the possibility of dysfunction of fallopian tubes and uterine muscle in DM1 [141]. About 20% of DM1 pregnancies terminated before 34 weeks, and only half of the pregnancies in patients with DM1 and 2 reached full completion [141,145]. More than one-third of the DM1 patients had to have cesarean section due to abnormal labor [141]. Interestingly, the preterm labors of DM patients mainly involved affected fetuses [144]. Due to the congenital DM1, polyhydramnios is present in about 20% of pregnant DM1 women, and the perinatal mortality is reported to be 15%, about 10 times of the general population [141,144]. Polyhydramnios and increased perinatal mortality are not seen in DM2 pregnancies; which is consistent with the fact that congenital DM2 has not yet been reported. Depolarizing neuromuscular blockers should be avoided during anesthesia as they have been reported to cause myotonic spasms, which may interfere with the patient's ventilation [146,147].

Facioscapulohumeral muscular dystrophy (FSHD) is a dominantly inherited myopathy with a prevalence estimated to be 1:20,000. FSHD is the third most common dystrophy after the dystrophinopathies and myotonic dystrophy [148]. Common initial manifestations include difficulty reaching above shoulder level due to weakness of the scapular fixators. Facial weakness is common, but often mild and asymptomatic. The other limb muscles become affected later in the course, and about 10–20% of the patients become wheelchair bound. Ocular and bulbar muscles are usually spared and respiratory weakness has been reported in about 1% [148,149]. About 95% of patients with FSHD have deletion of a repetitive element on 4q35 known as D4Z4 [148]. Around 25% of the pregnant patients with FSHD reported worsening of their muscle weakness, which is reversible in some, but not all of the patients after delivery [150,151]. The outcome of the pregnancy usually is favorable and comparable to the general population [150,151]. However, the second stage of the labor could be abnormal, potentially due to abdominal muscle weakness, as there is increased rate of operative vaginal deliveries and cesarean section in the parturient with FSHD [150,151].

Limb girdle muscular dystrophies (LGMD) are a heterogenous group of myopathies which result from a number of mutations that alter certain proteins of the sarcolemma, myocyte cytoplasmic enzymes, or nuclear membrane. They typically present with a slowly progressive weakness and atrophy of the limb girdle muscles starting in the first or second decades of life. In a study of nine patients with LGMD, five patients (55%) had exacerbation in their weakness during their pregnancies, which did not improve after the delivery [150]. This could be related to the difficulty coping with weight gain when the proximal lower limb muscles are very weak. Obstetric management of a patient with LGMD should be individualized, depending on the severity of muscle weakness. Although normal delivery can be considered in milder cases, significant weakness of the truncal and pelvic muscles may result in abnormal labor and increased rate of cesarean section [150,152]. Patients with significant respiratory muscle weakness and kyphoscoliosis should be treated with NPPV in the later stages of pregnancy and considered for elective cesarean section [153].

Neuraxial (rather than general) anesthesia has been preferred by some physicians, as complications such as malignant hyperthermia (MH) and rhabdomyolysis have rarely been reported with the use of suxamethonium and volatile anesthetics [153].

Muscle Channelopathies

Muscle channelopathies are a group of nondystrophic myopathies which are caused by mutations that result in malfunction of the muscle ionic channels. Depending on the type of the channel involved, they may manifest with myotonia, paramyotonia, periodic paralysis, or MH [154,155]. Genetic and phenotypic variability are common, and different phenotypes are reported even with the same mutation [154].

Myotonia congenita is caused by mutations in *CLCN1*, which encodes for the skeletal muscle chloride channel [154,156]. It can be dominantly or recessively inherited. Pregnancy can result in deterioration of the symptoms in myotonia congenita [156,157] and in rare cases, the symptoms present during a pregnancy [158,159]. The worsening of myotonic symptoms has been attributed to slight hyperpolarization of the muscle resting membrane potential in pregnant women [160]. Furthermore, a study by Fialho et al. [161] showed significant inhibition of the voltage-gated chloride channels in the *Xenopus* oocytes by progesterone and testosterone. The authors speculated that hormonal-induced inhibition of the chloride channels can potentially aggravate the myotonia during pregnancy. Pregnant women with myotonia congenita should avoid cold and intense pain which could aggravate myotonia. Normal vaginal delivery has been reported in gestations of women with myotonia congenita [162]; however, some have suggested elective cesarean section as they speculated that the stress of labor may result in exacerbation of the symptoms and that the stiffness could result in difficulty with vaginal delivery [163,164]. Depolarizing muscle relaxants must be avoided [162,164]. Suxamethonium was reported to cause severe masseter spasm in a patient who was subsequently diagnosed with myotonia congenita [165].

Mutations in the *SCN4A* which encodes for voltage-gated sodium channel $Na_v1.4$ result in dominantly inherited paramyotonia congenita, hyperkalemic periodic paralysis (hyperPP), and rarely, hypokalemic periodic paralysis (hypoPP) [154]. Similar to myotonia congenita, exposure to cold and depolarizing neuromuscular blockers must be avoided [166]. A patient with paramyotonia congenita was reported to have an abortion after exposure to cold [167]. HyperPP is a rare disease characterized by episodic focal or generalized muscle weakness, often precipitated by rest after strenuous exercise [154]. Myotonia may be present at the onset of the attacks, which last for minutes to an hour. A pregnant woman with hyperPP was reported to have complete disappearance of the attacks of weakness during the second and third trimesters of her pregnancy [168]. The parturient with hyperPP should have frequent monitoring of the serum potassium during labor and delivery.

HypoPP is the most common form of periodic paralysis. The most common mutations associated with hypoPP are those of *CACNA1S*, which encodes for α subunit of skeletal muscle calcium channel. Less commonly, hypoPP is caused by mutations in *SCN4A*. Episodes of weakness in hypoPP may be triggered by exercise and a carbohydrate-rich meal. The duration of the attacks is usually longer than those of hyperPP, lasting hours to days [154]. A previously undiagnosed patient with hypoPP had an episode of weakness that was induced by a glucose tolerance test during pregnancy [169]. The management of labor and delivery in hypoPP should include close monitoring of serum potassium and continuous potassium supplementation and avoidance of glucose-containing solutions [170]. A passive second stage of labor and assisted delivery by forceps also is suggested to prevent strenuous labor. General anesthesia and long-acting neuromuscular blockers may cause postdelivery weakness and should be avoided [171]. Epidural anesthesia will also decrease pain-induced hyperventilation and the catecholamine release, thereby potentially preventing hypokalemia secondary to these factors [170,171].

MH is a potentially lethal disease that is caused by mutations in the *RyR1*, which encode for the ryanodine receptors. There is increased entrance of calcium from the sarcoplasmic stores to the myoplasm when the patient is exposed to certain medications such as volatile anesthetics and neuromuscular depolarizing agents [155]. Due to the sustained muscle contraction, the patient develops hyperthermia, metabolic acidosis, rhabdomyolysis, and hyperkalemia if treatment with dantrolene is not rapidly started. Mutations of the *RyR1* are also associated with central core disease, some forms of multi-minicore disease, and centronuclear myopathy, and patients with these diseases also are predisposed to MH [155]. Close monitoring, avoiding the pharmacologic agents mentioned earlier, and sometimes prophylactic use of dantrolene are the mainstay of management, when general anesthesia is used for cesarean section [172–174].

Metabolic Myopathies

Fatty acid oxidation defects, glycogen storage diseases, and mitochondrial myopathies are the major subtypes of the metabolic myopathies. The data regarding metabolic myopathies in the parturient is limited to a number of case reports. The most common diseases that affect the fatty acid oxidation are carnitine palmitoyltransferase type II (CPT II) and carnitine deficiency. CPT II causes episodes of rhabdomyolysis after prolonged endurance-type activity, infections, or fasting. Labor may potentially precipitate hypoglycemia and rhabdomyolysis in patients with CPT II [175]; but there are a few case reports of normal delivery in these patients [175–178]. Rhabdomyolysis may occur in the labor or during the postpartum period. Therefore, intravenous glucose infusion and regular monitoring of the blood glucose during labor and in the postpartum are essential in the management of labor and delivery in women with CPT II [177,178]. Carnitine deficiency is another type of lipid pathway disorder which may cause a progressive myopathy with abnormal lipid storage, as well as myalgia, fatigue, and weakness during periods of high metabolic demand such as labor. Carnitine deficiency can be acquired and may be due to a variety of causes like malnutrition, renal tubular defects, sepsis, pregnancy, or medications such as valproic acid and azidothymidine. Mutations in the carnitine transporter (affecting OCTN2 protein) are the most commonly encountered genetic cause for carnitine deficiency [179]. Donnelly et al. reported a pregnant patient with genetic carnitine deficiency [180]. The patient was treated with intravenous carnitine

4 g/day, as well as glucose, and cesarean section was performed to avoid normal labor.

Glycogen storage diseases (GSD) result from a number of mutations in the enzymes involved in glycogen synthesis, glycogenolysis, and glycolysis. The myopathic forms of GSD may present with episodes of rhabdomyolysis or a progressive weakness due to a glycogen storage myopathy. McArdle disease presents with episodes of muscle cramps and pigmenturia after high-intensity exercise like weight lifting or climbing stairs. Normal delivery has been reported in a patient with McArdle disease [181]. Forceps application was necessary to deliver in that report, but abnormal labor was attributed to abnormal fetal presentation rather than inefficient uterine contractions. However, cesarean section has been performed in other patients to avoid active labor [182,183]. It has been shown that oral sucrose can improve the exercise tolerance in the patients with McArdle disease [184]; and treatment with intravenous glucose is recommended in the treatment of these patients during anesthesia or labor to prevent rhabdomyolysis [181,182,185].

Mitochondrial diseases are a heterogenous group of genetic disorders that affect the mitochondrial respiratory chain. They are usually caused by mutations affecting either the mitochondrial DNA (mtDNA) or the nuclear genes that are involved in the mitochondrial protein synthesis [186]. Mitochondrial myopathies have a predilection for the extraocular muscles, but the limb, truncal, and respiratory muscles can also be affected. Epidural anesthesia has been used in vaginal delivery to minimize the increase in oxygen consumption [187]. Uneventful pregnancy outcomes have been reported in patients with mitochondrial myopathy and respiratory muscle weakness [188,189]. NPPV and elective cesarean section were used in these patients. A patient with mitochondrial myopathy secondary to cytochrome oxidase deficiency was reported to have severe fatigue, muscle weakness, and respiratory compromise at the twentieth week of gestation following a respiratory tract infection [190]. She remained immobile during the pregnancy and underwent elective cesarean section, delivering a full-term infant.

Motor Neuron Diseases

Spinal muscular atrophy (SMA) refers to a heterogenous group of diseases characterized by progressive anterior horn cell degeneration. SMA is autosomal recessively inherited, and is classified as type I–III based on the age of the onset and the clinical course [191]. SMA I–III are caused by mutations in the survival motor neuron1 (*SMN1*) gene [191]. Type III is the milder phenotype with a more protracted clinical course. Proximal limb and respiratory muscle weakness and kyphoscoliosis are common in SMA. Patients with SMA should be advised not to get pregnant if they have significant respiratory muscle weakness. In a study of seventeen gestations in SMA patients, the muscle weakness deteriorated in eight, and weakness persisted after the delivery in five [192]. The pregnancy was complicated by premature labor, prolonged labor, or delayed postpartum recovery in 83% of the patients. Although patients with SMA may have normal vaginal deliveries, cesarean section should be considered if there is significant respiratory compromise, skeletal deformities, and pelvic floor weakness [84,193]. Use of neuraxial anesthesia may be technically complicated because of the chest wall deformities. Furthermore, depolarizing neuromuscular blockers must be avoided because of potential hyperkalemia (see Guillain Barre Syndrome); and nondepolarizing blockers have been associated with prolonged postoperative weakness and inadequate ventilation [194] and thus should be avoided.

Successful pregnancies have been rarely reported in patients with amyotrophic lateral sclerosis (ALS) [195–197]. Depending on the severity of the respiratory weakness, patients may have vaginal delivery or undergo cesarean section [196,197].

References

[1] Bekheirnia MR, Schrier RW. Pathophysiology of water and sodium retention: edematous states with normal kidney function. Curr Opin Pharmacol 2006;6:202–7.

[2] Ritchie JR. Orthopedic considerations during pregnancy. Clin Obstet Gynecol 2003;46:456–66.

[3] Goldsmith LT, Weiss G, Steinetz BG. Relaxin and its role in pregnancy. Endocrinol Metab Clin North Am 1995;24:171–86.

[4] Cormio C, Benelli A. The carpal tunnel syndrome. Irritation of the median nerve at the wrist in women during pregnancy. Minerva Med 1961;52:2645–7.

[5] Soferman N, Weissman SL, Haimov M. Acroparesthesias in pregnancy. Am J Obstet Gynecol 1964;89:528–31.

[6] Sax TW, Rosenbaum RB. Neuromuscular disorders in pregnancy. Muscle Nerve 2006;34:559–71.

[7] Tsen LC. Neurologic complications of labor analgesia and anesthesia. Int Anesthesiol Clin 2002;40:67–88.

[8] Kristiansson P, Svardsudd K, von Schoultz B. Serum relaxin, symphyseal pain, and back pain during pregnancy. Am J Obstet Gynecol 1996;175:1342–7.

[9] Schauberger CW, Rooney BL, Goldsmith L, Shenton D, Silva PD, Schaper A. Peripheral joint laxity increases in pregnancy but does not correlate with serum relaxin levels. Am J Obstet Gynecol 1996;174:667–71.

[10] Marnach ML, Ramin KD, Ramsey PS, Song SW, Stensland JJ, An KN. Characterization of the relationship between joint laxity and maternal hormones in pregnancy. Obstet Gynecol 2003;101:331–5.

[11] Warner MA, Warner DO, Harper CM, Schroeder DR, Maxson PM. Lower extremity neuropathies associated with lithotomy positions. Anesthesiology 2000;93:938–42.

[12] Usubiaga JE. Neurological complications following epidural anesthesia. Int Anesthesiol Clin 1975;13:1–153.

[13] Tafuri A, Alferink J, Moller P, Hammerling GJ, Arnold B. T cell awareness of paternal alloantigens during pregnancy. Science 1995;270:630–3.

[14] Jiang SP, Vacchio MS. Multiple mechanisms of peripheral T cell tolerance to the fetal "allograft". J Immunol 1998;160:3086–90.

[15] Russell AS, Johnston C, Chew C, Maksymowych WP. Evidence for reduced Th1 function in normal pregnancy: a hypothesis for the remission of rheumatoid arthritis. J Rheumatol 1997;24:1045–50.

[16] Adams Waldorf KM, Nelson JL. Autoimmune disease during pregnancy and the microchimerism legacy of pregnancy. Immunol Invest 2008;37:631–44.

[17] Wise RA, Polito AJ, Krishnan V. Respiratory physiologic changes in pregnancy. Immunol Allergy Clin North Am 2006;26:1–12.
[18] Cugell DW, Frank NR, Gaensler EA, Badger TL. Pulmonary function in pregnancy. I. Serial observations in normal women. Am Rev Tuberc 1953;67:568–97.
[19] Marx GF, Murthy PK, Orkin LR. Static compliance before and after vaginal delivery. Br J Anaesth 1970;42:1100–4.
[20] Gilroy RJ, Mangura BT, Lavietes MH. Rib cage and abdominal volume displacements during breathing in pregnancy. Am Rev Respir Dis 1988;137:668–72.
[21] Wallace JT, Cook AW. Carpal tunnel syndrome in pregnancy: a report of two cases. Am J Obstet Gynecol 1957;73:1333–6.
[22] Melvin JL, Burnett CN, Johnson EW. Median nerve conduction in pregnancy. Arch Phys Med Rehabil 1969;50:75–80.
[23] Turgut F, Cetinsahinahin M, Turgut M, Bolukbasi O. The management of carpal tunnel syndrome in pregnancy. J Clin Neurosci 2001;8:332–4.
[24] Ekman-Ordeberg G, Salgeback S, Ordeberg G. Carpal tunnel syndrome in pregnancy. A prospective study. Acta Obstet Gynecol Scand 1987;66:233–5.
[25] Ostensen M. Nonsteroidal anti-inflammatory drugs during pregnancy. Scand J Rheumatol Suppl 1998;107:128–32.
[26] Padua L, Aprile I, Caliandro P, Mondelli M, Pasqualetti P, Tonali PA. Carpal tunnel syndrome in pregnancy: multiperspective follow-up of untreated cases. Neurology 2002;59:1643–6.
[27] Roubal PJ, Chavinson AH, LaGrandeur RM. Bilateral radial nerve palsies from use of the standard birthing bar. Obstet Gynecol 1996;87:820–1.
[28] Buckley CW, Davis TR. Bilateral ulnar and radial nerve palsies as a complication of childbirth. Br Med J (Clin Res Ed) 1983;287:180.
[29] Pleet AB, Massey EW. Intercostal neuralgia of pregnancy. JAMA 1980;243:770.
[30] Samlaska S, Dews TE. Long-term epidural analgesia for pregnancy-induced intercostal neuralgia. Pain 1995;62:245–8.
[31] Kaplan PW. Neurologic disease in women. New York: Demos; 2006.
[32] Skeen MB, Eggleston M. Thoraconeuralgia gravidarum. Muscle Nerve 1999;22:779–80.
[33] Bell C. The nervous system of the human body. Rees, Orme, Brown and Green, London: Longman; 1830.
[34] Gillman GS, Schaitkin BM, May M, Klein SR. Bell's palsy in pregnancy: a study of recovery outcomes. Otolaryngol Head Neck Surg 2002;126:26–30.
[35] Kovo M, Sagi Y, Lampl Y, Golan A. Simultaneous bilateral Bell's palsy during pregnancy. J Matern Fetal Neonatal Med 2009;22:1211–3.
[36] Hilsinger Jr. RL, Adour KK, Doty HE. Idiopathic facial paralysis, pregnancy, and the menstrual cycle. Ann Otol Rhinol Laryngol 1975;84:433–42.
[37] Vrabec JT, Isaacson B, Van Hook JW. Bell's palsy and pregnancy. Otolaryngol Head Neck Surg 2007;137:858–61.
[38] Prescott CA. Idiopathic facial nerve palsy (the effect of treatment with steroids). J Laryngol Otol 1988;102:403–7.
[39] Shmorgun D, Chan WS, Ray JG. Association between Bell's palsy in pregnancy and pre-eclampsia. QJM 2002;95:359–62.
[40] Shapiro JL, Yudin MH, Ray JG. Bell's palsy and tinnitus during pregnancy: predictors of pre-eclampsia? Three cases and a detailed review of the literature. Acta Otolaryngol 1999;119:647–51.
[41] Ramsey MJ, DerSimonian R, Holtel MR, Burgess LP. Corticosteroid treatment for idiopathic facial nerve paralysis: a meta-analysis. Laryngoscope 2000;110:335–41.

[42] Park-Wyllie L, Mazzotta P, Pastuszak A, Moretti ME, Beique L, Hunnisett L, et al. Birth defects after maternal exposure to corticosteroids: prospective cohort study and meta-analysis of epidemiological studies. Teratology 2000;62:385–92.
[43] Yanagihara N, Hato N, Murakami S, Honda N. Transmastoid decompression as a treatment of Bell palsy. Otolaryngol Head Neck Surg 2001;124:282–6.
[44] Peitersen E. Bell's palsy: the spontaneous course of 2,500 peripheral facial nerve palsies of different etiologies. Acta Otolaryngol Suppl 2002;549:4–30.
[45] Fast A, Shapiro D, Ducommun EJ, Friedmann LW, Bouklas T, Floman Y. Low-back pain in pregnancy. Spine (Phila Pa 1976) 1987;12:368–71.
[46] Mantle MJ, Greenwood RM, Currey HL. Backache in pregnancy. Rheumatol Rehabil 1977;16:95–101.
[47] Bushnell LF. The postural pains of pregnancy parietal neuralgia of pregnancy. West J Surg Obstet Gynecol 1949;57:123–7.
[48] Rhodes P. Orthopaedic conditions associated with childbearing. Practitioner 1958;181:304–12.
[49] Spankus JD. The cause and treatment of low back pain during pregnancy. Wis Med J 1965;64:303–4.
[50] LaBan MM, Perrin JC, Latimer FR. Pregnancy and the herniated lumbar disc. Arch Phys Med Rehabil 1983;64:319–21.
[51] Alexander JT, McCormick PC. Pregnancy and discogenic disease of the spine. Neurosurg Clin N Am 1993;4:153–9.
[52] Brown MD, Levi AD. Surgery for lumbar disc herniation during pregnancy. Spine (Phila Pa 1976) 2001;26:440–3.
[53] Garmel SH, Guzelian GA, D'Alton JG, D'Alton ME. Lumbar disk disease in pregnancy. Obstet Gynecol 1997;89:821–2.
[54] LaBan MM, Rapp NS, von Oeyen P, Meerschaert JR. The lumbar herniated disk of pregnancy: a report of six cases identified by magnetic resonance imaging. Arch Phys Med Rehabil 1995;76:476–9.
[55] Druga R, Drugova B. Postpartal atraumatic sacral fracture. A case report and biomechanical comments. Ceska Gynekol 2008;73:192–5.
[56] Thein R, Burstein G, Shabshin N. Labor-related sacral stress fracture presenting as lower limb radicular pain. Orthopedics 2009;32:447.
[57] Lin JT, Lutz GE. Postpartum sacral fracture presenting as lumbar radiculopathy: a case report. Arch Phys Med Rehabil 2004;85:1358–61.
[58] Denis F, Davis S, Comfort T. Sacral fractures: an important problem. Retrospective analysis of 236 cases. Clin Orthop Relat Res 1988;227:67–81.
[59] Katirji B, Wilbourn AJ, Scarberry SL, Preston DC. Intrapartum maternal lumbosacral plexopathy. Muscle Nerve 2002;26:340–7.
[60] Whittaker WG. Injuries to the sacral plexus in obstetrics. Can Med Assoc J 1958;79:622–7.
[61] Terzi I. A case of hematoma of the iliopsoas in labor. Minerva Ginecol 1955;7:266–72.
[62] Rafi J, Muppala H. Conservative management of massive puerperal spontaneous onset retroperitoneal psoas muscle haematoma following normal vaginal delivery. J Obstet Gynaecol 2008;28:105–6.
[63] Gonik B, Stringer CA, Cotton DB, Held B. Intrapartum maternal lumbosacral plexopathy. Obstet Gynecol 1984;63:45S–6S.
[64] Kitchen C, Simpson J. Meralgia paresthetica. A review of 67 patients. Acta Neurol Scand 1972;48:547–55.
[65] Harney D, Patijn J. Meralgia paresthetica: diagnosis and management strategies. Pain Med 2007;8:669–77.

[66] Van Diver T, Camann W. Meralgia paresthetica in the parturient. Int J Obstet Anesth 1995;4:109–12.
[67] Paul F, Zipp F. Bilateral meralgia paresthetica after cesarian section with epidural analgesia. J Peripher Nerv Syst 2006;11:98–9.
[68] Roy S, Levine AB, Herbison GJ, Jacobs SR. Intraoperative positioning during cesarean as a cause of sciatic neuropathy. Obstet Gynecol 2002;99:652–3.
[69] Postaci A, Karabeyoglu I, Erdogan G, Turan O, Dikmen B. A case of sciatic neuropathy after caesarean section under spinal anaesthesia. Int J Obstet Anesth 2006;15:317–9.
[70] Sahai-Srivastava S, Amezcua L. Compressive neuropathies complicating normal childbirth: case report and literature review. Birth 2007;34:173–5.
[71] Adornato BT, Carlini WG. "Pushing palsy": a case of self-induced bilateral peroneal palsy during natural childbirth. Neurology 1992;42:936–7.
[72] Wong CA, Scavone BM, Dugan S, Smith JC, Prather H, et al. Incidence of postpartum lumbosacral spine and lower extremity nerve injuries. Obstet Gynecol 2003;101:279–88.
[73] Kofler M, Kronenberg MF. Bilateral femoral neuropathy during pregnancy. Muscle Nerve 1998;21:1106.
[74] Dar AQ, Robinson A, Lyons G. Postpartum femoral neuropathy: more common than you think. Anaesthesia 1999;54:512.
[75] Donaldson JO, Wirz D, Mashman J. Bilateral postpartum femoral neuropathy. Conn Med 1985;49:496–8.
[76] Nogajski JH, Shnier RC, Zagami AS. Postpartum obturator neuropathy. Neurology 2004;63:2450–1.
[77] Sorenson EJ, Chen JJ, Daube JR. Obturator neuropathy: causes and outcome. Muscle Nerve 2002;25:605–7.
[78] Warfield CA. Obturator neuropathy after forceps delivery. Obstet Gynecol 1984;64:47S–8S.
[79] Pirro N, Sastre B, Sielezneff I. What are the risk factors of anal incontinence after vaginal delivery? J Chir (Paris) 2007;144:197–202.
[80] Snooks SJ, Setchell M, Swash M, Henry MM. Injury to innervation of pelvic floor sphincter musculature in childbirth. Lancet 1984;2:546–50.
[81] Snooks SJ, Swash M, Mathers SE, Henry MM. Effect of vaginal delivery on the pelvic floor: a 5-year follow-up. Br J Surg 1990;77:1358–60.
[82] Young GL, Jewell D. Interventions for leg cramps in pregnancy. Cochrane Database Syst Rev 2000 CD000121
[83] Argov Z, de Visser M. What we do not know about pregnancy in hereditary neuromuscular disorders. Neuromuscul Disord 2009;19:675–9.
[84] Pugh CP, Healey SK, Crane JM, Young D. Successful pregnancy and spinal muscular atrophy. Obstet Gynecol 2000;95:1034.
[85] Yim R, Kirschner K, Murphy E, Parson J, Winslow C. Successful pregnancy in a patient with spinal muscular atrophy and severe kyphoscoliosis. Am J Phys Med Rehabil 2003;82:222–5.
[86] Bach JR. Successful pregnancies for ventilator users. Am J Phys Med Rehabil 2003;82:226–9.
[87] van Doorn PA, Ruts L, Jacobs BC. Clinical features, pathogenesis, and treatment of Guillain–Barré syndrome. Lancet Neurol 2008;7:939–50.
[88] Mori M, Kuwabara S, Fukutake T, Yuki N, Hattori T. Clinical features and prognosis of Miller Fisher syndrome. Neurology 2001;56:1104–6.
[89] Hughes RA, Cornblath DR. Guillain–Barré syndrome. Lancet 2005;366:1653–66.

[90] McKhann GM, Cornblath DR, Griffin JW, Ho TW, Li CY, Jiang Z, et al. Acute motor axonal neuropathy: a frequent cause of acute flaccid paralysis in China. Ann Neurol 1993;33:333–42.

[91] Asbury AK, Cornblath DR. Assessment of current diagnostic criteria for Guillain–Barré syndrome. Ann Neurol 1990;27(Suppl):S21–24.

[92] Van der Meche FG, Van Doorn PA, Meulstee J, Jennekens FG. Diagnostic and classification criteria for the Guillain–Barré syndrome. Eur Neurol 2001;45:133–9.

[93] Van Koningsveld R, Van Doorn PA, Schmitz PI, Ang CW, Van der Meche FG. Mild forms of Guillain–Barré syndrome in an epidemiologic survey in The Netherlands. Neurology 2000;54:620–5.

[94] Hadden RD, Karch H, Hartung HP, Zielasek J, Weissbrich B, Schubert J, et al. Preceding infections, immune factors, and outcome in Guillain–Barré syndrome. Neurology 2001;56:758–65.

[95] Hughes RA, Rees JH. Guillain–Barré syndrome. Curr Opin Neurol 1994;7:386–92.

[96] Rees JH, Soudain SE, Gregson NA, Hughes RA. *Campylobacter jejuni* infection and Guillain–Barré syndrome. N Engl J Med 1995;333:1374–9.

[97] Araki, T, Nakata, H, and Kusunoki, S. [Two cases of Guillain–Barré syndrome in late pregnancy]. Rinsho Shinkeigaku 2010;50:24–26.

[98] Mendizabal JE, Bassam BA. Guillain–Barré syndrome and cytomegalovirus infection during pregnancy. South Med J 1997;90:63–4.

[99] Luijckx GJ, Vles J, de Baets M, Buchwald B, Troost J. Guillain–Barré syndrome in mother and newborn child. Lancet 1997;349:27.

[100] Ropper AH. The Guillain–Barré syndrome. N Engl J Med 1992;326:1130–6.

[101] Cheng Q, Jiang GX, Fredrikson S, Link H, de Pedro-Cuesta J. Increased incidence of Guillain–Barré syndrome postpartum. Epidemiology 1998;9:601–4.

[102] Chan LY, Tsui MH, Leung TN. Guillain–Barré syndrome in pregnancy. Acta Obstet Gynecol Scand 2004;83:319–25.

[103] Ahlberg G, Ahlmark G. The Landry–Guillain–Barré syndrome and pregnancy. Acta Obstet Gynecol Scand 1978;57:377–80.

[104] Nelson LH, McLean Jr. WT. Management of Landry–Guillain–Barré syndrome in pregnancy. Obstet Gynecol 1985;65:25S–9S.

[105] Elovaara I, Apostolski S, van Doorn P, Gilhus NE, Hietaharju A, Honkaniemi J, et al. EFNS guidelines for the use of intravenous immunoglobulin in treatment of neurological diseases: EFNS task force on the use of intravenous immunoglobulin in treatment of neurological diseases. Eur J Neurol 2008;15:893–908.

[106] Kuller JA, Katz VL, McCoy MC, Hansen WF. Pregnancy complicated by Guillain Barré syndrome. South Med J 1995;88:987–9.

[107] Yamada H, Noro N, Kato EH, Ebina Y, Cho K, Fujimoto S. Massive intravenous immunoglobulin treatment in pregnancy complicated by Guillain–Barré syndrome. Eur J Obstet Gynecol Reprod Biol 2001;97:101–4.

[108] Hughes RAC, Swan AV, Cornblath DR, Hartung HP. Randomised trial of plasma exchange, intravenous immunoglobulin, and combined treatments in Guillain–Barré syndrome. Plasma exchange/sandoglobulin Guillain–Barré syndrome trial group. Lancet 1997;349:225–230.

[109] van der Meche FG, Schmitz PI. A randomized trial comparing intravenous immune globulin and plasma exchange in Guillain–Barré syndrome. Dutch Guillain–Barré study group. N Engl J Med 1992;326:1123–9.

[110] Stangel M, Kiefer R, Pette M, Smolka MN, Marx P, Gold R. Side effects of intravenous immunoglobulins in neurological autoimmune disorders—a prospective study. J Neurol 2003;250:818–21.

[111] Visser LH, Schmitz PI, Meulstee J, van Doorn PA, van der Meche FG. Prognostic factors of Guillain–Barré syndrome after intravenous immunoglobulin or plasma exchange. Dutch Guillain–Barré study group. Neurology 1999;53:598–604.
[112] Mabie WC. Peripheral neuropathies during pregnancy. Clin Obstet Gynecol 2005;48:57–66.
[113] Feldman JM. Cardiac arrest after succinylcholine administration in a pregnant patient recovered from Guillain–Barré syndrome. Anesthesiology 1990;72:942–4.
[114] Gronert GA, Theye RA. Pathophysiology of hyperkalemia induced by succinylcholine. Anesthesiology 1975;43:89–99.
[115] Koller H, Kieseier BC, Jander S, Hartung HP. Chronic inflammatory demyelinating polyneuropathy. N Engl J Med 2005;352:1343–56.
[116] Dalakas MC, Engel WK. Chronic relapsing (dysimmune) polyneuropathy: pathogenesis and treatment. Ann Neurol 1981;9(Suppl):134–45.
[117] Calderon-Gonzalez R, Gonzalez-Cantu N, Rizzi-Hernandez H. Recurrent polyneuropathy with pregnancy and oral contraceptives. N Engl J Med 1970;282:1307–8.
[118] d'Ambrosio G, de Angelis G. Guillain–Barré syndrome in pregnancy. Rev Neurol (Paris) 1985;141:33–6.
[119] McCombe PA, McManis PG, Frith JA, Pollard JD, McLeod JG. Chronic inflammatory demyelinating polyradiculoneuropathy associated with pregnancy. Ann Neurol 1987;21:102–4.
[120] Pestronk A, Chaudhry V, Feldman EL, Griffin JW, Cornblath DR, Denys EH, et al. Lower motor neuron syndromes defined by patterns of weakness, nerve conduction abnormalities, and high titers of antiglycolipid antibodies. Ann Neurol 1990;27:316–26.
[121] Chaudhry V, Escolar DM, Cornblath DR. Worsening of multifocal motor neuropathy during pregnancy. Neurology 2002;59:139–41.
[122] Nave KA, Sereda MW, Ehrenreich H. Mechanisms of disease: inherited demyelinating neuropathies—from basic to clinical research. Nat Clin Pract Neurol 2007;3:453–64.
[123] Bellina JH, Deming B. Charcot–Marie–Tooth disease and pregnancy: report of a case. J La State Med Soc 1973;125:393–5.
[124] Pollock M, Nukada H, Kritchevsky M. Exacerbation of Charcot–Marie–Tooth disease in pregnancy. Neurology 1982;32:1311–4.
[125] Rudnik-Schoneborn S, Rohrig D, Nicholson G, Zerres K. Pregnancy and delivery in Charcot–Marie–Tooth disease type 1. Neurology 1993;43:2011–6.
[126] Hoff JM, Gilhus NE, Daltveit AK. Pregnancies and deliveries in patients with Charcot–Marie–Tooth disease. Neurology 2005;64:459–62.
[127] Scull T, Weeks S. Epidural analgesia for labour in a patient with Charcot–Marie–Tooth disease. Can J Anaesth 1996;43:1150–2.
[128] Greenwood JJ, Scott WE. Charcot–Marie–Tooth disease: peripartum management of two contrasting clinical cases. Int J Obstet Anesth 2007;16:149–54.
[129] Doria A, Iaccarino L, Ghirardello A, Briani C, Zampieri S, Tarricone E, et al. Pregnancy in rare autoimmune rheumatic diseases: UCTD, MCTD, myositis, systemic vasculitis and Bechet disease. Lupus 2004;13:690–5.
[130] England MJ, Perlmann T, Veriava Y. Dermatomyositis in pregnancy. A case report. J Reprod Med 1986;31:633–6.
[131] Steiner I, Averbuch-Heller L, Abramsky O, Raz E. Postpartum idiopathic polymyositis. Lancet 1992;339:256.
[132] Rosenzweig BA, Rotmensch S, Binette SP, Phillippe M. Primary idiopathic polymyositis and dermatomyositis complicating pregnancy: diagnosis and management. Obstet Gynecol Surv 1989;44:162–70.

[133] Gutierrez G, Dagnino R, Mintz G. Polymyositis/dermatomyositis and pregnancy. Arthritis Rheum 1984;27:291–4.

[134] Silva CA, Sultan SM, Isenberg DA. Pregnancy outcome in adult-onset idiopathic inflammatory myopathy. Rheumatology (Oxford) 2003;42:1168–72.

[135] Vancsa A, Ponyi A, Constantin T, Zeher M, Danko K. Pregnancy outcome in idiopathic inflammatory myopathy. Rheumatol Int 2007;27:435–9.

[136] Emery AE. Carrier detection in sex-linked muscular dystrophy. J Genet Hum 1965;14:318–29.

[137] Moser H, Emery AE. The manifesting carrier in Duchenne muscular dystrophy. Clin Genet 1974;5:271–84.

[138] Barkhaus PE, Gilchrist JM. Duchenne muscular dystrophy manifesting carriers. Arch Neurol 1989;46:673–5.

[139] Geifman-Holtzman O, Bernstein IM, Capeless EL, Hawley P, Specht LA, Bianchi DW. Increase in fetal breech presentation in female carriers of Duchenne muscular dystrophy. Am J Med Genet 1997;73:276–8.

[140] Brook JD, McCurrach ME, Harley HG, Buckler AJ, Church D, Aburatani H, et al. Molecular basis of myotonic dystrophy: expansion of a trinucleotide (CTG) repeat at the 3' end of a transcript encoding a protein kinase family member. Cell 1992;68:799–808.

[141] Rudnik-Schoneborn S, Zerres K. Outcome in pregnancies complicated by myotonic dystrophy: a study of 31 patients and review of the literature. Eur J Obstet Gynecol Reprod Biol 2004;114:44–53.

[142] Ranum LP, Rasmussen PF, Benzow KA, Koob MD, Day JW. Genetic mapping of a second myotonic dystrophy locus. Nat Genet 1998;19:196–8.

[143] Day JW, Roelofs R, Leroy B, Pech I, Benzow K, Ranum LP. Clinical and genetic characteristics of a five-generation family with a novel form of myotonic dystrophy (DM2). Neuromuscul Disord 1999;9:19–27.

[144] Rudnik-Schoneborn S, Nicholson GA, Morgan G, Rohrig D, Zerres K. Different patterns of obstetric complications in myotonic dystrophy in relation to the disease status of the fetus. Am J Med Genet 1998;80:314–21.

[145] Rudnik-Schoneborn S, Schneider-Gold C, Raabe U, Kress W, Zerres K, Schoser BG. Outcome and effect of pregnancy in myotonic dystrophy type 2. Neurology 2006;66:579–80.

[146] Thiel RE. The myotonic response to suxamethonium. Br J Anaesth 1967;39:815–21.

[147] Mitchell MM, Ali HH, Savarese JJ. Myotonia and neuromuscular blocking agents. Anesthesiology 1978;49:44–8.

[148] Tawil R. Facioscapulohumeral muscular dystrophy. Neurotherapeutics 2008;5:601–6.

[149] Wohlgemuth M, van der Kooi EL, van Kesteren RG, van der Maarel SM, Padberg GW. Ventilatory support in facioscapulohumeral muscular dystrophy. Neurology 2004;63:176–8.

[150] Rudnik-Schoneborn S, Glauner B, Rohrig D, Zerres K. Obstetric aspects in women with facioscapulohumeral muscular dystrophy, limb-girdle muscular dystrophy, and congenital myopathies. Arch Neurol 1997;54:888–94.

[151] Ciafaloni E, Pressman EK, Loi AM, Smirnow AM, Guntrum DJ, Dilek N, et al. Pregnancy and birth outcomes in women with facioscapulohumeral muscular dystrophy. Neurology 2006;67:1887–9.

[152] Pash MP, Balaton J, Eagle C. Anaesthetic management of a parturient with severe muscular dystrophy, lumbar lordosis and a difficult airway. Can J Anaesth 1996;43:959–63.

[153] Allen T, Maguire S. Anaesthetic management of a woman with autosomal recessive limb-girdle muscular dystrophy for emergency caesarean section. Int J Obstet Anesth 2007;16:370–4.

[154] Ryan AM, Matthews E, Hanna MG. Skeletal-muscle channelopathies: periodic paralysis and nondystrophic myotonias. Curr Opin Neurol 2007;20:558–63.
[155] Platt D, Griggs R. Skeletal muscle channelopathies: new insights into the periodic paralyses and nondystrophic myotonias. Curr Opin Neurol 2009;22:524–31.
[156] Colding-Jorgensen E. Phenotypic variability in myotonia congenita. Muscle Nerve 2005;32:19–34.
[157] Hakim CA, Thomlinson J. Myotonia congenita in pregnancy. J Obstet Gynaecol Br Commonw 1969;76:561–2.
[158] Lacomis D, Gonzales JT, Giuliani MJ. Fluctuating clinical myotonia and weakness from Thomsen's disease occurring only during pregnancies. Clin Neurol Neurosurg 1999;101:133–6.
[159] Wu FF, Ryan A, Devaney J, Warnstedt M, Korade-Mirnics Z, Poser B, et al. Novel CLCN1 mutations with unique clinical and electrophysiological consequences. Brain 2002;125:2392–407.
[160] Forsum E, Forsberg AM, Nilsson E, Bergstrom J, Hultman E. Electrolytes, water, RNA, total creatine and calculated resting membrane potential in muscle tissue from pregnant women. Ann Nutr Metab 2000;44:144–9.
[161] Fialho D, Kullmann DM, Hanna MG, Schorge S. Non-genomic effects of sex hormones on CLC-1 may contribute to gender differences in myotonia congenita. Neuromuscul Disord 2008;18:869–72.
[162] Basu A, Nishanth P, Ifaturoti O. Pregnancy in women with myotonia congenita. Int J Gynaecol Obstet 2009;106:62–3.
[163] Butwick AJ, Riley ET. Successful spinal blockade in a parturient with myotonia congenita. Int J Obstet Anesth 2007;16:292–3.
[164] Farrow C, Carling A. Successful spinal blockade in a parturient with myotonia congenita. Int J Obstet Anesth 2007;16:89–90.
[165] Looi I, Bakar AA, Lim CH, Khoo TH, Samuel PE. Anaesthetists' nightmare: masseter spasm after induction in an undiagnosed case of myotonia congenita. Med J Malaysia 2008;63:423–5.
[166] Grace RF, Roach VJ. Caesarean section in a patient with paramyotonia congenita. Anaesth Intensive Care 1999;27:534–7.
[167] Chitayat D, Etchell M, Wilson RD. Cold-induced abortion in paramyotonia congenita. Am J Obstet Gynecol 1988;158:435–6.
[168] Finsterer J. Disappearance of episodic weakness during pregnancy in hyperkalemic periodic paralysis from the SCNA4 mutation T704M. Neurologist 2009;15: 289–90.
[169] Damallie KK, Drake JG, Block WA. Hypokalemic periodic paralysis in pregnancy after 1-hour glucose screen. Obstet Gynecol 2000;95:1037.
[170] Viscomi CM, Ptacek LJ, Dudley D. Anesthetic management of familial hypokalemic periodic paralysis during parturition. Anesth Analg 1999;88:1081–2.
[171] Melnick B, Chang JL, Larson CE, Bedger RC. Hypokalemic familial periodic paralysis. Anesthesiology 1983;58:263–5.
[172] Foster RN, Boothroyd KP. Caesarean section in a complicated case of central core disease. Anaesthesia 2008;63:544–7.
[173] Douglas MJ, McMorland GH. The anaesthetic management of the malignant hyperthermia susceptible parturient. Can Anaesth Soc J 1986;33:371–8.
[174] Lips FJ, Newland M, Dutton G. Malignant hyperthermia triggered by cyclopropane during cesarean section. Anesthesiology 1982;56:144–6.
[175] Slater PM, Grivell R, Cyna AM. Labour management of a woman with carnitine palmitoyl transferase type 2 deficiency. Anaesth Intensive Care 2009;37:305–8.

[176] Dreval D, Bernstein D, Zakut H. Carnitine palmitoyl transferase deficiency in pregnancy—a case report. Am J Obstet Gynecol 1994;170:1390–2.
[177] Mardirosoff C, Dumont L, Cobin L, Massaut J. Labour analgesia in a patient with carnitine palmityl transferase deficiency and idiopathic thrombocytopenic purpura. Int J Obstet Anesth 1998;7:134–6.
[178] Lilker S, Kasodekar S, Goldszmidt E. Anesthetic management of a parturient with carnitine palmitoyltransferase II deficiency. Can J Anaesth 2006;53:482–6.
[179] Treem WR, Stanley CA, Finegold DN, Hale DE, Coates PM. Primary carnitine deficiency due to a failure of carnitine transport in kidney, muscle, and fibroblasts. N Engl J Med 1988;319:1331–6.
[180] Donnelly CT, Hameed AB, Abdenur JE, Wing DA. Carnitine deficiency in pregnancy. Obstet Gynecol 2007;110:480–482.
[181] Cochrane P, Alderman B. Normal pregnancy and successful delivery in myophosphorylase deficiency (McArdle's disease). J Neurol Neurosurg Psychiatry 1973;36:225–7.
[182] Coleman P. McArdle's disease. Problems of anaesthetic management for Caesarean section. Anaesthesia 1984;39:784–7.
[183] Samuels TA, Coleman P. McArdle's disease and caesarean section. Anaesthesia 1988;43:161–2.
[184] Vissing J, Haller RG. The effect of oral sucrose on exercise tolerance in patients with McArdle's disease. N Engl J Med 2003;349:2503–9.
[185] Ellis FR. Inherited muscle disease. Br J Anaesth 1980;52:153–64.
[186] Vu TH, Hirano M, DiMauro S. Mitochondrial diseases. Neurol Clin 2002;20:809–39. vii-viii
[187] Blake LL, Shaw RW. Mitochondrial myopathy in a primigravid pregnancy. Br J Obstet Gynaecol 1999;106:871–3.
[188] Yuan N, El-Sayed YY, Ruoss SJ, Riley E, Enns GM, Robinson TE. Successful pregnancy and cesarean delivery via noninvasive ventilation in mitochondrial myopathy. J Perinatol 2009;29:166–7.
[189] Diaz-Lobato S, Gomez Mendieta MA, Moreno Garcia MS, Mayoralas-Alises S, Arpa Gutierrez FJ. Two full-term pregnancies in a patient with mitochondrial myopathy and chronic ventilatory insufficiency. Respiration 2005;72:654–6.
[190] Soccio PS, Phillips WP, Bonisteel P, Bennett KA. Pregnancy with cytochrome oxidase-deficient mitochondrial myopathy. Obstet Gynecol 2001;97:815–6.
[191] Wirth B. An update of the mutation spectrum of the survival motor neuron gene (SMN1) in autosomal recessive spinal muscular atrophy (SMA). Hum Mutat 2000; 15:228–37.
[192] Rudnik-Schoneborn S, Zerres K, Ignatius J, Rietschel M. Pregnancy and spinal muscular atrophy. J Neurol 1992;239:26–30.
[193] Carter GT, Bonekat HW, Milio L. Successful pregnancies in the presence of spinal muscular atrophy: two case reports. Arch Phys Med Rehabil 1994;75:229–31.
[194] McLoughlin L, Bhagvat P. Anaesthesia for caesarean section in spinal muscular atrophy type III. Int J Obstet Anesth 2004;13:192–5.
[195] Jacka MJ, Sanderson F. Amyotrophic lateral sclerosis presenting during pregnancy. Anesth Analg 1998;86:542–3.
[196] Sarafov S, Doitchinova M, Karagiozova Z, Slancheva B, Dengler R, Petri S, et al. Two consecutive pregnancies in early and late stage of amyotrophic lateral sclerosis. Amyotroph Lateral Scler 2009;10:483–6.
[197] Kawamichi, Y, Makino, Y, Matsuda, Y, Miyazaki, K, Uchiyama, S, and Ohta, H. Riluzole use during pregnancy in a patient with amyotrophic lateral sclerosis: a case report. J Int Med Res 2010;38:720–726.

10 Sleep Disorders and Pregnancy

Ahmet Ursavas

Uludag University Medical Faculty, Respiratory Medicine Department, Bursa, Turkey

In the United States, over one million pregnancies each year result in adverse outcomes such as pre-eclampsia, intrauterine growth restriction, and preterm delivery [1]. There are no defined risk factors for 50% of these pregnancies. Sleep disturbances are frequent complaints in pregnant women and this may be a specific contributor to adverse pregnancy outcomes [2]. The subject of sleep disorders in pregnancy will be discussed in this chapter as regular sleep pattern in pregnancy, sleep-related breathing disorders in pregnancy, and other sleep disorders in pregnancy.

Regular Sleep Duration and Pattern in Pregnancy

Sleep patterns in women present different characteristics than in men. Menstrual cycle, puberty, menopause, and hormonal, emotional, and body heat changes emerging in pregnancy affect the sleep [3]. Dynamic and physiologic changes affecting the functions of many organs and systems occur in pregnancy. Mechanical and hormonal changes occurring in pregnancy affect regular sleep routine, sleep duration, and pattern. Sleep has several functions in the human body. Although regular sleep pattern in human is well known, normal sleep duration differs in persons. Normal sleep duration is 4–11 h in adults. Of healthy adults, 75% sleep 6–8 h, 15% over 8 h, and 10% under 6 h. Sleep duration in society has been reported to have decreased 1.5–2 h on average compared to 40 years ago [4]. Sleep duration in pregnancy is variable. In general, sleep duration increases in the first gestational trimester, returns to normal in the second trimester, and decreases in the last trimester. In a study conducted by survey method in Finland, mean daily sleep durations during the pregnancy of the patient who slept a mean 7.8 h before pregnancy were defined as 8.2 h in the first trimester, 8.0 h in the second, and 7.8 h in the last trimester [5]. However, studies conducted by polysomnography application indicate the exact sleep durations of the pregnant women are 30 min less than their subjective statements. Polysomnography applied to pregnant patients at home has defined sleep duration that is 7.4 h in 11–12 gestational weeks, decreased to 6.9 h in the 36th gestational week.

Besides sleep duration, sleep pattern also presents changes in pregnancy. The factors causing this change can be discussed in two groups, hormonal and

Neurological Disorders and Pregnancy. DOI: 10.1016/B978-0-12-384911-3.00010-5

Table 10.1 Factors Affecting Quality and Stages of Sleep During Pregnancy

Positive Factors on Non-REM Sleep	Positive Factors on REM Sleep	Mechanical Factors Resulting in Arousals
Progesterone	Estrogen	Uterine contractions
Luteinizing hormone	Cortisol	Fetal movement
Prolactin		Stomach ache
		Frequency of urination
		Leg cramps
		Gastroesophageal reflux

mechanical factors. Estrogen, progesterone, and cortisol levels changing in pregnancy are the major hormonal factors affecting the sleep. Estrogen and progesterone progressively increase in pregnancy. Estrogen has been reported to decrease rapid eye movement (REM) sleep and progesterone to increase non-REM sleep. In rats with oophorectomy performed, REM sleep was defined to increase with decreasing of estrogen and to decrease with estrogen treatment [6]. Exogenous progesterone application leads to sedative effect and increase of the REM sleep in men and women. The sedative characteristic of progesterone has been associated with the effect of gamma aminobutyric acid A receptor agonist. Except estrogen and progesterone, cortisol levels that reached high levels in pregnancy decrease the REM sleep, luteinizing hormone increases non-REM sleep, and prolactin increases both REM and non-REM sleep [7,8]. Mechanical factors such as the growth of the fetus and the upcoming birth affect sleep in pregnancy in the last trimester of pregnancy. Uterine contractions, abdominal pain, frequent urination, leg cramps, and gastroesophageal reflux cause arousals during sleep, negatively affecting the sleep quality [9]. The factors affecting regular sleep in the pregnancy are seen in Table 10.1.

Sleep Deprivation in Pregnancy

Sleep Deprivation and Preterm Delivery

Insufficient sleep duration and poor sleep quality are considered to be endemic in modern society. Optimal sleep duration in pregnancy is not known. Insufficient sleep has been suggested to have effects on the health of mother and baby. Short sleep duration in pregnancy has been found to be associated with postpartum depression, preterm delivery, and the need for cesarean. When considering the general population, there is a significant correlation between short sleep duration and mortality. Possible reasons of this correlation are short sleep duration, impairing of the cognitive functions, increase in traffic and occupational accidents, and metabolic and endocrine dysfunctions [10,11]. Short sleep duration alone can increase the risk for preterm delivery. As previously described, residency studies among female physician trainees were associated with increased risk of preterm delivery [12]. In a study by Lee et al [13]., on polysomnography performed in the last four gestational weeks, a significant need for cesarean was seen in pregnant patients with a sleep duration under 6 h, compared to those with a sleep duration over 7 h.

Several studies with nonpregnant women indicate sleep disorders increase the level of inflammation indicators. In a study subjectively evaluating Pittsburgh sleep quality index and sleep diary, interleukin6 level was reported to be higher in the pregnant patient with sleep disorder defined in mid-pregnancy and last trimester [14]. Inflammatory cytokines play a crucial role in the onset mechanism of the delivery and in addition, they affect the preterm delivery etiopathogenesis. Prostaglandins have a major role in the onset and maintenance of uterine contractions [15]. Inflammatory cytokine concentrations in amniotic fluids have been reported to significantly increase in the pregnant patient with preterm delivery [16].

Sleep Deprivation and Postpartum Depression

Postpartum depression is defined as an episode of depression emerging within 4 weeks of delivery and lasting up to 6 months in duration. Previous studies suggest that the rate of the onset of depression increases threefold in the months after childbirth [17]. Postpartum depression is seen in approximately 10–15% of all women giving birth. Postpartum depression prevalence has been reported as levels of 40–50% in the high-risk pregnancy in terms of depression [17,18]. The main risk factors for postpartum depression are low socioeconomic class, lack of education, social isolation, poor family relations, unplanned pregnancy, preterm delivery, cesarean section, psychological stress, and previously experienced postpartum depression [18].

Sleep deprivation is a risk factor that is known to be associated with depression, but has not attracted enough attention. Past epidemiologic studies have described an association between sleep disturbance and depression [19]. Goyal et al. [20] followed 124 primiparous women from their last month of pregnancy through 3 months postpartum. In another study, Wolfson and colleagues examined self-reported depressive symptoms and sleep patterns from the late pregnancy to 1-year postpartum and observed an association between sleep patterns during the late pregnancy and depressive symptoms in the first few weeks of the postpartum period. Although both groups of women reported similar sleep patterns in the postpartum period, mothers who develop greater depressive symptoms at 2–4 postpartum weeks had significantly different sleep routines in late pregnancy compared to nondepressed mothers [21].

Various mechanisms for the development of postpartum depression have been suggested. The most accepted suggestion among these is the sudden drop of estrogen and progesterone hormones after birth that had progressively increased during the pregnancy period. However, various cytokines are also suggested to have a role in this situation. Changes occurring in cytokine levels due to sleep disturbances may play a role in the pathogenesis of depression by affecting neuorochemical transmission and/or the hypothalamic pituitary adrenal axis [22]. Effects of sleep deprivation in pregnancy are summarized in Figure 10.1.

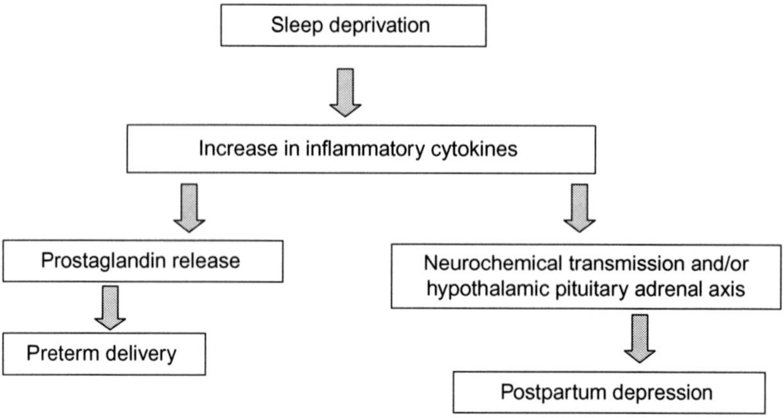

Figure 10.1 Effects of sleep deprivation in pregnancy.

Sleep-Disordered Breathing in Pregnancy

Sleep-Disordered Breathing

Sleep-disordered breathing (SDB) includes snoring, upper airway resistance syndrome, and obstructive sleep apnea (OSA). OSA is characterized by repetitive collapse of the upper airway during sleep, resulting in obstruction of airflow and oxygen desaturation, which cause arousal from sleep. OSA is a common disorder affecting at least 2–4% of the adult population [23]. The prevalence of OSA is estimated to be 5–6% among women of reproductive age [24].

Apnea is defined as the complete cessation of airflow for a minimum of 10 s. A $\geq$30% reduction of airflow associated with $\geq$4% drop in oxygen saturation, or alternatively a $\geq$50% reduction of airflow associated with $\geq$3% drop in oxygen saturation, or associated with an electroencephalogram arousal is considered hypopnea according to American Academy of Sleep Medicine manual scoring system. The average number of apnea–hypopnea per hour is called apnea–hypopnea index (AHI). OSA is diagnosed when a patient has clinical symptoms in conjunction with an AHI $>$5 events per hour [25].

Both epidemiologic and sleep clinic-based studies indicate that OSA is more common in men than in women. There are a number of pathophysiologic differences to suggest why men are more prone to the disease than women. Although the exact mechanisms are unknown, differences in obesity, upper airway anatomy, breathing control, hormones, and aging are all thought to play a role [26]. Ninety-three percent of women with moderate-to-severe OSA were not clinically diagnosed in the Wisconsin sleep cohort study [27]. The diagnosis of OSA starts with a sleep history that typically is obtained in one of three setting; first as part of routine health maintenance evaluation, second as part of evaluation of symptoms of OSA, and third as part of the comprehensive evaluation of patients at high risk of OSA. Symptoms and signs most suggestive of OSA include habitual snoring, witnessed apneas, gasping and choking sensations during sleep, large neck, obesity, and hypertension.

The classic OSA presentation and major symptoms may not be in female OSA patients. Female OSA patients referred for evaluation at sleep clinic more frequently, insomnia, nocturnal palpitation, depression, lack of energy, night sweats, fibromyalgia, irritable bowel syndrome, compared to men with OSA [28].

Effect of Pregnancy on SDB

Several physiologic changes that alter the functions of many organs and systems occur during pregnancy. Some of these changes may provide protection from SDB, whereas others may put women at risk. Anatomic changes such as progressive weight gain and the enlarging uterus up toward the diaphragm 3–4 cm, subcostal angle increases, and thorax transverse diameter increases by 2 cm, combined with the supine position during sleep may reduce functional residual capacity and predispose women to OSA [29].

A number of hormonal rhythms, some of which influence sleep, are altered by pregnancy. Estrogen and progesterone are progressively increasing in pregnancy and affect sleep. High levels of estrogen and progesterone are required to maintain pregnancy. Along with estrogen and progesterone, the changes occurring during pregnancy in prostaglandin and cortisol levels may also have an impact on the SDB physiology [29,30]. Reduced upper airway dimensions during pregnancy have been demonstrated. Nasal zone is responsible for 50% of upper airway resistance. Estrogen induces changes in the airway mucosa consisting of hypersecretion, hyperemia, nasopharyngeal mucosal edema, and vasomotor rhinitis which can predispose to increased upper airway resistance, snoring, and upper airway obstructive events [31]. Nasal obstruction has been shown to be an independent risk factor for OSA in the adult population [32]. A study reported nasal congestion and rhinitis symptoms in 42% of the subjects at the 36th week of gestation. In fact, rhinitis symptoms have been reported to be higher even during the luteal phase of the menstrual cycle [33]. Another factor that both protects against and is conducive to OSA is the elevated progesterone level that occurs during pregnancy. Progesterone enhances respiratory center sensitivity to CO_2, thereby up-regulating ventilatory drive and minute ventilation. This hyperventilation reduces arterial $PaCO_2$ to a nadir of about 30 mmHg but blood pH and PaO_2 remains normal. The increased respiratory drive protects against upper airway occlusion by enhancing responsiveness of upper airway dilator muscles to chemical stimuli during sleep. Furthermore, progesterone itself has been shown to increase upper airway dilator muscle electromyographic activity [34,35]. On the contrary, increased ventilatory drive with resultant respiratory alkalosis has been predisposed to central apnea. Another effect of increased ventilatory drive is increased diaphragmatic activity. This can lead to greater negative inspiratory pressure and increased tendency for upper airway collapse [36]. The factors increasing snoring and apnea frequency in pregnancy are summarized in Figure 10.2.

SDB in Pregnant Women

The prevalence of SDB during pregnancy is unknown. There are several studies on snoring and other symptoms of OSA during pregnancy, all confirming an increase in OSA symptoms among pregnant women compared to prepregnancy status or

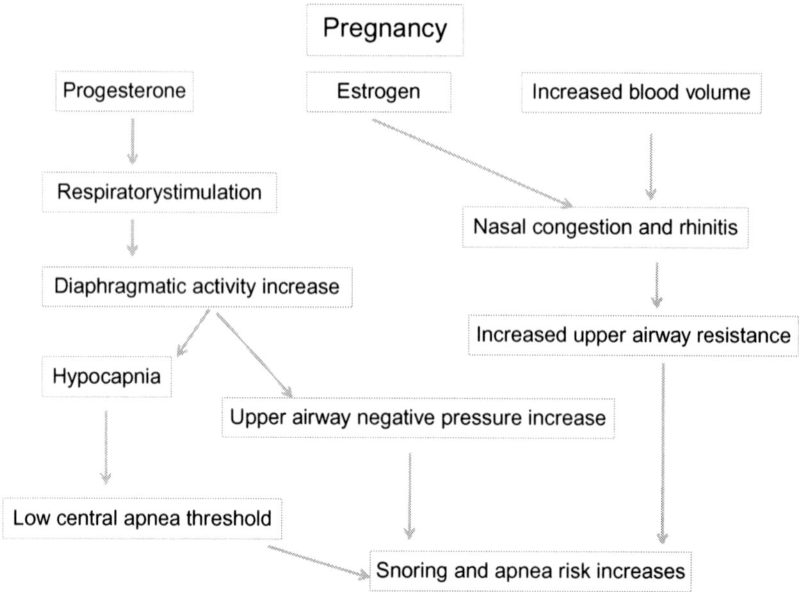

Figure 10.2 The factors increasing snoring and apnea frequency in pregnancy.

nonpregnant women [37–41]. Many studies were based on questionnaires and were limited by a lack of polysomnographic confirmation of OSA.

The incidence of snoring in a US population of healthy pregnant women was found to be 14%, significantly greater than the 4% incidence found in age-matched nonpregnant population [37]. In a similar study carried out by Franklin et al. [38] in Sweden, 502 pregnant women were asked to complete a questionnaire. They found that during the last week of pregnancy, 23% of the women reported snoring every night. Only 4% reported snoring before their pregnancy. Guilleminault et al. [41] investigated 267 pregnant women in a two-stage study. All subjects underwent ambulatory monitoring of their sleep with a six-channel recorder at the 6-month prenatal visit. Prepregnancy snoring prevalence was reported to be 3.7%, while it was observed to be 11.8% during the last trimester. In the second stage of the study, 26 subjects underwent polysomnography, 13 based on symptoms, blood pressure values, and the ambulatory monitoring results; and 13 chosen at random from the group. Abnormal respiratory patterns were detected but none of the subjects were determined to have apnea or hypopnea. Age, obesity, and smoking predispose to snoring and other sleep-related breathing disorders. The prevalence of habitual snoring in middle-aged French males was reported at 32%. Age, neck circumference, tobacco consumption, excess weight, and large soft palate were independently associated with snoring [42]. Resta et al. [43] investigated the prevalence of snoring and OSA in obese subjects. They showed that neck circumference in men and body mass index (BMI) in women were the strongest predictors of the severity of OSA. Maasilta et al. [40] recruited 11 obese and 11 control women. Overnight polysomnography was performed in early and late pregnancy. They showed that early and late pregnancy AHIs, oxygen desaturations, arousal indexes, and snoring times were significantly higher in the obese pregnant women as compared to the nonobese pregnant controls. The results of a large questionnaire study indicate that age, smoking during pregnancy, and weight before delivery were independent risk factors for habitual snoring in pregnancy, according to logistic regression analysis. Furthermore, neck circumference is higher in habitual snorers when compared to nonhabitual snorers in univariable analysis [44].

SDB, Gestational Hypertension, and Pre-eclampsia

SDB has been proposed as a risk factor for adverse maternal and fetal outcomes such as fetal heart rate abnormalities, fetal growth retardation, fetal death, pregnancy-induced hypertension (gestational hypertension), pre-eclampsia, pulmonary hypertension, and gestational diabetes. Some studies also suggested that SDB was associated with adverse pregnancy outcomes; however, other studies did not indicate significant association. These inconsistent results may be due to the fact that most of the studies were of small sample size and had an absence of polysomnographic data [45].

The National Heart, Lung, Blood Institute working group defines gestational hypertension as a new onset of systolic blood pressure ⩾140 mmHg or a diastolic blood pressure ⩾90 mmHg after mid-pregnancy. When associated with proteinuria, it is called pre-eclampsia [46]. Gestational hypertension complicates 6–8% of pregnancies [47]. OSA is an independent risk factor for hypertension in the general population. Observational studies indicate that untreated OSA is associated with an increased risk of prevalent hypertension, whereas prospective studies of normotensive cohorts suggest that OSA may increase the risk of incident hypertension in the nonpregnant adult population [48]. Nocturnal blood pressure values are higher when compared with daytime values in pre-eclampsia and diurnal variations are observed [49][47]. Moreover, diurnal variations are observed in hypertension in such patients as well. Therefore, an association between pre-eclampsia and SDB has been postulated. Risk factors for pre-eclampsia include nulliparity, pre-existing hypertension, diabetes, obesity, dyslipidemia, depression, renal disease, asthma, history of gestational hypertension, multifetal gestation, insulin resistance, thrombophilia, living in high altitude, collagen vascular disease, and hydatidiform mole [50]. There is some evidence that maternal snoring is a poor prognostic factor for the mothers who have a greater risk of hypertension and pre-eclampsia [51]. Izci et al. [52] investigated 167 healthy pregnant, 82 pre-eclamptic pregnant, and 160 nonpregnant women. They reported that 32% of control, 55% of pregnant, and 85% of pre-eclamptic women snored. Franklin et al. [38] reported that snoring pregnant women had a two-fold (odds ratio of 2.03) greater incidence of hypertension and pre-eclampsia than did nonsnorers. In another study, snoring was a risk factor for gestational hypertension with an adjusted odds ratio of 1.82 after adjustments for prepregnancy BMI, weight gain during pregnancy, smoking, alcohol, age, and neck circumference [53]. Snoring was a risk factor for gestational hypertension but not pre-eclampsia, and neck circumference was an independent risk factor for gestational hypertension and pre-eclampsia, according to logistic regression analysis in a case–control study [44]. A recent study of 1000 subjects indicated that factors used in the regression analysis included age, BMI, diabetes, chronic hypertension, multifetal gestations, smoking, and renal disease. Symptoms of SDB were associated with a higher likelihood of pregnancy-induced hypertension and pre-eclampsia (OR 2.38, 95% CI 1.4–4.1); gestational diabetes (OR 2.1, 95% CI 1.3–3.4); and unplanned cesarean sections (OR 3.80 95% CI 2.2–6.7) after multivariable regression analysis [54]. In conclusion, snoring during pregnancy may be an important finding, as it has been associated with gestational hypertension and pre-eclampsia.

OSA during pregnancy was first reported in 1978 by Joel-Cohen et al. [55]. After this case report, there are several studies about OSA during pregnancy consisting largely of case reports, questionnaire, or small sample size case–control studies. Subsequent case–control studies using overnight recordings were used. In the first case–control study, Connolly et al. [56] enrolled 15 healthy and 15 pre-eclamptic pregnant women along with 15 nonpregnant women in their study. The subjects were monitored overnight for blood pressure and respiration. They were also monitored with an oximeter. While none of the subjects was found to have significant sleep apnea syndrome, pre-eclamptic pregnant women were observed with significant inspiratory flow limitation. Episodic inspiratory flow limitation observed in upper airway resistance syndrome was brief and resulted in arousal. However, these subjects were observed with long episodes of minutes at a time. Champagne et al. [57] performed tests involving 17 pregnant women with gestational hypertension and 33 pregnant women without hypertension. The crude odds ratio for the presence of OSA given the presence of gestational hypertension was 5.6. The odds ratio was 7.5 (95% CI 3.5–16.2), based on a logistic regression model with adjustment for maternal age, gestational age, prepregnancy BMI, prior pregnancies, and previous live births.

While it now appears clear that there is an association between the existence of SDB and hypertension during pregnancy, the primary causal abnormality has not been proved. Increased edema in the upper airway resulting from the generalized vascular changes found in pre-eclampsia may precipitate SDB [36]. Upper airway diameters of 37 pre-eclamptic and 13 nonpre-eclamptic pregnant women in the third trimester, as well as 50 nonpregnant women were measured by using acoustic reflection method and then compared. Upper airway diameters in pre-eclamptic pregnant women were observed to be significantly narrower than those of the nonpregnant women and those of the nonpre-eclamptic pregnant women [58]. However, it has been speculated that intermittent maternal hypoxia induced by SDB could cause placental ischemia, triggering oxidative stress, and endothelial activation. Oxidative stress and endothelial activation are implicated in the pathogenesis of gestational hypertension [45,59]. The relationship between snoring, OSA, gestational hypertension, and pre-eclampsia is shown in Figure 10.3.

SDB and Gestational Diabetes Mellitus

SDB may be a risk factor for gestational diabetes. Several epidemiologic and experimental studies showed that chronic partial sleep loss is associated with increased

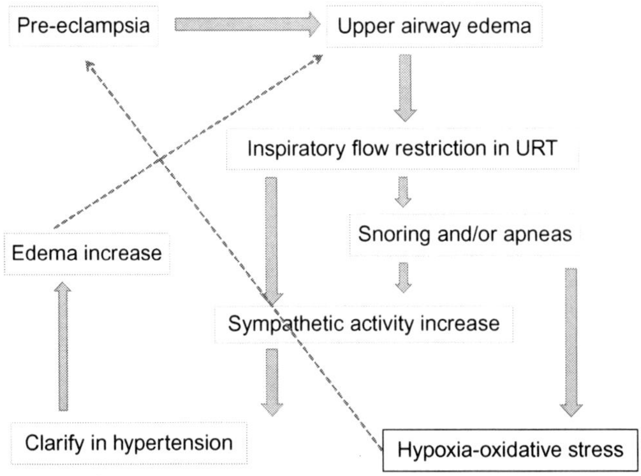

Figure 10.3 The relationship among snoring, OSA, and pre-eclampsia.

risk of obesity and obesity-related disorders such as impaired glucose tolerance. The estimated OSA prevalence in diabetic cohort is 17.5% (24.7% in men, 10.3% in women). OSA is associated with prevalent glucose intolerance and insulin resistance even after adjustment for confounders, especially obesity in the general population [60]. Although the exact mechanisms underlying these associations have yet to be elucidated, evidence from experimental studies suggests that insufficient habitual snoring and sleep apnea result in metabolic and neuroendocrine alteration. Moreover, there has been data that long-term intermittent hypoxia and sleep fragmentation increase sympathetic activity, which in turn leads to disorders of glucose metabolism [61]. The oxygen desaturation index (number of episodes of reduction in oxygen saturation by >4%, per hour of sleep) is a better predictor of insulin resistance than BMI [62]. There are very little data about how insufficient sleep and SDB during gestation contribute to increased risk of medical complications of pregnancy, including gestational diabetes mellitus. Youssef et al. [63] analyzed through 2003 health care cost utilization project nationwide inpatient data of all pregnant women. Controlling for race, gender, and obesity, OSA conferred twice the likelihood of having gestational diabetes. A recent cohort study of 1290 women was interviewed during early pregnancy. After adjusting for maternal age and ethnicity, gestational diabetes mellitus risk was increased among women sleeping ≤4 h compared with those sleeping 9 h/night. Snoring was associated with a 1.86-fold increased risk of gestational diabetes mellitus. The risk of gestational diabetes mellitus was elevated particularly among overweight women who snored [64].

SDB in Pregnancy and Fetal Outcome

The clinical fetal outcome of SDB during pregnancy remains controversial. Some early reports suggest that it may represent a new risk factor to intrauterine growth restriction and lower Apgar scores at birth [36]. However, other studies did not precisely support this association [65].

Repetitive episodes of obstructive respiratory events during sleep give rise to cyclic episodes of maternal hypoxemia. It is also known that hypoxia is observed in pregnant women particularly in the last trimester due to physiologic changes occurring in the respiratory system. It has been reported that PaO_2 levels dropped below 90 mmHg in the supine position in 25% of pregnant women in the last trimester. As hypoxia can occur even during wakefulness, a minor alteration in respiration pattern during sleep may impair maternal and fetal oxygenation severely [66]. Previous studies conducted on pregnant subjects living in higher altitudes or those with hypoxia due to pulmonary parenchyma demonstrated that maternal hypoxia led to retarded fetal development [67]. Experimental rat studies revealed that prenatal hypoxia impaired the development of the chemoafferent pathway, as well as the ventilatory and metabolic responses to hypoxia [68]. Gozal et al. [69] demonstrated that newborns of pregnant rats exposed to intermittent hypoxia, a hallmark of sleep apnea syndrome, had lower birth weight when compared with newborns of pregnant rats exposed to normoxia. The same study also established that normoxic ventilation was higher in newborn rats whose mothers had been exposed to intermittent hypoxia.

Questionnaire-based investigations were performed to address the association between snoring and fetal outcome. The results of these studies are contradictory. Franklin et al. [38] established impaired fetal development in 8 (7.1%) of the 113 pregnant women with habitual snoring and 10 (2.6%) of the 379 pregnant women with no habitual snoring. The difference was statistically significant, indicating that snoring was a risk factor for intrauterine growth restriction and low Apgar scores. In contrast, Loube et al. [37] reported that pregnant women who were snorers did not have deliveries resulting in infants with evidence of an increase in compromised outcomes. A recent questionnaire study also indicated that there was no significant relationship between snoring and fetal outcome [70]. Polysomnography and fetal heart monitoring-based studies were also performed to investigate fetal outcome in pregnant OSA patients. A case–control study included 57 pregnant women with confirmed OSA and 114 healthy pregnant controls. OSA patients had more pre-eclampsia (19.3% versus 7.0%) and preterm births (29.8% versus 12.3%). Controlling for comorbid conditions, OSA was associated with an increased risk of preterm birth (OR 2.6), mostly secondary to pre-eclampsia (63%). Cesarean delivery (OR 8.1) and OSA were associated with maternal morbidity (OR 4.6) [71]. Sahin et al. [72] simultaneously investigated the polysomnography and nonstress test (NST) records of 35 pregnant women. OSA was diagnosed in four, of which three with adequate NST had fetal heart decelerations associated with maternal desaturation. Apgar scores and birth weights were lower for the four women with confirmed OSA. However, a similar recent study indicated that no association was observed between fetal heart rate monitoring abnormalities and OSA parameters [73]. However, there are some studies that did not find association, and preliminary reports suggest that OSA may cause fetal deceleration and lower birth weight and Apgar scores.

Evaluation and Treatment of OSA in Pregnancy

There are no specific guidelines for screening pregnant women for OSA because the data are limited in this population. The incidence of SDB in normal and complicated pregnancy is not defined. Most symptoms of OSA are nonspecific and may overlap normal pregnancy symptoms such as fatigue, sleepiness, or insomnia [65]. In pregnancy, the Berlin questionnaire poorly predicts OSA [73]. Consequently, the decision to investigate and treat must be individualized according to intensity and spectrum of symptoms, impact on quality of life, risk of accidents, comorbidities, concomitant disease, and acceptability of diagnostic testing [45,65]. Some authors recommended that excessive daytime sleepiness, loud snoring, and witnessed apneas in pregnant women should be evaluated by overnight polysomnography (evidence C) [74]. However, others have proposed that the indication for polysomnography in pregnant women probably should be expanded to include those with hypertension, pre-eclampsia, previous babies with unexplained intrauterine growth restriction, persistant insomnia, or hypersomnia associated with snoring and obesity (evidence C) [35,44]. Several studies indicated that nocturnal polysomnography was successfully performed in pregnant women. Sleep studies in pregnant women can be applied similarly to nonpregnant women [41,45].

Treatment guidelines for pregnant women with OSA are similar to that of the general population. In nonpregnant OSA patients, a number of treatment options are available, including various types of positive airway pressure (PAP) therapy, oral appliances, surgery, and conservative approach. All pregnant women should follow conservative precautions, such as avoiding weight gain, sleeping in a lateral position, elevating the head end of the bed, treating nasal obstruction with external nasal dilators, inhaling corticosteroids, avoiding allergens in the context of allergies, and restraining the use of sedatives and alcohol. Oral appliances usually are not initiated during pregnancy because of the delay required for optimization of therapy. It may be an option in patients who cannot tolerate PAP. Moreover, if treatment is already adjusted before pregnancy, it should be continued. Upper airway surgical therapies are not recommended routinely due to increased surgical risk during pregnancy [45,65].

Continuous positive airway pressure (CPAP) remains the predominant therapy for the treatment of patients with OSA and has been shown to resolve SDB levels and improve several clinical outcomes. CPAP is conventionally delivered via a nasal mask at a fixed pressure that remains constant throughout the respiratory cycle. CPAP's proposed mechanism of action is as a pneumatic splint that maintains the patency of the upper airway in a dose-dependent fashion (Figure 10.4). CPAP therapy is currently indicated for the treatment of moderate-to-severe OSA and for patients with mild OSA and associated symptoms, and/or associated cardiovascular disease [75]. From the summary of case reports and small sample size studies, evidence showed that CPAP was safe and well tolerated during pregnancy. No adverse events were reported among pregnant women with OSA who were treated with nasal CPAP therapy [76,77]. In a case series of twelve pregnant women with OSA (seven diagnosed before pregnancy and five diagnosed in the first trimester of pregnancy) in whom CPAP was initiated before early pregnancy, there was an

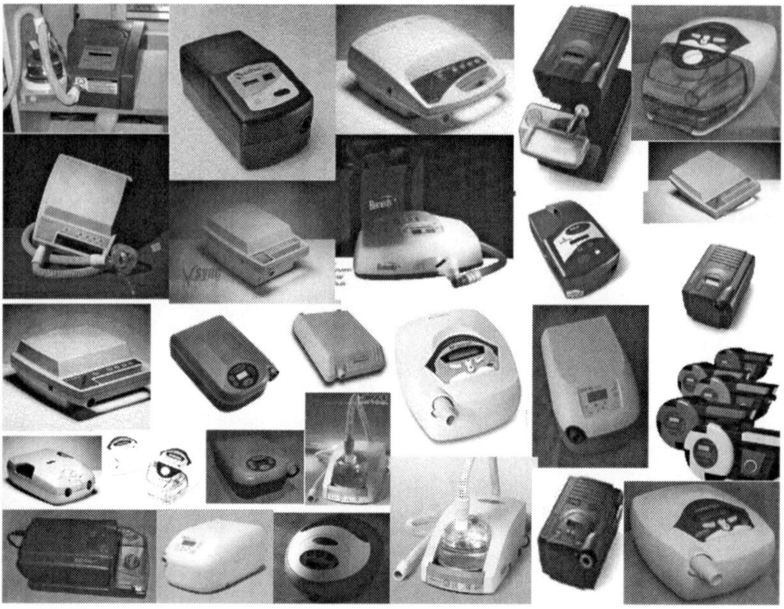

Figure 10.4 CPAP devices.

improvement OSA symptom, all babies were healthy, and side effects were not different than the ones observed in other CPAP users [78]. Some studies found nasal CPAP to be particularly useful in reducing nocturnal blood pressure increments in women with pre-eclampsia. Guilleminault and colleagues investigated the possibility of using nasal CPAP early in pregnancy for prevention of pre-eclampsia. In the first study, 12 women with either chronic hypertension or obesity were recruited in the first trimester to utilize CPAP throughout pregnancy. All of the women were able to utilize CPAP throughout pregnancy. There were some small differences in episodes of tachypnea when CPAP was used, but none of the chronic hypertensive patients developed pre-eclampsia or needed to increase their dosage of antihypertensive medication. One of the obese patients developed pre-eclampsia [79]. Only one randomized controlled trial of CPAP among pregnant women was retrieved. This study compared the addition of nasal CPAP treatment to standard prenatal care or to standard prenatal care alone in hypertensive women treated with alpha-methyldopa during early pregnancy. Subjects were randomized to receive either CPAP with standard prenatal care (treatment group) or standard prenatal care alone (control group) with routine obstetric follow-up. Nocturnal polysomnography was performed in all patients randomized to the treatment group for initial CPAP titration. In the control group (n=9), a progressive rise in blood pressure with a corresponding increase in alpha-methyldopa doses was observed, beginning at the sixth month of pregnancy. There was also an increase in the number of nonscheduled postnatal visits during the first postpartum month. Pre-eclampsia occurred in one subject; the remaining eight patients had normal pregnancies and infant deliveries. In the treatment group

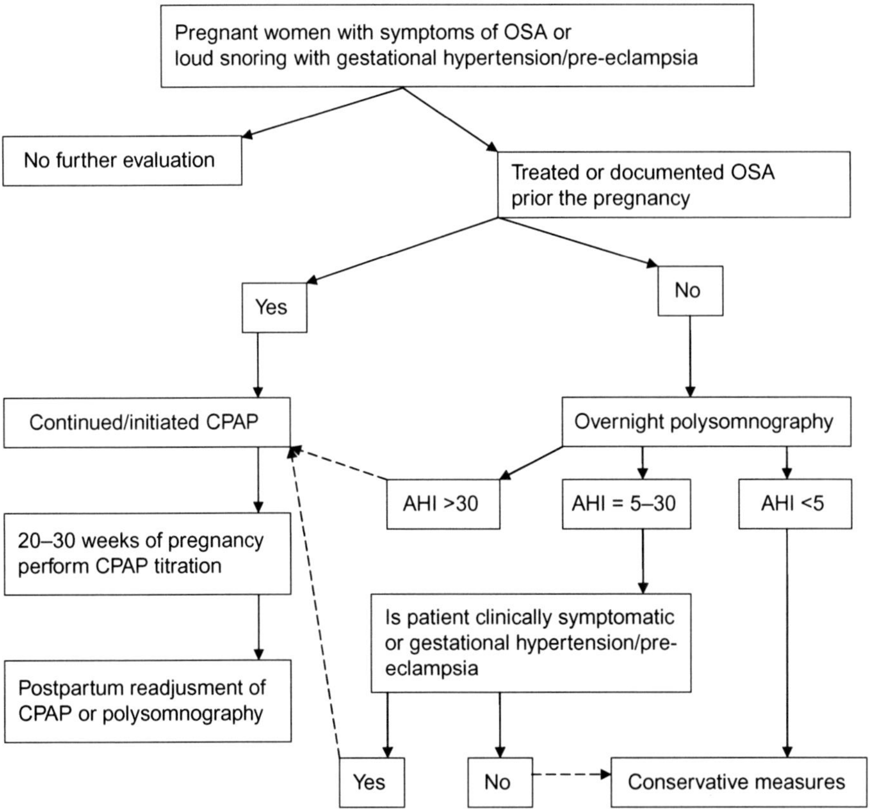

Figure 10.5 Recommendations for the evaluation and treatment of pregnant women suspected of having SDB.
Source: Modified from [45].

($n = 7$), blood pressure was noted to decrease significantly as compared to the control group with associated decreases in doses of antihypertensive medications at 6 months of gestation. All treated patients experienced uncomplicated pregnancies and delivered infants with higher Apgar scores at 1 min postdelivery compared to those of controls [80]. Because delivery is associated with a decrease in severity of OSA, some reports recommended performing a postpartum polysomnography once weight is stabilized [57,81]. Recommendations for the evaluation and treatment of pregnant women suspected of having SDB are shown in Figure 10.5.

Other Sleep Disorders in Pregnancy

Other sleep disorders that have been reported to occur and in some cases were triggered or worsened by pregnancy are periodic leg movements (PLM), leg cramps, restless legs syndrome (RLS), sleepwalking, night terror, and narcolepsy. The true incidence of other sleep disorders in pregnancy is unknown [35].

According to the International Classification of Sleep disorders, RLS and leg cramps are classified as sleep-related movement disorders [82]. Leg cramps are intense painful muscle contractions affecting the foot, calf, or both while falling asleep. However, leg cramps can cause awakenings. It is common in the general population, affecting up to 95% of exercising college students, 35–60% of the elderly, and up to 30% of pregnant women [83]. Many causes can be lead to leg cramps in the general population such as inactivity, excessive exercise, hypomagnesemia, hypocalcemia, hyponatremia, structural disorders, dehydration, metabolic, and vascular or neurologic disorders. However, etiopathogenesis of leg cramps during pregnancy is unknown and it may be idiopathic [84]. The best treatment for leg cramps during pregnancy may be oral magnesium before sleep. The evidence of this treatment is weak. Magnesium is an essential mineral for optimal metabolic function. Research has shown that the mineral content of magnesium in food sources is declining, and that magnesium depletion has been detected in persons with some chronic diseases [85]. One meta-analysis reviewed five trials involving 352 pregnant who had leg cramps. The only placebo-controlled trial of calcium treatment showed no evidence of benefit. Trials comparing sodium chloride with placebo (OR 0.54, 95% CI 0.23–1.29) and calcium with sodium chloride (OR 1.23, 95% CI 0.47–3.27) showed no evidence of benefit. Placebo-controlled trials of multivitamin with mineral supplements (OR 0.23, 95% CI 0.05–1.01) and magnesium (OR 0.18, 95% CI 0.05–0.60) provided some suggestion of benefit [86]. In conclusion, Hensley [87] recommended that once a serious disorder has been ruled out and the diagnosis of leg cramps has been made, reassurance can be offered that this disorder is benign, albeit disturbing. Supplemental magnesium at bedtime might provide relief.

RLS is a sensorimotor disorder characterized by a distressing urge to move the legs and sometimes also other parts of the body, usually accompanied by a marked sense of discomfort or pain in the leg or other affected body part such as upper extremities, chest, and face; it can be unilateral and bilateral [88]. RLS is triggered by rest or inactivity, and its symptoms are temporarily relieved or suppressed by movement. The disorder can be relatively mild or may have profoundly disruptive effects on a patient's sleep and daily life. It may be either idiopathic (primary RLS, which often has a familial component) or secondary, occurring in conjunction with other medical conditions, particularly iron-deficiency anemia, pregnancy, or end-stage renal disease [88,89]. Although not completely understood, a deficiency of dopamine appears to be part of the etiology of RLS. Iron is an integral enzyme necessary for dopamine production. Low body stores of iron may negatively affect brain iron metabolism and dopamine production, as noted by the resolution of symptoms when dopaminergic agents or iron are administered. The three major reversible secondary forms of RLS (pregnancy, end-stage renal disease, and iron-deficiency anemia) are associated with iron insufficiency [90,91]. A recent questionnaire-based prospective cohort study attempted to investigate the prevalence and patterns of sleep disturbances during pregnancy. In this study, the percentage of patients who met diagnostic criteria for RLS increased from 17.5% at recruitment to 31.2% in the third trimester. Overall poor sleep quality, as defined by a Pittsburgh Sleep Quality Index score greater than 5, became significantly more common as pregnancy progressed (39.0% compared with 53.5%) [92]. One prospective observational study indicated that reduced sleep duration in pregnancy is associated with longer labors and an increased rate of operative delivery [93]. It appears that a loss of sleep during pregnancy from RLS could adversely impact functionality during daytime hours and perhaps length and mode of delivery [87]. Because RLS may be the only clinical indication of iron deficiency, clinicians should determine the serum ferritin level in all patients with RLS, especially those with a history of gastrointestinal blood loss, disorders, or medications predisposing to gastrointestinal blood loss, menorrhagia, frequent blood donation, or recent onset or worsening of symptoms. If the serum ferritin level concentration is in the abnormal range for the specific laboratory (usually <20 mcg/L) or percent iron saturation is low (generally <20%), a cause of iron deficiency should be pursued and replacement treatment instituted. A serum ferritin concentration lower than 45–50 mcg/L has been associated with an increased severity of RLS, and therapy can be attempted in patients with levels in this range on a case-by-case basis. A common regimen is 325 mg of ferrous sulfate 3 times a day in combination with 100–200 mg of vitamin C with each dose to enhance absorption [88]. The treatment of RLS is to establish two components, pharmacologic and nonpharmacologic therapy. For patients with mild RLS, nonpharmacologic treatments should be tried before prescribing medications that may have unwanted side effects, especially in pregnant women. Treatments such as improved nutrition, exercise, and respecting good sleep hygiene are often emphasized. The first step is to avoid nicotine, caffeine, alcohol, dopamine antagonists, most antidepressants, antihistamines, and most antinausea agents [93]. Certain foods, such as ice cream (fairly common) and carbohydrates (especially white flour), may worsen RLS and should be avoided if the patient finds these foods to be a problem. The best nonpharmacologic treatments probably are those activities that the patient has already identified as being helpful in reducing his or her symptoms of RLS. These treatments include physical activity, particularly involving the limbs (stretching exercises just before bedtime tend to be helpful); very hot or, less commonly, very cold baths or even alternating hot and cold baths; or any mental activity that is very engrossing for the patient (e.g., video games, computer programming, painting, needlepoint, or active conversation). Sleep hygiene is important. The woman needs to retire and rise from bed at the same time every day. The first choice of pharmacologic treatment in nonpregnant women is dopaminergic agents. Although dopaminergic agents are FDA pregnancy category C, the companies warn against use during pregnancy due to potential teratogenic risks. Low-dose opioids could be considered to help the patient sleep through the night. Although benzodiazepines are FDA pregnancy category D/X, they could be used cautiously [88,94,95].

Published reports of narcolepsy are rare. Interaction between pregnancy and narcolepsy–cataplexy is unknown. Theoretically, narcolepsy is primarily treated with stimulants and REM-sleep suppressant. REM-inhibiting effect of estrogen and cortisol can be beneficial in pregnancy. Currently, there are two reports in the literature of pregnant narcoleptics with cataplexy undergoing cesarean delivery. Ping et al. [96] reported a woman who attempted a vaginal delivery experienced cataplectic attacks consisting of limb weakness and lack of verbal responsiveness for a few minutes following each uterine contraction. The patient had difficulty proceeding with a vaginal delivery, and a cesarean delivery was performed. Williams et al. [97] reported a woman with narcolepsy, cataplexy, and glutaric aciduria type II with increasingly frequent cataplectic attacks as she approached 37 weeks' gestation. The clinical manifestations of this patient's cataplexy were not described; the patient underwent elective cesarean delivery. In narcoleptic patients with clinically significant cataplexy, given the risk of labor-induced cataplexy and difficulty progressing through a vaginal delivery, elective cesarean delivery should be carefully considered by the patient in consultation with both her sleep physician and her obstetrician. No well-controlled studies of pregnant women who are using stimulants have been performed. The potential teratogenicity of modafinil is unknown; therefore, the most cautious advice would be to discontinue the medication during conception and pregnancy [98]. No stimulant for the treatment of narcolepsy has been proved to be safe during pregnancy. The pregnancy safety category for modafinil and methylphenidate is undefined; amphetamine is class C, and sodium oxybate is class B. The decision to continue or withhold medications for narcolepsy should be made by an informed patient, weighing the risks and benefits outlined [99].

Sleepwalking and night terrors are complex behaviors occurring in slow-wave non-REM sleep. These sleep disorders occurring during pregnancy and exacerbated by the condition have also been reported. There are two case reports in the literature. Pregnancy could predispose to sleepwalking and night terror by the latter mechanism. This is probably exemplified by a woman with a childhood history of sleepwalking who had recurrence during her two pregnancies. She received no treatment, and in both instances, sleepwalking ceased after delivery [100]. A second case report concerned a pregnant woman with night terror who experienced worsening night terrors during the third week of pregnancy. She experienced a spontaneous abortion, after which her night terror ceased [101]. Diazepam and imipramine can be safely used for sleepwalking and night terrors during pregnancy.

References

[1] Lurnley J. Defining the problem: the epidemiology of preterm birth. BJOG 2003; 110(Suppl. 20):3–7.

[2] Okun ML, Roberts JM, Marsland AL, Hall M. How disturbed sleep may be a risk factor for adverse pregnancy outcomes—a hypothesis. Obstet Gynecol Sur 2009;64:273–80.

[3] St-Onge MP, Perumean-Chaney S, Desmond R, Lewis CE, Yan LL, Person SD, et al. Gender differences in the association between sleep duration and body composition: The Cardia Study. Int J Endocrinol 2010;2010:726071

[4] Schoenborn CA, Adams PE. Health behaviors of adults. United States 2005–2007. Vital Health Stat 2010;245:1–132.

[5] Hedman C, Pohjosvaara T, Tolonen U, et al. Effect of pregnancy on mothers' sleep. Sleep Med 2002;3:37–42.

[6] Lee KA. Alteration in sleep during pregnancy and postpartum: a review 30 years of research. Sleep Med Rev 1998;2:231–42.
[7] Colvin GB, Whitmoyer DI, Sawyer GH. Circadian sleep wakefulness patterns in rats after ovariectomy and treatment with estrogen. Exp Neurol 1969;25:616–25.
[8] Friess E, Tagaya H, Trachsel L, et al. Progesterone induced changes in sleep in male subjects. Am J Physiol 1997;272:E885–891.
[9] Santiago JR, Nolledo MS, Kinzler W, Santiago TV. Sleep and sleep disorders in pregnancy. Ann Intern Med 2001;134:396–408.
[10] Hublin C, Partinen M, Koskenvuo M, Kaprio J. Sleep and mortality: a population based 22-year follow-up study. Sleep 2007;30:1245–53.
[11] Banks S, Dinges DF. Behavioral and physiological consequences of sleep resriction. J Clin Sleep Med 2007;3:519–28.
[12] Klebanoff MA, Shiono PH, Rhoads GG. Outcomes of pregnancy in a national sample of resident physicians. N Engl J Med 1990;323:1040–5.
[13] Lee KA, Gay CL. Sleep in late pregnancy predict length of labor and type of delivery. Am J Obtetr Gynecol 2004;191:2041–6.
[14] Okun ML, Hall M, Coussons-Read ME. Sleep disturbances increase interleukin-6 production during pregnancy: implication for pregnancy complication. Reprod Sci 2007;14:560–7.
[15] Mitchell MD, Romero RJ, Edwin SS, Trautman MS. Prostaglandins and parturition. Reprod Fertil Dev 1995;7:623–32.
[16] Arntzen KJ, Kjollesdal AM, Halgunset J, Vatten L, Austgulen R. TNF, IL-1, IL-6, IL_8 and soluble TNF receptor in relation to chorioamnionitis and premature labor. J Perinat Med 1998;26:17–26.
[17] Gale S, Harlow BL. Postpartum mood disorders: a review of clinical and epidemiological factors. J Phychosom Obstet Gynaecol 2003;24:257–66.
[18] Lusskin SI, Pundiak TM, Habib SM. Perinatal depression: hiding in plain sight. Can J Psychiatry 2007;52:479–88.
[19] Dennis CL, Ross L. Relationship among infant sleep patterns, maternal fatigue, and development of depressive symptomatology. Birth (Berkeley, CA) 2007;8:215–21.
[20] Goyal D, Gay CL, Lee KA. Pattern of sleep disruption and depressive symptoms in new mothers. J Perinat Neonatal Nurs 2007;21:123–9.
[21] Wolfson AR, Crowley SJ, Anwer U, Bassett JL. Changes in sleep patterns and depressive symptoms in first time mothers: last trimester to 1-year postpartum. Behav Sleep Med 2003;1:54–67.
[22] Chang JJ, Pien GW, Duntley SP, Macones GA. Sleep deprivation during pregnancy and maternal and fetal outcomes: Is there a relationship. Sleep Med Rev 2010;14:107–14.
[23] Epstein LJ, Kristo D, Strollo PJ, et al. Clinical guideline for evaluation, management and longterm care of obstructive sleep apnea in adults. J Clin Sleep Med 2009;5:263–77.
[24] Young T, Patla M, Dempsey J, et al. The occurrence of sleep disorders breathing among middle-aged adults. N Engl J Med 1993;328:1230–5.
[25] Iber CAIS, Chesson A, Quan SF. AASM manual for the scoring of sleep and associated events: rules, terminology and technical specifications, 1 st ed. Westchester, IL: American Academy of Sleep Medicine; 2007.
[26] Lin CM, Davidson TM, Ancoli-Israel S. Gender differences in obstructive sleep apnea and treatment implications. Sleep Med Rev 2008;12:81–96.
[27] Young T, Evans L, Finn L, Patla M. Estimation of the clinically diagnosed proportion of sleep apnea syndrome in middle aged men and women. Sleep 1997;20:705–6.

[28] Ye L, Pien GW, Ratcliffe SJ, Weaver TE. Gender differences in obstructive sleep apnea syndrome and treatment response to continuous positive airway pressure. J Clin Sleep Med 2009;5:512–8.

[29] Ursavas A, Karada M. Sleep breathing disorders in pregnancy. Tuberk Toraks 2009;57:237–43.

[30] Elkus R, Popovich Jr. J. Respiratory physiology in pregnancy. Clin Chest Med 1992;13:555–65.

[31] Izci B, Vennelle M, Liston WA, Dundas KC, et al. Sleep-disorders breathing and upper airway size in pregnancy and post-partum. Eur Respir J 2006;27:321–7.

[32] Tagaya M, Nakata S, Yasuma F, et al. Pathogenetic role of increased nasal resistance in obese patients with obstructive sleep apnea syndrome. Am J Rhinol Allergy 2010;24:51–4.

[33] Stubner UP, Gruber D, Berger UE, et al. The influence of female sex hormones on nasal reactivity in seasonal allergic rhinitis. Allergy 1999;54:865–71.

[34] Popovic RM, White DP. Upper airway muscle activity in normal women: influence of hormonal status. J Appl Physiol 1998;84:1055–62.

[35] Santiago J, Nolledo MS, Kinzler W, Santiago TV. Sleep disorders breathing in pregnancy. Ann Intern Med 2001;134:396–408.

[36] Edwards N, Middleton PG, Blyton DM, Sullivan CE. Sleep disorders breathing and pregnancy. Thorax 2002;57:555–8.

[37] Loube MD, Poceta S, Morales MC, et al. Self reported snoring in pregnancy: association with fetal outcome. Chest 1996;109:885–9.

[38] Franklin KA, Holingren PA, Jönsson F, et al. Snoring, pregnancy-induced hypertension, and growth retardation of the fetus. Chest 2000;117:137–41.

[39] Pien GW, Fife Di Pack AI, Nkwuo JE, Schwab RJ. Changes in symptoms of sleep disordered breathing during pregnancy. Sleep 2005;28:1299–305.

[40] Maasilta P, Bachour A, Teramo K, et al. Sleep-related disordered breathing during pregnancy in obese women. Chest 2001;120:1448–554.

[41] Guilleminault C, Querra-Salva M, Chowdhuri S, Poyares D. Normal pregnancy, daytime sleeping, snoring and blood pressure. Sleep Med 2000;1:289–97.

[42] Teculescu D, Hannhart B, Cornette A, et al. Prevalance of habitual snoring in a sample of French males. Role of "minor" nose–throat abnormalities. Respiration 2001;68:365–70.

[43] Resta O, Foschino-Barbora MP, Legari G, et al. Sleep related breathing disorders, loud snoring and excessive daytimer sleepiness in obese subjects. Int J Obes Relat Metab Disord 2001;25:669–75.

[44] Ursavas A, Karadag M, Nalcı N, Ercan I, Gozu RO. Self reported snoring, maternal obesity and neck circumference as a risk factor for pregnancy induced hypertension and preeclampsia. Respiration 2008;76:33–9.

[45] Vencata C, Venkatesbiab SB. Sleep disordered breathing during pregnancy. J Am Board Fam Med 2009;22:158–68.

[46] Helewa ME, Burrows RF, Smith J, et al. Report of the Canadian Hypertension Society Consensus Conference: definition, evaluation, and classification of hypertensive disorders in pregnancy. CMAJ 1997;157:715–25.

[47] Roberts JM, Redman JW. Pre-eclampsia more than pregnancy induced hypertension. Lancet 1993;342:1447–51.

[48] Calhoun DA. Obstructive sleep apnea and hypertension. Curr Hypertens Rep 2010;12:189–95.

[49] Beilin LJ, Deacon J, Michael CA, et al. Diurnal rhythms of blood pressure, plasma renin activity, angiotensin II and catecholamines in normotensive and hypertensive pregnancies. Clin Exp Hypertens 1983;B2:271–93.

[50] Cudihy D, Lee RV. The pathophysiology of preeclampsia: current clinical concept. J Obstet Gynaecol 2009;29:576–82.
[51] Gislason T, Benediktsdottir B, Björnsson JK, et al. Snoring hypertension and the sleep apnea syndrome: an epidemiologic survey of middle aged woman. Chest 1993;103:1147–51.
[52] zci B, Martin SE, Dundas KC, et al. Sleep complaints: snoring and daytime sleepiness in pregnant and preeclamptic women. Sleep Med 2005;6:163–9.
[53] Perez-Chada D, Vidala AJ, O'Flaharty ML, et al. Snoring, witnessed sleep apneas and pregnancy induced hypertension. Acta Obstet Gynecol Scand 2007;86:788–92.
[54] Bourjeily G, Raker CA, Chalhoub M, Miller MA. Pregnancy and fetal outcomes of symptoms of sleep-disordered breathing. Eur Respir J 2010;36:849–55.
[55] Joel-Cohen SJ, Schoenfeld A. Fetal response to periodic sleep apnea: a new syndrome in obstetrics. Eur J Obstet Gynecol Reprod Biol 1978;8:77–81.
[56] Connolly G, Razak ARA, Hayanga A, et al. Inspiratory flow limitation during sleep in pre-eclampsia: comparison with normal pregnant and nonpregnant women. Eur Respir J 2001;18:672–6.
[57] Champagne K, Schwartzman K, Opatrny L, et al. Obstructive sleep apnea and its association with gestational hypertension. Eur Respir J 2009;33:559–65.
[58] zci B, Riha RL, Martin SE, et al. The upper airway in pregnancy and pre-eclampsia. Am J Respir Crit Care Med 2003;167:137–40.
[59] Yinon D, Lowenstein L, Suraya S, et al. Preeclampsia is associated with sleep disordered breathing and endothelial dysfunction. Eur Respir J 2006;27:328–33.
[60] Lam DC, Lui MM, Lam JC, Ong LH, Lam KS, Ip MS. Prevalence and recognisation of obstructive sleep apnea in Chinese with Tip 2 diabetes mellitus. Chest 2010;138:1101–7.
[61] Peltier AC, Consens EB, Sheikh K, Wang L, Song Y, Russel JW. Autonomic dysfunction in obstructive sleep apnea is associated with impaired glucose regulation. Sleep Med 2007;8:149–55.
[62] Saaresranta T, Polo O. Sleep-disordered breathing and hormones. Eur Respir J 2003;22:161–72.
[63] Youssef HF, Dombrovskiy VY, Santiago TV, Nolledo MS. Sleep apnea is associated with gestational diabetes mellitus and pregnancy induced hypertension. Am J Respir Crit Care Med 2007;175:A996.
[64] Qui C, Enquobahrie D, Frederick IO, et al. Glucose intolerance and gestational diabetes risk in relation to sleep duration and snoring during pregnancy: a pilot study. BMC Women's Health 2010;10:17.
[65] Champagne KA, Kimoff RJ, Barriga PC, Schwartzman K. Sleep disordered breathing in women of childbearing age during pregnancy. Indian J Med Res 2010;131:285–301.
[66] Awe RJ, Nicotra B, Newson TD, Viles R. Arterial oxygenation and alveolar-arterial gradients in term pregnancy. Obstet Gynecol 1979;53:182–6.
[67] Bernstein I, Gabbe SG. Intrauterine growth restriction. In: Gabbe SG, Niebyl JR, Simpson JL, editors. Obstetrics: normal and problem pregnancies (3rd ed.). New York, NY: Churchill Livingstone; 1996. p. 863–86.
[68] Peyronnet J, Roux JC, Geloen L, et al. Prenatal hypoxia impairs the postnatal development of neural and functional chemo afferent pathway in rat. J Physiol 2000;524:525–37.
[69] Gozal D, Reeves SR, Row BW, et al. Respiratory effects of gestational intermittent hypoxia in the developing rat. Am J Respir Crit Care Med 2003;167:1540–7.
[70] Ayrım A, Keskin EA, Özol D, Onaran Y, Yıldırım Z, Kafali H. Influence of self reported snoring and witnessed sleep apnea on gestational hypertension and fetal outcome in pregnancy. Arch Gynecol Obstet 2009;1327–32.

[71] Louis JM, Auckley D, Sokol RJ, Mercer BM. Maternal and neonatal morbidities associated with obstructive sleep apnea complicating pregnancy. 2010;202:261e1–5.
[72] Sahin FK, Köken G, Co ar E, et al. Obstructive sleep apnea in pregnancy and fetal outcome. In J Gynaecol Obstet 2008;100:141–6.
[73] Olivarez SA, Maheshwari B, McCarthy M, et al. Prospective trial on obstructive sleep apnea in pregnancy and fetal heart rate monitoring. Am J Obstet Gynecol 2010;202(557):e1–7.
[74] Pien GW, Schwab RJ. Sleep disorders during pregnancy. Sleep 2004;27:1405–17.
[75] Freedman N. Treatment of obstructive sleep apnea syndrome. Clin Chest Med 2010;31:187–201.
[76] Kowall J, Clark G, Nino Murcia G, et al. Precipitation of obstructive sleep apnea during pregnancy. Obstet Gynecol 1989;74:453–5.
[77] Brain KA, Thornton JG, Sarkar A, Johnson AO. Obstructive sleep apnea and fetal death: successful treatment with continuous positive airway pressure. BJOG 2001;108:543–4.
[78] Guilleminault C, Kreutzer M, Chang JL. Pregnancy, sleep-disordered breathing and treatment with nasal continuous positive airway pressure. Sleep Med 2004;5:43–51.
[79] Guilleminault C, Palombini L, Poyares D, Takaoka S, Huynh NT, El-Sayed YY. Early intervention with nasal CPAP in pregnant women with risk factors for preeclampsia: preliminary findings. Sleep Med 2007;9:9–14.
[80] Poyares D, Guilleminault C, Hachul H, Fujita L, Takaoka S, Tufik S, et al. Hypertension during pregnancy, chronic snoring, and early nasal CPAP intervention. Sleep Med 2007;9:15–21.
[81] Edwards N, Blyton DM, Hennessy A, Sullivan CE. Severity of sleep disordered breathing improves following parturition. Sleep 2005;8:737–41.
[82] American Sleep Disorders Association, Diagnostic Classification Steering Committee The international classification of sleep disorders: diagnostic coding manual, 2nd ed. Westchester, IL: American Academy of Sleep Medicine; 2006. 119 Pocket version
[83] Miller TM, Layzer RB. Muscle cramps. Muscle Nerve 2005;32:431–42.
[84] Walters AS. Clinical identification of the simple sleep related disorders. Chest 2007;131:1260–6.
[85] Guerrera MP, Volpe SL, Mao JJ. Therapeutic uses of magnesium. 2009;80:157–62.
[86] Young GL, Jewell D. Intervention for leg cramps in pregnancy. Cochrane Database Syst Rev 2002:1. CD000121
[87] Hensley JG. Leg cramps and restless leg syndrome during pregnancy. J Midwifery Womens Health 2009;54:211–8.
[88] Allen R, Picchiette D, Henning W, Trenkwalder C, Walters A, Montplaisi J. Restless leg syndrome: diagnostic criteria, special considerations and epidemiology. A report from the restless leg syndrome diagnosis and epidemiologic workshop at the National Institutes of Health. Sleep Med 2003;4:101–9.
[89] Kushida C. Clinical presentation, diagnosis and quality of life issues in restless legs syndrome. Am J Med 2007;120(1 Suppl. 1):S4–12.
[90] Guyton AC, Hall JE. Textbook of medical physiology, 11th ed. Philadelphia, PA: Elsevier Saunders; 2006.
[91] Sun ER, Chen CA, Ho G, Earley C, Allen RP. Iron and restless leg syndrome. Sleep 1998;21:381–7.
[92] Facco FL, Kramer J, Ho KH, Zee PC, Grobman WA. Sleep disturbances in pregnancy. Obstet Gynecol 2010;115:77–83.
[93] Paulson GW. Restless legs syndrome. How to provide symptom relief with drug and nondrug therapies. Geriatrics 2000;55:35–8. 43–4, 7–8

[94] Sibler MH, Ehrenber BL, Allen RP, Buchfuhrer MJ, et al. An algorithm fort he management of restless legs syndrome. Mayo Clinic Proc 2004;79:916–22.
[95] Hening WA. Current guidelines and standarts of practice for restless lags syndrome. Am J Med 2007;120(1 Suppl. 1):22–7.
[96] Ping LS, Yat FS, Kwok WY. Status cataplecticus leading to the obstetric complication of prolonged labor. J Clin Sleep Med. 2007;3:56–7.
[97] Williams SF, Alvarez JR, Pedro HF, Apuzzio JJ. Glutaric aciduria type II and narcolepsy in pregnancy. Obstet Gynecol. 2008;111:522–4.
[98] Littner M, Johnson SF, McCall WV, et al. Practice parameters for the treatment of narcolepsy: an update for 2000. Sleep 2001;24:451–66.
[99] Hoque R, Chesson AL. Conception, pregnancy, delivery and breastfeeding in a narcoleptic patients with cataplexy. J Clin Sleep Med 2008;4:601–3.
[100] Berlin RM. Sleep walking disorders during pregnancy: a case report. Sleep 1998;11:298–300.
[101] Synder S. Unusual case of sleep terror in a pregnant woman. Am J Psychiatry 1986;143:391.